# The Handbook of Clinical Intervention with Young People who Sexually Abuse

*The Handbook of Clinical Intervention with Young People who Sexually Abuse* provides an authoritative, critical and up-to-date overview of the growing body of empirical and theoretical knowledge in this field and clearly demonstrates how this knowledge guides evidence-based practice.

Previously neglected subjects such as female sexual offenders and offenders with intellectual disabilities are dealt with sensitively along with thought-provoking discussion of key subjects including:

- Essentials of effective treatment programmes
- Relapse prevention
- Psychiatric disorder and adolescent offending
- Work with families of young people who sexually abuse
- The psychophysiological assessment of juvenile offenders
- Preparing services and staff to work with young people who sexually abuse

Practical guidelines from acknowledged international experts with extensive experience of research and clinical practice are provided. This book will be invaluable to all those working with young people who engage in sexually abusive behaviour.

**Gary O' Reilly** is Deputy Director of the Doctoral Programme in Clinical Psychology at University College Dublin.
**William L. Marshall** is Emeritus Professor of Psychology and Psychiatry at Queen's University, Canada.
**Alan Carr** is Director of the Doctoral Programme in Clinical Psychology at University College Dublin.
**Richard C. Beckett** is a Consultant Forensic Clinical Psychologist in Oxford.

# The Handbook of Clinical Intervention with Young People who Sexually Abuse

Edited by Gary O' Reilly,
William L. Marshall, Alan Carr and
Richard Beckett

Psychology Press
Taylor & Francis Group
HOVE AND NEW YORK

First published 2004 by Brunner-Routledge
27 Church Road, Hove, East Sussex BN3 2FA

Simultaneously published in the USA and Canada
by Brunner-Routledge
29 West 35th Street, New York NY 10001

*Brunner-Routledge is an imprint of the Taylor & Francis Group*



Typeset in Times by RefineCatch Limited, Bungay, Suffolk
Printed and bound in Great Britain by Biddles Ltd, Guildford and King's Lynn
Paperback cover design by Lisa Dynan



This publication has been produced with paper manufactured to strict
environmental standards and with pulp derived from sustainable forests.

*British Library Cataloguing in Publication Data*
A catalogue record for this book is available from the British Library

*Library of Congress Cataloging-in-Publication Data*
Handbook of clinical intervention with young people who sexually abuse /
edited by Gary O'Reilly . . . [et al.].—1st ed.
p. ; cm.
Includes bibliographical references and index.
ISBN 1–58391–125–1 (hardback :alk.paper)—ISBN 1–58391–126–X (pbk.:alk.
paper)
1. Teenage sex offenders. 2. Teenage sex offenders—Rehabilitation.
3. Teenage sex offenders—Mental health services.
[DNLM: 1. Sex Offenses—prevention & control—Adolescent.
2. Adolescent Behavior—psychology. 3. Sex Behavior—psychology—
Adolescent. WM 611 H23585 2004] I. O' Reilly, Gary. II. Title.
RJ506.S48H363 2004
616.85'83'00835—dc22 2003026243

ISBN 1–58391–125–1 hbk
ISBN 1–58391–126–X pbk

About half way between West Egg and New York the motor road hastily joins the railroad and runs beside it for a quarter of a mile, so as to shrink away from a certain desolate area of land. This is a valley of ashes – a fantastic farm where ashes grow like wheat into ridges and hills and grotesque gardens; where ashes take the forms of houses and chimneys and rising smoke and, finally, with a transcendent effort, of ash-grey men who move dimly and already crumbling through the powdery air.

F. Scott Fitzgerald, *The Great Gatsby**

# Contents

# Figures

# Tables

# Contributors

**Professor Sharon K. Araji**, Department of Sociology, University of Alaska, Anchorage, Alaska, USA

**Professor Howard Barbaree**, Centre for Addiction and Mental Health & the University of Toronto, Toronto, Canada.

**Professor Judith Becker**, Department of Psychology, University of Arizona, Arizona, USA.

**Kurt M. Bumby**, Missouri Division of Youth Services, Missouri, USA.

**Professor Ruud Bullens**, HARVELD Institute, Holland.

**Professor Alan Carr**, Doctoral Programme in Clinical Psychology, University College Dublin, Ireland.

**Yvonne Duane**, Department of Child and Family Psychiatry, Mater Misericordiae University Hospital, Dublin, Ireland.

**Kevin Epps**, Forensic Child and Adolescent Mental Health Service Team, Reaside Clinic, Birmingham, UK.

**Yolanda Fernandez**, Queens University, Kingston, Canada.

**Dawn Fisher**, Llanarth Court Hospital, Raglan, South Wales, UK.

**Robert E. Freeman-Longo**, New Hope Treatment Centres, South Carolina, USA.

**Nancy Halstenson Bumby**, Department of Psychiatry, University of Missouri-Columbia School of Medicine, Missouri, USA

**Cathi Harris**, Special Commitment Centre, McNeil Island, Washington, USA.

**Professor John Hunter**, Department of Psychology, University of Virginia, Virginia, USA.

**Professor Raymond A. Knight**, Department of Psychology, Brandeis University, Waltham, Massachusetts, USA

**Calvin M. Langton**, Centre for Addiction and Mental Health & the University of Toronto, Toronto, Canada.

**Professor William L. Marshall**, Queens University, Kingston, Canada.

**Tony Morrison**, Independent Child Care Trainer Consultant and Practitioner, Rochdale, UK.

**David O' Callaghan**, G-MAP Programme, Manchester, UK.

**Gary O' Reilly**, Doctoral Programme in Clinical Psychology, University College Dublin, Ireland.

**Bobbie Print**, G-MAP Programme, Manchester, UK.

**Declan Sheerin**, Regional Child and Family Service, North Eastern Health Board, Drogheda, Ireland.

**Jerry Thomas**, Independent Family Practitioner, Memphis, Tennessee, USA.

**James R. Worling**, SAFE-T Program, Thistletown Regional Centre, Toronto, Ontario, Canada.

**A. Ph. Van Wijk**, HARVELD Institute, Holland.

# Preface

This volume is intended for researchers and practitioners working with young people who engage in sexually abusive behaviour. It places this work within three contexts: Firstly, the context of what the empirical literature tells us of this population, their developmental and family experiences. Secondly, within a clinical context: What do experienced clinicians tell us about best practice approaches to assessment and intervention? Finally, within a systemic context: raising questions concerning the needs of staff working in this area and system needs regarding the effectiveness of intervention with young people in preventing further offending. This book is intended to be a stepping-stone to evidence-based practice through a review of what is known about this population, the provision of clear descriptions of best practice guidelines, combined with an attempt to signpost the direction that much-needed outcome research needs to take. We hope it will be helpful to practitioners in attaining their goal of reducing sexual assault through effective intervention with young people who by virtue of their past sexually abusive behaviour have a potential for further harm to others but by virtue of their youthfulness and other strengths have a potential for a safe and productive life.

GO'R<br>WLM<br>AC<br>RB

# Acknowledgements

There are a great number of people whose support we would like to acknowledge in preparing this book.

From the North Eastern Health Board: Dr Declan Sheerin, Dr Maria Lawlor, Mairead Dempsey, Petua Marshall, Rose Bentley, Mark Yalloway, Catriona McGregor, Yvonne Cahill, Nuala Crosse, Austin Waters, Denis Callaghan, Roisin Maguire, Alan Doran, Alan Dibble, and Nuala Doherty.

Paul Murphy from the Irish Prison Service has been an unwavering and substantial supporter in efforts to complete this book and other work – Thank you. We would also like to express our thanks to Des O' Mahaony and Anthony Cotter.

Dr Peter Reid, Dr Mary Belton, Dr Patrick Walsh and Pat Conroy from St John of Gods Services in Ireland are also owed a substantial debt of gratitude for their help.

We would like to thank our colleagues in the Department of Psychology at University College Dublin, particularly Muriel Keegan, Dr Barbara Dooley, Dr Muireann McNulty, Professor Ciaran Benson and Dr Geraldine Moane.

We are grateful to each of the authors who generously and patiently contributed chapters to this book.

Finally to our families and friends, thank you.

# Editors' note

There are many different phrases that have been used to describe those who engage in sexually abusive behaviour, such as, young people who sexually abuse, juvenile sexual offenders and juvenile sexual abusers. We have left it open to each author to use the term that reflects the context of their work. Throughout this book a number of authors illustrate points with reference to case material. In each instance, names and important details have been changed to protect the privacy of those concerned, or fictional but realistic case examples have been used.

# Part 1

# Foundations for practice

Chapter 1

# Preadolescents and adolescents

## Evaluating normative and non-normative sexual behaviours and development

*Sharon K. Araji*

### Introduction

In discussing sexual development in both children and adolescents, Bukowski *et al.* (1993, p. 87) ask, "What is healthy sexual development?" In response, they argue that descriptions of the goals of sexual development are unclear and have relied heavily on abstractions. As such, they say that little guidance has been provided with respect to identifying what constitutes healthy or unhealthy sexual development. They continue by saying that specifying the goals of healthy sexual development is a very difficult task because the development consists of factors that are subjective, interpersonal and socially embedded and vary as a function of age, sex and culture. Distinguishing between normative and non-normative sexual behaviours and development among preadolescents and adolescents is like drawing lines in the sand. Definitions shift across individuals, professionals, groups, organizations, communities, social institutions, societies and situations. While there are some cases that most would agree involve crossing the line between normative, non-normative and even criminal sexual behaviours, others are less clear. This is apparent from reflecting on the two cases below, both of which were reported in the media.

*Case One:* In Alaska three boys aged eleven, twelve and thirteen were apprehended by police and charged with first degree sexual assault for the forcible raping of a five-year-old girl. Police indicated that the boys used objects, although the specifics were not disclosed. The three boys chased the young girl, caught her, held her on the ground, took off her pants, and took turns raping her. This "gang rape" took place in a wooded area near the victim's home and came to light in a therapy session. All three boys had a record with social services or the law before this incident.

*Case Two:* A six-year-old, first grader in Lexington, North Carolina, was barred from his class for one day because he kissed a classmate on the cheek. He said he did it because "he liked her and she asked him to". A teacher saw the incident differently and reported that the girl had complained. As a result, school officials said the boy had broken school rules against sexual harassment. They later lowered the charge to a violation of a general school rule that prohibited "unwarranted and unwelcome touching of one student by another" (Zoglin, 1996).

In comparing these two cases, most would agree that Case One involves non-normative, abusive and even criminal sexual behaviours. In Case Two, fewer would agree that the boy engaged in a sexually deviant or a non-normative act for a six-year-old. His parents certainly did not and neither did many of the townspeople.

The obvious question for professionals who come into contact with cases such as these is, "What are the factors that can be used to determine when the sexual behaviours of children cross the line from normative to non-normative or criminal behaviours?" From a sociological perspective, there are several reasons why professionals need to develop guidelines to distinguish between the sexual behaviours exhibited by preadolescents and adolescents. First, guidelines are of particular interest as societies develop and become increasingly multicultural. Second, they are also necessary so that youth are not labelled as deviants if their behaviours are normative, but only when their behaviours can be clearly defined as non-normative, abusive or criminal.

### Aims of this chapter

The purpose of this chapter is to review relevant information that helps identify sexual behaviours considered normal, normative, non-normative, deviant or criminal for preadolescents and adolescents. This will be accomplished by reviewing the literature on the sexual behaviour and development of preadolescents and adolescents who experience sexual behaviour problems. Following this review, the commonalties and differences between the descriptions for these two age groups will be examined. A synthesis and analysis will then be offered and implications for clinical practice and social policies will be outlined. Finally, guidelines will be provided that can help assess problematic sexual behaviours.

## Defining concepts

### *Preadolescence and adolescence*

There is a tendency to attach chronological ages to differentiate preadolescents from adolescents. Biologically, the event that is used to separate these two phases in the lifecycle is puberty; the time in life marked by the onset of physical changes that make reproduction possible (e.g. menstruation and ejaculatory responses) (Martinson, 1991). However, over the years, trying to match ages with puberty has become problematic. Since the 1840s the secular trend in the characteristics of the population of young people reaching puberty (Bullough, 1981) decreased from about seventeen years of age to about twelve-and-a-half or thirteen-and-a-half years in the 1980s (Eveleth and Tanner, 1990). This downward trend appears to be continuing into the twenty-first century.

The earlier onset of puberty increases the difficulties of differentiating behaviours considered normal and normative from those considered abnormal or non-normative. Recognizing the issues associated with defining the concepts of "preadolescence" and "adolescence" for purposes of this chapter we still need to come up with some definitions. As much of the literature reviewed uses the age of twelve to separate these two groups, this will be used as a guide. As a heuristic tool, preadolescents will be defined as children twelve years of age and under and adolescents as youth who are teenagers.

### *Normal and normative sexual behaviours and development*

It is helpful to discuss concepts that are sometimes used interchangeably when describing sexual behaviours and development among preadolescents and adolescents. The concepts of "normative" or "appropriate" tend to be used when sexual behaviours are defined in a socio-cultural way, that is to indicate what is considered the norm in a given society, culture or group. Those who use the term normative are likely to be sociologists, professionals in the area of social work, administrators, and those associated with the justice system. These researchers or practitioners are likely to use "deviant" or "criminal" to describe preadolescents' and adolescents' sexual behaviours that lie outside the realm of social norms or laws.

In contrast to the concepts of normative or appropriate, the term 'normal' frequently describes sexual behaviours that occur as a result of the natural human biological and physiological development process. Those who use the term normal tend to work in areas related to medicine, psychology, sex education or child development. This group of professionals uses terms such as pathological or abnormal sexual behaviours to indicate that something has happened to disturb or alter sexual behaviours that would be expected as a part of the normal sexual development process. To compare these two perspectives, a child psychologist may consider exploratory sexual behaviours in young children as normal because it has been observed across societies and history as part of the natural developmental process. Those following a cultural or sociological perspective, however, may define certain exploratory behaviours as deviant or inappropriate if they go against group, religious or social norms.

## Sexual behaviour and development

### *Normative preadolescent sexual behaviour and development*

While sociologists have been late to enter discussions about the sexual development of youth, the sociological perspective is necessary even in a clinical setting because sexual behaviours are embedded in the broader context of interpersonal, social and cultural factors. It is only within this context that sexual behaviours and development come to be defined as normal, normative, deviant or criminal. As we will see, sexual behaviours and sexual development cannot be understood apart from physiological, cognitive, emotional, interpersonal, environmental and cultural factors that facilitate or hinder the developmental process.

Comprehensive reviews of research on preadolescents' normal, normative, non-normative and abusive sexual behaviours are fairly recent. Araji (1997) completed an extensive review of the many attempts to differentiate for preadolescents, normal, normative and appropriate sexual development from abnormal, non-normative and deviant/criminal development. Selected examples from this review are presented in Table 1.1. As can be seen, some practitioners and researchers are more comprehensive in their descriptions of normal or appropriate sexual behaviours as well as in differentiating by age groups within the preadolescent category, (e.g. Cunningham and MacFarlane, 1991; Gil, 1993).

An overview of the information in Table 1.1 provides some clues as to what various experts in the area of childhood and preadolescent sexual development view as normal or normative. As can be seen, very early sexual behaviours include only random and exploratory behaviours primarily involving the self. The behaviours tend to be touching self and others, genital play, masturbation, poking, watching, and showing interest in bathroom functions. Children may insert fingers or objects into body openings but stop when it hurts. The primary motivations appear to be exploration and curiosity.

As children grow older, they begin to imitate what they observe in their environment. This may involve playing doctor, house or mimicking sexual activities (see Gil, 1993; Cunningham and MacFarlane, 1991, in Table 1.1). At these early ages interpersonal imitative actions include kissing, holding

*Table 1.1* Normal, normative and appropriate sexual behaviours and development in preadolescents

| *Practitioners/researchers* | *Description of sexual behaviours and development* | | |
|---|---|---|---|
| *Rutter (1971)* | Erections may occur in young male infants. Orgasmic-like responses may be seen in males as young as 5 months. Thigh rubbing may occur with female preschoolers. Exhibitionism, voyeurism with other children and adults, sexual exploration games, asking about sex, genital interest, genital play, and masturbation (more pronounced in males) are normal for children 2 to 5 years of age.<br>During prepubescent years, masturbation gradually increases, as does heterosexual play (10% at 7 years of age to 80% at age of 13); homosexual play also increases (observed in 25% to 30% of 13-year-old boys). | | |
| *Money and Ehrhardt (1972) and Achenbach and Edelbrook (1983)* | Children ages 3 to 6 can exhibit flirtations, seductive behaviours and imitations of parents, older siblings, television and so on. During latency, they exhibit inhibitions and demand more privacy in response to learning cultural standards. | | |
| *Gil (1993)* | *Preschool (birth–4 years)*<br>Randomly touches/rubs own genitals. Watches, pokes others' bodies. Shows genitals. Interested/asks about bathroom functions. Uses dirty language. Plays house. Plays doctor (imitative). May insert fingers, objects/stops with pain. | *Young school age (age 5–7)*<br>Touches self (specific not only random). Watches, asks. Inhibited (becomes more private). Repulsed by/or drawn to opposite sex. Tells dirty jokes. Plays house. Kissing, holding hands. May mimic/practise sexual activities. | *Latency/preadolescent (age 8–12)*<br>Touches self/others. Mooning. Exhibitionistic. Kissing/dating. Petting. Touches others' genitals. Dry humping. Digital or vaginal intercourse. Oral sex in preadolescents (or adolescents). |
| *Johnson and Feldmeth (1993)* | *Behaviours:* Sex play, exploration involving touching and initiating gender roles. Sample behaviours include peeking, touching or exposing, auto-stimulation, kissing, hugging, peeking, touching or exposing genitals or both to other children, sometimes simulated intercourse. (Intercourse is rare and found in only 2% or 3% of children 12 years of age or less.) | | *Affect regarding sexuality:* Silly/giggly/light-hearted; perhaps parental- or religious-induced guilt.<br><br>*Response to discovery:* Shyness, embarrassment. |

| *Practitioners/researchers* | *Description of sexual behaviours and development* | | |
|---|---|---|---|
| | *Intensity:* Balanced, can stop and start at will.<br>*Sexual arousal:* Arousal/no arousal.<br>*Motivation:* Curiosity. Exploration. Needs to be like friends. Mimic what is seen in real life or on television. Sexual stimulation. | | *Planning:* Spontaneous/planned.<br>*Coercion:* Mutual involvement.<br>*Relationship to others involved in sexual behaviours:* Siblings (foster, natural, or step); friends.<br>*Age difference:* Similar age.<br>*Interpersonal relationship characteristics:* All kinds. |
| *Ryan, Blum, Sandau-Christopher, Law, Weher, Sundine, Astler, Teske and Dale (1993)* | Genital or reproduction conversation with peers or similar-age siblings.<br>Playing doctor. "You show me yours, I'll show you mine" with peers or siblings.<br>Occasional masturbation without penetration.<br>Kissing, flirting.<br>Dirty words or jokes within cultural or peer group norm. | | |
| *Cunningham and MacFarlane (1991)* | *Ages 0–5*<br>Masturbation as self-soothing behaviour.<br>Touching self or others is exploratory or results from curiosity.<br>Sexual behaviours are done without inhibition.<br>Intense interest in bathroom activities of others.<br>May verbalize about toilet functions. | *Ages 6–10*<br>Continues to fondle and touch own genitals and masturbate.<br>Becomes more secretive about self-touching.<br>Interest in others' bodies.<br>Becomes more "game playing" than exploratory curiosity – for example, "I'll show you mine, you show me yours."<br>Playing doctor.<br>Boys may begin comparing size of penis. | *Ages 10–12*<br>Masturbation continues.<br>Focused on establishing relationships with peers.<br>Engages in sexual behaviour with peers – for example, kissing, fondling and sexual penetration.<br>Most sexual activity is heterosexual but may be homosexual. |

| | | | |
|---|---|---|---|
| | Exhibition of genitalia as means of curiosity.<br>Responds quickly to adult limit-setting and redirection concerning sexual behaviours.<br>Sexual behaviours represent only one aspect of general curiosity about their bodies, others' bodies, and world around them.<br>Touching others is exploratory, not coercive.<br>Sexual exploration begins during this stage. | Develops extreme interest in sex, sex words, and dirty jokes.<br>Begins to seek information/pictures that explain body functions.<br>Swearing begins.<br>Touching may involve stroking or rubbing. | May be interested in others' bodies, especially the opposite sex; that may be in the form of looking at photos or published materials.<br>Sexual experiences are heterosexual, although homosexual experiences are common for this age group. |

hands, and exploratory sexual behaviours with others such as "I'll show you mine, if you show me yours." Males may compare penis size. As children move into the end of preadolescence, some practitioners (such as Cunningham and MacFarlane, 1991; Gil, 1993) view as normal or normative more advanced sexual activities such as fondling others' genitals, dry humping, and even various types of sexual intercourse and oral sex. Most practitioners and researchers argue, however, that intercourse and oral sex are uncommon in preadolescents and in the young adolescent population, as well. Preadolescents' sexual experiences may be either homosexual or heterosexual and include a wide variety of participants such as siblings and friends. As children move closer to late preadolescence and into adolescence, normative interactions become increasingly heterosexual in response to societal norms.

Regardless of the types of sexual interactions, researchers generally agree that for behaviour to be considered normal or normative, children should be of similar ages and participation should be mutual. While sexual activities may be spontaneous or planned, they should be balanced with respect to other activities such as sports, school activities and scouting, among others. Sexual arousal may or may not be present, and it is not considered to be the primary motive for engaging in sexual behaviours. The affect associated with sexual activities in the early stages of preadolescence are characterized as light-hearted and are associated with silliness and giggly behaviours. As children age during the preadolescent stage they may express shyness or embarrassment if they are discovered. This is a reaction to the societal norms learnt from interactions in their environment.

The families, subcultures and cultures in which children live will influence the extent to which these behaviours and social interactions are considered normative or non-normative. For example, if children grow up in sexually repressive homes where sex is seen as "dirty", any sexual behaviours presented in Table 1.1 may be viewed as non-normative. On the other hand, if children grow up in families where there are no sexual boundaries within or outside the family or in homes that are sexually charged, it may be normative for them to participate in the full range of behaviours shown in Table 1.1 regardless of age. Similarly, the restrictiveness or permissiveness of cultures will influence the degree to which behaviours described in Table 1.1 are viewed as normal, normative or non-normative (see Arnett, 2001).

### *Non-normative preadolescent sexual behaviour and development*

Table 1.2 describes behaviours, emotions, motives and interactions that would no longer be considered normal or normative for preadolescent children. Using Cunningham and MacFarlane's (1991) typology as an example, it is obvious that some practitioners view behaviours such sexual penetration, and genital kissing, as normal in late preadolescence but not when it is being

*Table 1.2* Non-normative and abusive sexual behaviours in preadolescents

| *Practitioners/researchers* | *Non-normative sexual behaviours→* | *Abusive sexual behaviours* | |
|---|---|---|---|
| *Friedrich, Urquiza and Beilke (1986)* | Sexual preoccupation and masturbation significantly more evident. Behaviours may persist even after therapy. | | |
| *Friedrich and Luecke (1988)* | Decrease in public sexual behaviour not apparent. | | |
| *Friedrich, Grambsch, Koverola, Hewitt, Damon, Lemond and Broughton (1989)* | Behaviours that would be unusual in non-sexually abused children 2 to 12 years of age: attempting intercourse, inserting objects in vagina or rectum, and touching breasts of adults more than once or on an incidental basis. | | |
| *Johnson and Feldmeth (1993)* | *Sexually reactive behaviours* | *Extensive mutual sexual behaviours* | *Children who molest* |
| | *Behaviours:* For children in this group, genitals may be a focus of their development. Frequently, sexual activity includes only self-masturbation, insertion of objects, and exposing.<br>Sexual behaviours often represent repetition and compulsion related to previous overstimulating sexuality.<br>May engage in sexual behaviours with others. | *Behaviours:* May participate in wide range of adult sexual behaviours including oral intercourse. More persuasive and focused sexual behaviour pattern than seen in sexually reactive children. | *Behaviours:* Sexual behaviours are similar to those of previous group. Children's thoughts and actions have a pervasively sexual nature. |
| | *Intensity of sexual behaviours:* Focus on sexuality is out of balance in relation to peer group. | *Intensity of sexual behaviours:* Persuasive need for reassurance through sexual contact. | *Intensity of sexual behaviours:* Preoccupation with sex. Sexualizes most contacts with people and things; sexual behaviours are consistent and persistent, not isolated events, and have compulsive and aggressive qualities. |

| *Practitioners/researchers* | *Non-normative sexual behaviours→* | *Abusive sexual behaviours* | |
|---|---|---|---|
| | *Sexual arousal:* Arousal/no arousal. | *Sexual arousal:* Arousal/no arousal. | *Sexual arousal:* Arousal/no arousal. |
| | *Motivation:* Anxiety reduction; posttraumatic stress reaction; reduce confusion or make sense of sexual misuse or victimization; recapitulate previous unassimilated, uncontainable, sexual over-stimulation; decrease physiological arousal; sexual stimulation; use sex as a tool for making friends. | *Motivation:* Coping mechanism to decrease isolation or loneliness or neediness. Decrease boredom; and/or depression. Make life more bearable. Stabilize sense of self. Provide an attachment figure. Create a connection to otherwise hostile world. Decrease physical arousal, sexual stimulation. | *Motivation:* Decrease anxiety, fear, loneliness, anger, abandonment fears, or other strong unpleasant internal sensations; reduce confusion; recapitulation of previous physical, sexual or emotional over-stimulation; decrease physiological arousal paired with early or ongoing stress or both; posttraumatic stress reaction; sibling rivalry; compulsive sexual drive; sexual stimulation. |
| | *Affect regarding sexuality:* Anxiety, shame, guilt, fear, confusion. | *Affect regarding sexuality:* Needy, confused, sneaky; "What's the big deal" attitude. | *Affect regarding sexuality:* Anxiety, anger, aggression, rage, confusion. |
| | *Response to discovery:* May be surprised (if discovered at time of sexual behaviour), upset and confused or afraid. | *Response to discovery:* Denies or blames other child or does not see problem with the sexual behaviour. | *Response to Discovery:* Acts aggressively and angrily blames other child or person who caught them or both; denies behaviour. |
| | *Planning:* Spontaneous/impulsive. | *Planning:* Planned. | *Planning:* Planned/explosive. |
| | *Coercion:* Generally no discussion prior to behaviour occurring. If discussion, no coercion. | *Coercion:* Agreement at conscious or unconscious level, not coercive. | *Coercion:* Threats/bribes/trickery, manipulation, coercion. |

| | | |
|---|---|---|
| *Relations to others involved in sexual behaviours:* Siblings (foster, natural, or step). Accessible children. May approach adults. | *Relations to others involved in sexual behaviours:* Mutual sibling incest (foster, natural, or step) and/or willing children. Sex may become a stable aspect of relationship. | *Relations to others involved in sexual behaviours:* Forced sibling incest (foster, natural, or step) or vulnerable children. May be directed at adults. |
| *Age difference:* Similar age. | *Age difference:* Similar age. | *Age difference:* Younger, same age, or older (0–12-year age difference). |
| *Interpersonal relationship:* May be isolated, unsure, wary of involvements. | *Interpersonal relationship:* Distrusts adults as caregivers – expects to be hurt. Unattached. Relies on sexual relationships for emotional strength. Prone to victimization by adults who take advantage of child's neediness and confusion. | *Interpersonal relationship:* Tend to have behaviour problems at home and at school. Few outside interests. Few, if any, friends. Lacks problem-solving and coping skills. Very limited social skills and relationships with people of any age. No reliable way to get approval. |
| *Family environment:* Possibly sexually abusive or other abuses. Liberal views. Lacks emotional support and cohesion between family members. Environment may expose children to pornography or be overly sexualized. | *Family environment:* Possible polyabuse in family history. Parents/caretakers emotionally distant and unsupportive. Extramarital affairs occurring in family. Overt and covert sexuality in home. Poor boundaries. | *Family environment:* Psychiatric disorders. Criminal justice problems. Parental violence. Mostly single-parent families. Environments tend to lack boundaries, be sexually charged, and have a history of physical abuse between caretakers. Parents frequently have history of sexual, physical, emotional and substance abuse. |

| *Practitioners/researchers* | *Non-normative sexual behaviours→* | *Abusive sexual behaviours* | |
|---|---|---|---|
| | *Possible etiological factors:* Recent or ongoing sexual abuse, emotional abuse, trauma or sexualization. Pornography. History of sexual abuse in family. Overt sexual lifestyle in home. | *Possible etiological factors:* Sexual, emotional or physical abandonment, or all three. Neglect. Extramarital liaisons of parents. Inadequate early bonding to caretakers. Physiological or hormonal problems. Sexually abused in a group. Lack of adult attachments. Continuous out of home placements. | *Possible etiological factors:* Intense rivalry for attention between siblings. Lack of positive emotional relationships. Physiological/ hormonal problems. Trauma-induced neurobiological changes. Pairing of sex/anger, aggression/ anxiety. Sexual, emotional or physical abuse, or all three. Neglect/abandonment. Inherited vulnerabilities. Violence in family history. Sexualized relationships. Sexualized environment in family. Poor boundaries. Caretakers with many unmet needs. |
| *Cunningham and MacFarlane (1991)* | *Ages 0–5*<br>Curiosity about sexual behaviour becomes obsessive preoccupation.<br>Behaviour involves injury to self.<br>Children's behaviour involves coercion, threats, secrecy, aggression, violence or developmentally inappropriate (precocious) acts.<br>Unequal power base and exploitative regarding age, size, power, authority and lack of consent. | *Ages 6–10*<br>Sexual penetration.<br>Genital kissing.<br>Oral copulation.<br>Simulated intercourse. | *Ages 10–12*<br>Highly unusual for this age group to be involved in sex play with younger children. |

| | | | |
|---|---|---|---|
| *Ryan, Blum, Sandau-Christopher, Sundine, Astler, Law, Weher, Teske and Dale (1993)* | *Yellow Flag*<br>Preoccupation with sexual themes, especially sexually aggressive.<br>Attempting to expose others' genitals (e.g. pulling others' skirts up and pants down).<br>Sexually explicit or precocious conversation with peers.<br>Sexual graffiti (especially chronic or impacting individuals).<br>Sexual teasing/embarrassment of others.<br>Single occurrences of peeping/exposing/obscenities/pornographic interest/frottage.<br>Preoccupation with masturbation.<br>Mutual masturbation/group masturbation.<br>Simulating foreplay with dolls or peers with clothing on (e.g. petting and French kissing). | *Red Flag*<br>Sexually explicit conversation with significant age difference.<br>Touching genitals of others.<br>Degradation/humiliation of self or others with sexual themes.<br>Forced exposure of others' genitals.<br>Inducing fear/threats of force.<br>Sexually explicit proposals/threats including written notes.<br>Repeated or chronic peeping/exposing/obscenities/pornographic interests/frottage.<br>Compulsive masturbation/task interruption to masturbate.<br>Masturbation including vaginal or anal penetration.<br>Simulating intercourse with dolls. | *"No Question"*<br>Oral, vaginal, anal penetration of dolls, children, and animals.<br>Forced exposure of others' genitals.<br>Simulating intercourse with peers with clothing off.<br>Any genital injury or bleeding not explained by accidental cause. |

performed by children in early or mid-preadolescence. Rather than using age as a criterion for deciding what is normal or normative sexual behaviours for preadolescence, Ryan *et al.* (1993) use the concepts of "Yellow Flag", "Red Flag" and "No Questions" to indicate a progression of non-normative to abusive sexual behaviours.

The information in Table 1.2 indicates that sexual behaviours cross the line from normal or normative when they are no longer in balance with other activities in preadolescents' lives. The sexual activities become patterned rather than isolated events and children become preoccupied or obsessed with sexual activities. As children begin to engage in sexual behaviours they know are inappropriate, they become secretive. If caught by parents, caretakers or others their typical response is to deny it if they can; if not, to blame others. In sum, as children begin to engage in sexual behaviours they know are wrong, they begin to develop defensive strategies to protect themselves.

As evidenced in Table 1.2, sexually abusive or aggressive behaviours represent the extreme end of the sexual behaviour and development continuum. These sexual behaviours are far too advanced for children twelve years of age and younger. The behaviours have an aggressive quality, involving use of force, coercion (social or physical), and secrecy. As previously noted, the sexual acts represent patterned rather than isolated events (see Ryan *et al.*, 1993; Johnson and Feldmeth, 1993). The sexual behaviours may be opportunistic, but many are planned, calculated and predatory. Sexually deviant behaviours exist in combination with other antisocial behaviours such as those associated with conduct and oppositional disorders. Furthermore, sexually abusive behaviours continue even when intervention occurs. Children who exhibit these extreme behaviours are very resistant to treatment.

Repeated or chronic behaviours such as peeping, exposing or pornographic interests are also viewed as non-normative and not part of the normal sexual development of preadolescent children. Further, any behaviours that inflict harm on the self or others, are viewed as not only non-normative, but also abusive. The normal or normative motives for engaging in sexual behaviours are no longer confined to curiosity and exploration. Johnson and Feldmeth (1993) provide a detailed description of deviations from normal motivations, suggesting that engaging in sexual behaviours is no longer exploratory in nature, but serves as a coping mechanism for satisfying unmet needs that are manifest in feelings of loneliness, isolation, anxiety, fear, and other affective states.

The information provided in Table 1.2 suggests the sexual behaviours increasingly involve children or others who are viewed as vulnerable. This may be relative to size, age, cognitive or physical abilities, or social status. Language becomes sexually explicit with children who are of significantly younger ages. The beginnings of sexual harassment may be seen in the form of sexual teasing or embarrassment of others (see Ryan *et al.*, 1993). Threatening language, both verbal and non-verbal, may also be used. The affect associated with sexual behaviours is no longer light-hearted, but rather it takes on negative qualities such as anxiety, guilt, fear, confusion, anger and rage (see Johnson and Feldmeth, 1993).

Several programmes, most notably Hindman's (1994) "It's About Childhood", add a dimension not included in the programmes discussed in Table 1.2. In this programme, if a youth (under age 18) engages in sexual behaviours that have non-normative characteristics, and the child knows the behaviour is inappropriate and associated with punishment (i.e. the child is viewed as culpable), the behaviour is viewed as a criminal act. This view gives new meaning to sexually abusive and aggressive behaviours by children. That is, if the sexual behaviour is defined as criminal, it would be processed through the criminal justice system and the child would be labelled criminal. This view is very controversial among those who work with preadolescents and even adolescents.

### *Classification comparisons*

Table 1.3 provides a summary of preadolescent sexual behaviours that are considered not only deviant but abusive. It also provides associated risk factors. As can be seen, the sexual behaviours and development are far advanced from what is considered normal. These behaviours involve the use of force, coercion, secrecy and bribery and are repetitive, patterned and may be compulsive and obsessive. Little self-control is evident and little empathy for victims is shown. Sexual behaviours may be opportunistic, but increasingly become calculated and predatory. The behaviours are associated with feelings of anger, rage, fear, shame and confusion. The motivations may be related to power and control issues or be a means of coping with unmet needs. Children engaged in sexually abusive behaviours may have histories of abuse, and their family environments, as well as their outside environments, are conducive to sexually deviant as well as other antisocial activities. Some of these behaviours are criminal. Finally, the labels or conceptualizations of these children's behaviours can have far-reaching intervention outcomes. For example, Hindman's (1994) approach, compared with other programmes described in Table 1.1, would increase the chances of children ending up in the criminal justice system.

### *Summary of preadolescent sexual development*

The material presented in Tables 1.1, 1.2 and 1.3, coupled with the above discussion, demonstrate that preadolescents engage in a variety of sexual acts alone and with others. These range from sexual behaviours considered normal or normative to those considered problematic, inappropriate, deviant, abusive, aggressive or even criminal. As can be seen from Tables 1.1 and 1.2 there is some agreement among researchers and practitioners concerning

*Table 1.3* Non-normative and/or sexually abusive behaviours for preadolescents and associated risk factors: a summary

| *Characteristics of non-normative or sexually abusive behaviours* | *Emotions demonstrated by sexually abusive children* |
|---|---|
| Sexual behaviours are developed far beyond those expected for age of abuser. May include oral copulation, vaginal and oral intercourse, or forcible penetration of anus or vagina with fingers or other objects.<br>Sexual behaviours have aggressive/abusive quality involving use of force, coercion, secrecy, or all three. Behaviours may involve self, but generally involve others.<br>Coercion may be of two types: use of physical force, or threat to use weapon, injury to victim(s), and/or sexual acts that may be sadistic or ritualistic in nature and/or use of social threats (e.g. "I won't be your friend any more"), bribes, trickery, persuasion, intimidation, peer pressure, and so on.<br>Types of secrecy are used to deny victim(s) – through abuser's use of coercion – the right to disclose their experience and serves to protect sexual aggressor.<br>Sexual behaviours increase over time, become repetitive or obsessive or both, become compulsive, and are patterned rather than isolated events.<br>When another is involved, sexual behaviours are planned, calculated and predatory – exceed opportunistic sexual activities.<br>Sexual behaviours may be associated with other antisocial behaviours such as conduct disorders, oppositional disorders, etc.<br>Sexual behaviours continue despite intervention.<br>Under the "It's About Childhood" programme, the sexual behaviour may be considered criminal; that is, if culpability is high (the abuser knows the behaviour is non-normative and is associated with negative consequences), it will be considered to have criminal intent. | Abusers demonstrate deep feelings of anger, rage, fear, shame and loneliness. Practitioners and researchers, such as Johnson and Feldmeth (1993) and Friedrich (1990), argue that these emotions are paired with aggression. Abusers lack empathy for victims.<br>*Abuse histories*<br>Sexual aggressors may been sexually abused.<br>All have been abused in some way – sexually, physically, emotionally, or all three. Many have been neglected.<br>*Abuser–victim relationship: power and control*<br>Abusers choose victims they believe have less power and control and who appear weaker and vulnerable. Defining characteristics include difference in age (2–5 years), size, status, intelligence, cognitive development, handicapped, unmet needs, and so on.<br>Victims may be siblings, other children living in the home, schoolmates, or other acquaintances. Victims may be older than abuser, but abuser has some type of authority or power over victim.<br>Victims usually do not give informed consent.<br>*Environments*<br>Living arrangements lack sexual boundaries; highly sexualized environments that may include frequent exposure to pornography; abusive environments; parents or caretakers are substance abusers or demonstrate other parental dysfunctions.<br>Outside home environments conducive to socializing children into sexually abusive/aggressive activities. |

| | |
|---|---|
| *Motives for sexually aggressive behaviours*<br>Need to reduce negative feelings of fear, anger and loneliness.<br>Need for power and application of coercion. | *Treatment outcomes*<br>Considering all groups of children with sexual behaviour problems and disturbances, sexually abusive/aggressive children are most resistant to treatment.<br>Sexually abusive/aggressive children are in need of intensive specialized treatment. |
| *Self-control*<br>Sexually abusive/aggressive children demonstrate little self-control as related to their sexual behaviour. | |

specific sexual behaviours that can be characterized as normal/normative, non-normative and abusive, although there exists a variety of labels that are used when describing these behaviours. The labels tend to vary by discipline or perspective of the practitioners or researchers.

While there is not yet a definitive set of symptoms that clearly distinguishes children who engage in either normal, normative or non-normative sexual behaviours (see Beitchman *et al.*, 1991; Conte and Schuerman, 1987; Kendall-Tackett *et al.*, 1993), the typologies discussed here are useful because they provide a range of sexual behaviours and associated social, psychological and environmental factors that can help assess whether preadolescents' sexual behaviours are normal/normative or abnormal/deviant and even the direction future sexual development may take. In closing this section, it should be obvious that sexual behaviours and development during preadolescence will influence sexual development during adolescence. Indeed, as Steele and Ryan (1991) note, the origins of sexually deviant behaviour lie in childhood experiences. Likewise, the origins of adolescents' normal and normative sexual development begin in these early years.

### *Normative adolescent sexual behaviour and development*

Many marked changes related to size, shape and functioning of the body, emotional, cognitive, self-concept and interpersonal relationships occur as adolescents make the transition from preadolescence (Lerner and Galambos, 1998). Structural changes related to sexual development include growth of the penis and testes and lengthening of the vagina. With the onset of puberty youth experience changes related to reproduction; girls experience menstruation, boys begin the production of seminal fluid and ejaculation occurs. As physical and structural changes take place, adolescence is a time when many young men and women encounter their first interpersonal sexual experiences. It is within this context, similar to preadolescence, that many of the sexual behaviours and sexual development become defined as normative, deviant or criminal.

There is a body of literature (Gagnon, 1972; Simon and Gagnon, 1969) that provides information regarding the sequence of sexual behaviours that unfold during adolescence, although as noted previously, there are sex, racial and cultural differences. In general, males and African-Americans are likely to engage in the developmental sexual processes earlier than Caucasians and females. The sexual development of Asian-Americans appears to occur later than either African-Americans or Caucasians (Santrock, 2001).

Table 1.4 outlines sexual behaviours and development that many researchers consider normal or normative for adolescents. While information provided in this table is only an abbreviated listing of sources, the ideas set forth are generally representative of the body of research on this topic. According to Santrock (2001) by the end of adolescence the majority of youth have

*Table 1.4* Progression of normal and normative sexual behaviours and development in adolescents

| *Source of information* | *Description of sexual behaviours and development* |
|---|---|
| *Schofield (1965)* | 1. Sexual desires and urges<br>2. Sexual attraction to others<br>3. Dating<br>4. Holding hands<br>5. Kissing<br>6. Touching<br>7. Sexually fondling other person<br>8. Sexual intercourse |
| *Conger and Galambos (1997, ch. 6)*<br>*Santrock (2001, ch. 11)*<br>*Bukowski, Sippola and Brender (1993)* | 1. First sexual behaviours take place alone, especially true for males.<br>2. Masturbation (boys). Begin by age 13. 90% masturbate by age 19. Occurs frequently. Average is about 5 times per week.<br>3. Masturbation (girls). 60–70% masturbate by age 20. Occurs less frequently than among boys.<br>4. Kissing.<br>5. Necking (mutual touching and fondling above the waist).<br>6. Petting (mutual touching and fondling below the waist).<br>7. Sexual intercourse (highly irregular pattern after first experience).<br>8. Oral sex. Occurs later than first experience of sexual intercourse. |
| *Santrock (2001, pp. 357–365)* | 1. Sexual interest/sexual arousal.<br>2. Masturbation (most frequent outlet). More common among males and frequency is greater for males than females.<br>3. Ejaculation (wet dreams) in most males by 12–13 years of age.<br>4. (a) Heterosexual continuum of sexual development:<br>• Kissing (males 13.9 years; females 15 years).<br>• French kissing (males 14.6 years; females 15.5 years).<br>• Touching breasts (males 14.6 years; females 16.2 years).<br>• Touching penis (males 15.7 years).<br>• Touching vagina (males 15.4 years; females 16.4 years).<br>• Sexual intercourse (males 16.3 years; females 17 years).<br>• Oral sex (males 16.9 years; females 17.8 years).<br>4. (b) Homosexual continuum of sexual development:<br>• Exclusively heterosexual behaviours.<br>• Mostly heterosexual but occasional homosexual behaviours.<br>• Largely heterosexual but more occasional homosexual contacts.<br>• Equal amounts of heterosexual and homosexual behaviours. |

| Source of information | Description of sexual behaviours and development |
|---|---|
| | • Mostly homosexual but more than incidental heterosexual behaviours.<br>• Mostly homosexual with occasional heterosexual behaviours.<br>• Exclusively homosexual behaviours.<br>4. (c) Bisexual development. Very rare (about 1% of the population). |

progressed through the sexual behaviours shown in Table 1.4 although by the age of nineteen one in five have not yet experienced intercourse.

Information in Table 1.4 demonstrates that many of the sexual behaviours are similar to those considered normal/normative for preadolescents. This includes behaviours such as masturbation for both males and females; similar to preadolescents, masturbation is more common among males as is the frequency of such behaviour. Sexual interest, sexual arousal, kissing, sexual intercourse and oral sex are also considered normal or normative for adolescents. Interestingly, as can be seen in Table 1.4, those who study the period of adolescence view sexual intercourse and oral sex as behaviours that should not occur until later in the sequence of normal adolescent sexual development.

Those writing about adolescents view the behaviours shown in Table 1.4 as representing a normal progression of sexual behaviours and development for this age group. But if one compares Table 1.1 and Table 1.4, it can be concluded that some preadolescents would have gone through this progression of sexual developments prior to ever reaching adolescence, and some practitioners such as Gil (1993) and Cunningham and MacFarlane (1991) view this as normal. However, it is not clear what the qualitative and quantitative factors are that would cause kissing, for example, to be considered normative for adolescents but not for preadolescents. One answer seems to lie in determining the motivation for kissing. According to Ryan and Blum (1994), opposite-sex interactions prior to puberty tend to be more exploratory and social. After puberty behaviours such as kissing, flirting and foreplay (touching, fondling) are more goal-oriented toward intimacy, sexual arousal and orgasm.

With respect to heterosexual, homosexual or bisexual behaviours, both preadolescents and adolescents may be involved with a variety of partners. Early preadolescent experiences with either or both sexes seem once again to be primarily centred around experimentation and curiosity. As children move through preadolescence and become aware of social norms, these behaviours are likely to become more heterosexual during adolescence when there is more emphasis on developing a sexual identity.

Other qualitative and quantitative factors that differentiate similarly labelled sexual behaviours for preadolescents and adolescents are the frequency and the private–public nature of sexual behaviours. It is considered more acceptable for adolescents as compared to preadolescents to display their intimate affection for one another publicly, such as embracing and kissing one another. For younger children this would not be seen as acceptable unless it demonstrated only imitation or friendship and lacked sexual and intimate connotations. Similarly, there is more tolerance for private intimate sexual activities among adolescents as they move toward the next stage in the lifecycle, adulthood.

Most current researchers and professionals involved in the study of adolescents' sexual development agree that the process is multifaceted (Brooks-Gunn and Paikoff, 1993; Graber, Brooks-Gunn and Galen, 1999). Brooks-Gunn and Paikoff (1997) provide a list of five developmental issues that can help professionals determine whether adolescents' sexual development appears normative or is associated with factors that may lead to abnormal, non-normative or deviant sexual development. This list includes the following.

*Timing of sexual experiences:* Brooks-Gunn and Paikoff (1997) are of the opinion that young adolescents should not have sexual intercourse. Their reasoning is that young adolescents are less likely to engage in protected sex, increasing the possibility of pregnancy and also, it might be said, sexually transmitted diseases. Also, they believe young adolescents are emotionally and cognitively unable to understand and cope with sexuality's intense, varied feelings and complex meanings. Along similar lines, Bingham and Crockett (1996) found that the earlier in adolescence that boys and girls engage in sexual intercourse, the more likely they are to show adjustment problems.

*Timing of behaviours associated with sexual maturation:* Brooks-Gunn and Paikoff (1997) contend that early maturation for girls is associated with having sexual intercourse. Further, it is associated with early dating, having older friends, being pursued by older males, wanting less supervision by parents and spending more time in private activities that exclude adult supervision. Graber, Britto and Brooks-Gunn (1999) conclude that special attention should be given to early-maturing girls as they are sexually vulnerable.

*Co-occurrence of health-related behaviour:* Brooks-Gunn and Paikoff (1997) argue that early sexual maturity is not only linked to engaging in sexual intercourse but also is associated with early drinking, smoking, having unprotected sex, drug use, delinquency and school-related problems. These authors view early sexual maturation as placing adolescents on a precarious developmental course that can propel them into non-normative sexual activities and, additionally, other deviant or even criminal behaviours.

*Gender and sexuality:* Brooks-Gunn and Pikoff (1997) argue that young adolescent girls may be involved in sexual activities that are involuntary or happen in social settings where male dominance plays a role. One of the reasons these researchers suggest this can happen is that sexual scripts are often different for males and females.

*Context of sexual behaviour:* Brooks-Gunn and Paikoff (1997) note that sexual behaviours and development are influenced by the environments in which adolescents interact. These include factors such as poverty, neighbourhoods, school characteristics, peer group norms and varied cultural contexts. Males, African-Americans, lower socio-economic groups and inner-city youth appear to be the most sexually active, while Asian-Americans seem most restrictive (Clark *et al.*, 1984; Feldman *et al.*, 1999; Santrock, 2001).

Conger and Galambos (1997) report that for younger adolescents, more conservative sexual behaviour is associated with being politically conservative and religiously oriented. They also report that having conservative families and peers slow down the progression and frequency of sexual activity, especially in the area of sexual intercourse and beyond (see also Lerner and Galambos, 1998).

If we compare the ideas about normal sexual behaviours and development set forth by Brooks-Gunn and Paikoff (1997) with our earlier discussions on normative and non-normative sexual behaviours and development of preadolescents, it is clear that these authors do not agree with Gil (1993) and Cunningham and MacFarlane (1991), who view sexual intercourse in the latency period (ages 8–12) as part of the normal sexual development of preadolescents. In fact, looking at Table 1.4, most professionals who work with adolescents or study the period of adolescence, view sexual intercourse as a behaviour that should occur only late in the progression of adolescent sexual development. One possible explanation for these discrepancies is that some practitioners and researchers only focus on the preadolescent stages of sexual development while others only focus on adolescents. Each group, then, provides only part of the total picture of the normative sexual development of young people.

### Non-normative adolescent sexual behaviour and development

In the previous section we discussed broad categories of behaviours that can include at-risk sexual behaviours and individual and environmental factors that can increase the risk of engaging in these behaviours. Table 1.5 provides a more comprehensive picture of the specific types of sexual activities and accompanying risk factors that professionals and researchers have identified. These accompanying factors include emotions, motivations, abuse histories, power and control issues, and problems with self-esteem, as well as the individual and contextual factors discussed in the previous section.

As can be seen in Table 1.5, there are some types of non-normative or sexually deviant behaviours that are similar to those discussed for preadolescents, such as rape or sexual behaviours that involve the use of bribes, secrets, tricks or surprises. Because adolescents are expected to be more cognitively advanced than preadolescents, they are expected to be more aware of the standards and consequences associated with engaging in behaviours such as unprotected sexual activities that can lead to sexually transmitted diseases and premarital pregnancies. Hence, when they engage in these behaviours it is considered more socially irresponsible and non-normative than when preadolescents are involved in unprotected sexual activities. Likewise, behaviours that bring harm to the self, others or society are not only considered non-normative for adolescents, but also may be viewed as criminal.

Non-normative behaviours may also include a variety of paraphilic interests or activities. In a study of adult sexual offenders, Abel *et al.* (1993) reported that of 1,025 paraphiliacs seen in outpatient clinics, many of the paraphilic interests developed during adolescence. Transvestism had the earliest age of onset, occurring at thirteen (13.6) years of age. Fetishism, bestiality, voyeurism, obscene phone calls, masochism and sadism began in late adolescence (16 to 19 years). The impact of the family environment on these behaviours was noted, as almost all clients came from families that were incestuous and sexually abusive.

Behaviours that involve the use of force, coercion and manipulation are considered not only deviant, but also criminal. Likewise, overt or covert unwanted sexual advances are considered non-normative or criminal. Behaviours such as date rape and sexual harassment may be motivated by needs for power and control. On a sociological level, power and control may be defined in terms of significant age, size, social status discrepancies, or other factors that place the perpetrator in an authority position over the victim. As Table 1.5 indicates, types of affect or needs that contribute to deviant sexual behaviours include feelings of emptiness, anger, confusion, anxiety or lack of empathy for victims.

It appears likely that adolescents who engage in deviant sexual activities come from highly dysfunctional families where family members may have histories of abuse. Outside the family, these adolescents may be involved in peer groups that are conducive to not only sexual deviance but other types of deviant behaviour such as excessive drinking, drug use, delinquency and school-related problems (see Steele and Ryan, 1991). However, this is not always the case. Some adolescents who engage in deviant sexual behaviours are popular among their peers and are high achievers in academics and sports (Araji, 2000).

## Recommendations for reducing at risk behaviours

Based on the previous discussion it is clear that normal, normative or deviant sexual behaviours do not develop in a vacuum. They are influenced by both

*Table 1.5* Non-normative or sexually abusive behaviours for adolescents and associated risk factors: a summary

| *Characteristics of non-normative or sexually abusive behaviours* | *Abuse histories* |
|---|---|
| *Behaviours*<br>• Behaviours that stand out as abnormal or non-normative – e.g. unprotected sexual activity, promiscuity, teen-pregnancy, transmission of sexual diseases.<br>• Behaviours that have a negative or harmful effect on self or others or the environment – e.g. prostitution, paraphilic interests such as transvestism, fetishism, bestiality, voyeurism, masochism and sadism.<br>• Behaviours that involve the use of surprise, force, threat or coercion such as date or acquaintance rape.<br>• Behaviours that involve the use of bribes, manipulation, trickery, persistent persuasion or intimidation.<br>• Overt and covert sexual acts that are unwanted by the recipient – e.g. sexual harassment or stalking.<br>*Emotions*<br>• Feelings of emptiness or loneliness due to earlier neglect, abuse or other disruptions in life.<br>• Lack of empathy.<br>• Anger, confusion and anxiety. | *Abuse histories*<br>• Sexually abusive adolescents may have a history of various types of abuse including neglect, and emotional, physical or sexual abuse.<br>*Abuser–victim relationships*<br>• Characterized by power and control.<br>• Victims are chosen based on perceived weaknesses and vulnerability – those over whom the abuser perceives having power and control.<br>• Characteristics may include significant differences in age, size, status and cognitive development.<br>*Environments*<br>• Early exposure to sexual behaviour or activity.<br>• Living environments may lack sexual boundaries and norms.<br>• Homes may be overly permissive, overly restrictive or exploitative – e.g. sex is an exchange commodity. Home lives may be characterized by various dysfunctions such as abusing parents, substance abuse, maladaptive coping mechanisms, poor communication, lack of attachment and supervision. |

| | |
|---|---|
| *Motives*<br>• Need to reduce negative feelings of fear, anger, loneliness or emptiness.<br>• Need for power and control.<br>• Need to raise low self-esteem. | • May experience frequent exposure to erotic or pornographic material, unsafe sex.<br>• Outside home environments and peer associations conducive to sexually and non-sexually deviant behaviours – e.g. excessive drinking, drug use, abuse, delinquency and school-related problems. Especially apparent in minority and socially disadvantaged groups where neighbourhoods and communities may be characterized by poverty, and urban, high-density living arrangements.<br>• Frequent moves and other disruptive environmental factors. |

Source: Material used in developing this table comes from Steele and Ryan (1991, pp. 83–100); Conger and Galambos (1997); Santrock (2001, pp. 381–383); Abel *et al.* (1993, pp. 104–115); Lerner and Galambos (1998); Ryan *et al.* (1993); and Ryan and Blum (1994).

individual and environmental factors for both preadolescents and adolescents. Further, deviant sexual acts appear to be part of a constellation of other at-risk behaviours such as substance abuse, school problems and delinquency. This was obvious in Case Study One discussed earlier.

Much of the literature reviewed in this chapter indicates that early sexual maturation, or early exposure to non-normative or abnormal sexual activities, are key factors that can lead youth toward non-normative, deviant or even criminal sexual acts. With respect to helping adolescents develop healthy sexuality and avoid at-risk behaviours, Brooks-Gunn and Paikoff (1997) offer a set of recommendations that are aimed at adolescents' sexual practices. These include:

- Practising sexual abstinence, yet feeling good about one's body.
- Engaging in sexual intercourse with another individual in late adolescence or early adulthood in the context of committed relationships.
- Using safe-sex practices.
- Practising pre-intercourse behaviours with others in early adolescence, which can be followed by sexual intercourse in late adolescence or early adulthood.

The next set of recommendations focuses on what society can do to assist in the normal and normative sexual development of both preadolescents and adolescents.

*Assessment of individuals' protective and at-risk behaviours* It is apparent from material presented in this chapter that most practitioners agree that the onset of early puberty is a biological or individual characteristic that exposes a young person to a constellation of behaviours that can lead not only to unwise sexual behaviours but also to exposure to sexual harassment, date rape and adjustment problems. Early exposure to sexual activities such as incest can lead to non-normative sexual behaviours as well as problems in school or juvenile delinquency. Other at-risk individual factors include unmet needs, inability to feel and express empathy, and non-normative power and control issues. Being male, African-American, and living in high-density poor urban areas also increase the risk of early exposure to sexual behaviours and development. Some protective factors include reaching puberty at the average age and experiencing normal cognitive, emotional and physical development.

*Assessment of environmental protective and at-risk factors* Protective environmental factors include having families and peers who are conservative and religious, but not extremely so. Both adolescents and preadolescents benefit from families with whom they have positive attachments and where there is adequate supervision. Families and communities that take an interest in providing an atmosphere of healthy sexual development also serve as a protection against unwanted pregnancies, acquaintance rape, sexual harassment and the spread of sexually transmitted diseases.

Environments that place preadolescents and adolescents at risk of abnormal or non-normative sexual behaviours and development include those that demonstrate overly restrictive or permissive sexual attitudes, that expose children to abusive behaviours, alcohol and drug misuse, pornography, delinquent and criminal activities, and that provide few opportunities for the development of healthy self-conceptions and feelings.

*Early identification and intervention for at-risk behaviours* Parents, teachers, clinicians and other professionals must be knowledgeable about what constitutes normal and normative behaviours and the individual and environmental factors that provide warning signs that youth are on deviant developmental pathways. These risk factors must be identified early and appropriate interventions applied. As noted in the discussion of preadolescents' non-normative sexual behaviours, once behaviours become patterned they are more resistant to treatment. This is also true for associated risk behaviours such as alcohol and drug abuse, predatory behaviours, school failures and other delinquent or criminal acts.

Individualized attention may be clinical or may involve socially attaching a youth to a responsible adult such as someone in the "Big-Brother, Big-Sister" programme. Social skills training enables youth to cope with and resist potentially negative influences from families, peers and the media. Given the cultural role of the family, parents must be involved at all levels: prevention, intervention and treatment. However, we must not ignore the fact that many families are the cause of children being unable to experience normal sexual development as well as the development of other negative behaviours, self-conceptions and feelings (see Engles *et al.*, 1999). If siblings or peers are part of the problem, then they also need to be part of the solution (see Engles *et al.*, 1999; Ennett and Bauman, 1994; Epstein, 1983). Clinicians, as well as concerned schools and families, cannot by themselves bring about changes that may be helpful in social institutions such as the media. For example, it is difficult for parents and schools to teach sexual abstinence in a society when the media bombards young people with sexual messages. Youth who live in industrial and post-industrial nations are confronted on a daily basis with sexual material and messages that are not conducive to normal sexual development. Moreover, with technological advances such as videos and the internet, they can be exposed to every type of sexually abusive, deviant and criminal behaviour (Araji, 2000). This is true even in sexually restrictive societies.

Collaborative work is necessary so that all parts of the world are working in harmony to promote the healthy sexual development of young people. The need for such collaboration is nowhere more evident than in African countries where large percentages of the populations are contracting, spreading and dying from Aids. This is especially true among the young people.

### *Review and assessment considerations*

This chapter has reviewed sexual behaviours and development for preadolescents and adolescents that are considered normal, normative, deviant and even criminal. What has emerged is that many of the sexual behaviours that appear in descriptions of normal sexual development for adolescents are also considered normal sexual development for preadolescents. However, many scholars writing about adolescent sexual development, in contrast to those writing about preadolescent development, would be opposed to viewing sexual intercourse and oral sex as normal sexual behaviours for preadolescents. In fact, many scholars of adolescence view early expressions of sexual behaviours that occur outside the realm of curiosity, exploration and imitation, as inappropriate. It is suggested that the examination of adolescent and preadolescent sexual development should not be studied separately, but should be viewed as a continuum. It is becoming increasingly clear that many deviant behaviours expressed during adolescence have their origins in preadolescent experiences and this is similarly true for normal and normative sexual development.

This chapter has also demonstrated that both individual and environmental factors influence the sexual development of preadolescents and adolescents, either positively or negatively. Individual factors include the onset of puberty, motivations and affect, as well as beliefs and feelings about self and others. Environmental factors include the influence of family, peers and school, and exposure to substance use, sexualized language and erotic and pornographic material.

It has further been shown that normal or deviant sexual development is associated with other behaviours such as the use or abuse of substances, various conduct disorders, school problems and delinquent and criminal actions. Preadolescents or adolescents who have been exposed to these problems may also be at risk of engaging in sexually deviant behaviours. It is a well-known fact, for example, that acquaintance or date rape is associated with alcohol or substance use (Barnett *et al.*, 1997).

Based on this knowledge, parents and professionals would be well-advised to work together to ensure that children have access to both personal and environmental tools that will allow for healthy sexual development and the development of related behaviours such as responsible use of alcohol, protection against pregnancy and sexually transmitted diseases, school success, and other actions that lead toward healthy and productive lives. In short, sexual development of preadolescents and adolescents does not occur in a vacuum. The development of each young person is influenced by many individual and environmental factors.

In concluding this chapter, some questions are offered that parents, clinicians and other professionals can use as a general guide for determining whether sexual behaviours are problematic. These questions can be applied to all age groups, families, communities and societies. Some of these questions are derived from Ryan and Blum (1994).

- Is the behaviour putting the individual at risk of physical harm, disease or exploitation?
- Is the behaviour interfering with the individual's overall development, learning, or social or family relationships?
- Is the behaviour putting others at risk of physical harm, disease or exploitation?
- Is the behaviour interfering with the developmental behaviours, learning and social or family relationships of others?
- Is the behaviour violating a rule or a law?
- Is the behaviour causing the individual to feel confused, embarrassed, guilty, or negative about him/herself?
- Is the behaviour causing others to feel uncomfortable, confused, embarrassed, guilty, or negative about themselves?
- Is the behaviour abusive because it involves a lack of consent, a lack of equality, or some type of coercion or force?
- Is the behaviour dysfunctional for the development of healthy relationships?
- Is the behaviour destructive to the family, peer groups, school, community or society?

The more questions that are answered in the affirmative, the more problematic one should consider the developmental patterns, and how the questions are answered will determine the types of intervention, treatment and prevention programmes that may be implemented.

## Conclusions

The purpose of this chapter was to address the challenging task of differentiating normal and normative sexual development from abnormal, deviant or even criminal development for preadolescents and adolescents. It became clear that the process of sexual development is embedded within physical, social, cognitive, emotional and motivational developments. Further, whether preadolescents and adolescents proceed down the paths of normal or deviant sexuality is very much related to other behavioural developments occurring simultaneously. These include individual behaviours such as use or abuse of alcohol or drugs, school failures or successes, and the development of social skills. The conclusion that emerged is that discussions of the development of normal or deviant sexual behaviours must be studied within the contexts of individual and environmental factors. For the benefit of youth, their families, communities and societies, the information provided in this chapter should be useful in identifying risk factors as well as protective factors that can be used in prevention, intervention and treatment programmes.

Preadolescent and adolescent sexual development should be studied as a continuum. Most researchers, practitioners, social planners and members of the justice system, agree that normal and abnormal sexual behaviours of adolescents (and even adults) have their origins in development during preadolescence. This knowledge, however, is frequently ignored. The information provided in this chapter should serve as a departure for subsequent work on the study of sexual development during preadolescence and adolescence. Many, but not all of the behaviours that scholars and practitioners consider normal sexual development for preadolescents, are very similar to what is considered normal sexual development for adolescents (compare Tables 1.1 and 1.4). We need to articulate those motives, cognitions, affects, situations and other factors that can be used to clearly differentiate normal from and abnormal sexual behaviours for both preadolescents and adolescents. It is not sufficient to identify "kissing", for example, as part of the normal development for both groups. We must develop a continuum that demonstrates the associated factors that allow us to define behaviours such as kissing as normal or abnormal for each group. We have the information to complete this task, but it has not been developed into a comprehensive continuum that stretches from preadolescence through adolescence.

*Acknowledgement*

Thanks are extended to Marina Makarova for assistance with typing this manuscript.

## References

Abel, G. G., Osborn, C. A., and Twigg, D. A. (1993). Sexual assault through the lifespan: Adult offenders with juvenile histories. In H. E. Barabee, W. L. Marshall and S. M. Hudson (eds), *The Juvenile Sex Offender*. New York: Guilford Press, pp. 104–117.

Achenbach, T. M., and Edelbrook, C. (1983). *Manual for Child Behaviour Checklist and Revised Child Behaviour Profile*. Burlington: University of Vermont Department of Psychiatry.

Araji, S. K. (1997). *Sexually Aggressive Children: Coming to Understand Them*. Thousand Oaks, CA: Sage.

Araji, S. K. (2000). Serial offenders: Child sexual abusers, a review and update. In L. B. Schlesinger (ed.), *Serial Offenders: Current Thought, Recent Findings, Unusual Syndromes*. New York: CRC Press.

Arnett, J. J. (2001). *Adolescence and Emerging Adulthood*. New Jersey: Prentice Hall.

Barnett, O., Miller-Perrin, C., and Perrin, R. (1997). *Family Violence across the Life-span*. Thousand Oaks, CA: Sage.

Beitchman, J., Zucker, K., Hood, J., DaCosta, G. A., and Akman, A. J. (1991). A review of the short-term effects of child sexual abuse. *Child Abuse and Neglect, 15*, 537–556.

Berliner, L., Manaois, O., and Monastersky, C. (1986). *Child Sexual Behavior Disturbance: An Assessment and Treatment Model*. Seattle, WA: Harborview Sexual Assault Center.

Bingham, C. R., and Crockett, L. J. (1996). Longitudinal adjustment patterns of boys and girls experiencing early, middle, and late sexual intercourse. *Developmental Psychology, 32*, 647–658.

Brooks-Gunn, J., and Paikoff, R. L. (1993). Sex is a gamble, kissing is a game: Adolescent sexuality and health promotion. In S. G. Millstein, A. C. Petersen and E. O. Nightingale (eds), *Promoting the Health of Adolescents*. New York: Cambridge University Press.

Brooks-Gunn, J., and Paikoff, R. L. (1997). Sexuality and development transitions during adolescence. In J. Schulenberg, J. Maggs and K. Hurrelmann (eds), *Health Risk and Developmental Transitions during Adolescence*. New York: Cambridge University Press.

Bukowski, W. M., Sippola, L., and Brender, W. (1993). Where does sexuality come from? Normative sexuality from a developmental perspective. In H. E. Barabee, W. L. Marshall and S. M. Hudson (eds), *The Juvenile Sex Offender*. New York: Guilford Press.

Bullough, V. L. (1981). Age at menarche: A misunderstanding. *Science, 213*, 365–366.

Cassell, C. (1984). *Swept Away: Why Women Fear Their Own Sexuality*. New York: Simon & Schuster.

Clark, S. D., Zabin, L. S., and Hardy, J. B. (1984). Sex, contraception, and parenthood: Experience and attitudes among urban black young men. *Family Planning Perspectives, 16*, 77–82.

Conger, J. J., and Galambos, N. L. (1997). *Adolescence and Youth*. New York: Longman.

Conte, J. R., and Schuerman, J. R. (1987). Factors associated with an increased impact of child sexual abuse. *Child Abuse and Neglect, 11*, 201–211.

Cunningham, C., and MacFarlane, L. (1991). *When Children Molest Children: Group Treatment Strategies for Young Sexual Offenders*. Orwell, VT: Safer Society Press.

Ellis, N. (1991). An extension of the Steinberg accelerating hypothesis. *Journal of Early Adolescence, 11*, 221–235.

Engles, R. C. M. E., Knibbe, R. A., de Vries, H., Drop, M. J., and van Breukelen, G. J. P. (1999). Influences of parental and best friends' smoking and drinking on adolescent use: A longitudinal study. *Journal of Applied Social Psychology, 29*, 337–361.

Ennett, S., and Bauman, K. (1994). The contribution of influence and selection to adolescent peer group homogeneity: The case of adolescent cigarette smoking. *Journal of Personality and Social Psychology, 67*, 653–663.

Entwistle, D. (1990). Schools and the adolescent. In S. Feldman and G. Elliott (eds), *At the Threshold: The Developing Adolescent*. Cambridge, MA: Harvard University Press.

Epstein, J. (1983). Selecting friends in contrasting secondary school environments. In J. Epstein and N. Karweit (eds), *Friends in School*. New York: Academic Press.

Epstein, J. S., Pratto, D. J., and Skipper, J. K. (1990). Teenagers, behavioural problems, and preferences for heavy metal and rap music: A case study of a Southern middle school. *Deviant Behaviour, 11*, 381–394.

Eveleth, P. B., and Tanner, J. M. (1990). *Worldwide Variation in Human Growth*, 2nd edn. Cambridge: Cambridge University Press.

Feldman, S. S., Turner, R. A., and Araujo, K. (1999). Interpersonal context as an influence on the sexual timetables of youth: Gender and ethnic effects. *Journal of Research on Adolescence, 9*, 25–52.

Friedrich, W. N. (1990). *Psychotherapy of Sexually Abused Children and their Families*. New York: Norton.

Friedrich, W. N., and Luecke, W. J. (1998). Young school-age sexually aggressive children. *Professional Psychology: Research and Practice, 19(2)*, 155–164.

Friedrich, W. N., Urquiza, A. J., and Beilke, R. (1986). Behavior problems in sexually abused young children. *Journal of Pediatric Psychology, 11*, 47–57.

Friedrich, W. N., Grambsch, P., Koverola, C., Hewitt, S., Damon, L., Lemond, T., and Broughton, D. (1989). "The Child Sexual Behaviour Inventory: Normative and Clinical Findings". Unpublished manuscript.

Gagnon, J. H. (1972). The creation of the sexual in early adolescence. In J. Kagan and R. Coles (eds), *Twelve to Sixteen: Early Adolescence*. New York: Norton.

Gagnon, J. H. (1973). Scripts and the coordination of sexual conduct. *Nebraska Symposium on Motivation, 21*, 27–59.

Gil, E. (1993). Age-appropriate sex play versus problematic sexual behaviors. In E. Gil and T. C. Johnson (eds), *Sexualised Children: Assessment and Treatment of Sexualised Children and Children who Molest*. Rockville, MD: Launch Press.

Graber, J. A., Britto, P. R., and Brooks-Gunn, J. (1999). What's love got to do with it? Adolescents' and young adults' beliefs about sexual and romantic relationships. In W. Furman, C. Feiring and B. B. Brown (eds), *Contemporary Perspectives on Adolescent Relationships*. New York: Cambridge University Press.

Graber, J. A., Brooks-Gunn, J., and Galen, B. R. (1999). Betwixt and between: Sexuality in the context of adolescent transitions. In R. Jessor (ed.), *New Perspectives on Adolescent Risk Behaviour*. New York: Cambridge University Press.

Hindman, J. (1994). *JCA-Juvenile Culpability Assessment*, 2nd edn. Ontario, OR: Alexandria.

Johnson, T. C., and Feldmeth, J. R. (1993). Sexual behaviors: A continuum. In E. Gil and T. C. Johnson (eds), *Sexualised Children: Assessment and Treatment of Sexualised Children who Molest*. Rockville, MD: Launch Press.

Kendall-Tackett, K. A., Williams, L. M., and Finkelhor, D. (1993). Impact of sexual abuse on children: A review and synthesis of recent empirical studies. *Psychological Bulletin, 113(1)*, 164–180.

Kinsey, A. C., Pomeroy, W. B., and Martin, C. E. (1948). *Sexual Behavior in the Human Male*. Philadelphia: W. B. Saunders.

Kinsey, A. C., Pomeroy, W. B., Martin, C. E., and Gebhard, P. (1953). *Sexual Behavior in the Human Female*. Philadelphia: W. B. Saunders.

Lerner, R. M., and Galambos, N. L. (1998). Adolescent development: Challenges and opportunities for research, programmes, and policies. *Annual Review Psychology, 49*, 413–446.

Martinson, F. M. (1991). Normal sexual development in infancy and early childhood.

In G. D. Ryan and S. L. Lane (eds), *Juvenile Sex Offending: Causes, Consequences, and Correction*. Lexington, MA: Lexington Books.
Martinson, F. M. (1994). *The Sexual Life of Children*. Westport, CT: Bergin & Garvey.
Money, J., and Ehrhardt, A. A. (1972). *Man and Woman, Boy and Girl*. Baltimore, MD: Johns Hopkins University Press.
Okami, P. (1992). Child perpetrators of sexual abuse: The emergence of a problematic deviant category. *Journal of Sex Research, 29(1)*, 109–140.
Pithers, W., Gray, A. S., Cunningham, C., and Lane, S. (1993). *From Trauma to Understanding*. Brandon, VT: Safer Society Programme & Press.
Pitt, D. (2000). Study: More teenagers into drugs, smoking; other risk factors down. *Moscow-Pullman Daily News*, 9 June, p. 4A.
Rutter, M. (1971). Normal psychological development. *Journal of Child Psychology and Psychiatry, 2*, 259–283.
Ryan, G., and Blum, J. (1994). *Childhood Sexuality: A Guide for Parents*. Denver: Kempe Children's Center, University of Colorado Health Sciences Center.
Ryan, G., Blum, J., Sandau-Christopher, D., Law, S., Weher, F., Sundine, C., Astler, L., Teske, J., and Dale, J. (1993). *Understanding and Responding to the Sexual Behavior of Children: Trainer's Manual*. Denver: Kempe Children's Center, University of Colorado Health Sciences Center.
Santrock, J. W. (2001). *Adolescence*. Boston: McGraw Hill.
Schofield, M. (1965). *The Sexual Behavior of Young People*. Boston: Little, Brown.
Sgroi, S. M., Bunk, B. S., and Wabrek, C. J. (1998). Children's sexual behaviors and their relationship to sexual abuse. In S. M. Sgroi (ed.), *Vulnerable Populations And Treatment of Sexually Abused Children and Adult Survivors*. Lexington, MA: Lexington Books.
Simon, W., and Gagnon, J. H. (1969). On psychosexual development. In D. Goslin (ed.), *Handbook of Socialization Theory and Research*. New York: Rand McNally.
Steele, B., and Ryan, G. (1991). Deviancy: Development gone wrong. In G. D. Ryan and S. L. Lane (eds), *Juvenile Sex Offending: Causes, Consequences and Correction*. Lexington, MA: Lexington Books.
Utah Task Force of the Utah Network on Juveniles Offending Sexually (1996). *The Utah Report on Juvenile Sex Offenders*. Salt Lake City: Author.
Zoglin, R. (1996). A kiss isn't just a kiss. *Time*, 6 October.

Chapter 2

# A review of theoretical models of sexual offending

*Gary O' Reilly and Alan Carr*

## Introduction

This chapter reviews the main theoretical ideas that have emerged in the literature concerning sexual offending. The models described here are specific descriptions of the development of sexually abusive behaviour and its maintenance rather than a recasting of the traditional theoretical paradigms within psychology (such as behaviourist theory or psychoanalytic theory) to explain sexual offending. Initially many of the specific models were concerned with the development of sexual offending behaviour among adults. However, over time theorists have expanded their conceptual thinking to incorporate ideas on the development of sexually abusive behaviour in adolescents and children. A common theme that emerges in this literature is that sexually abusive behaviour can be understood as reflective of a developmental pathway in life that often begins in childhood with experiences of emotional, physical and sexual abuse. These experiences unfold a number of potential developmental trajectories including healthy recovery, prolonged experiences of personal distress, and in some instances, the emergence of individual psychological characteristics, when combined with situational and cultural factors, that lead to a vulnerability to engage in sexually abusive behaviour. Most theorists have based their models on some combination of three key ingredients. These are (i) observations based on clinical experience of working with adults, adolescents and children who engage in sexually abusive behaviour; (ii) existing empirical findings concerning people who abuse others; and (iii) other theoretical models. An important challenge exists regarding the need for stringent a priori empirical research to evaluate each model in terms of its value in understanding the development of sexually abusive behaviour and its implications for sound assessment and intervention. One aspect of many of the models that has an as yet unproven potential value is that they imply different typologies that could be applied to people who engage in sexually abusive behaviour. It is conceivable that those in different typological categories may require and respond differently to various forms of assessment and intervention. This is one of the many ideas that requires the attention of researchers in this field.

## Finkelhor's model of sexual offending

Finkelhor (1984) outlines a model that has two key elements. The first is an attempt to summarise as four factors the main theoretical and empirical ideas existing at that time regarding adult sexual offenders and their behaviour (known as the four factor model). The second is an attempt to describe a blue-print of common factors that precede the perpetration of a specific sexual offence (known as the four preconditions model). In many descriptions of Finkelhor's work these two separate models have often been collapsed into one.

### *Finkelhor's four factor model*

Finkelhor describes four factors that he believes provide an overarching framework to "summarize, synthesize and integrate" (1984, p. 33) the large amount of theoretical and research ideas that attempt to explain the development of sexually abusive behaviour. Finkelhor does not intend his four factors to provide an exhaustive list of those factors that precipitate and contribute to the development of sexually abusive behaviour. Instead he intends it to be a useful framework for summarising different research and theoretical ideas that can be added to as appropriate. His framework also allows competing and complementary ideas about an aspect of the development of sexually assaultive behaviour to be considered, tested and refined under the umbrella of a single factor. In developing his four factor model Finkelhor is attempting to develop a framework that could to be used to explain the variety and complexity of perpetrators of sexual abuse against children. Consequently the usefulness of this aspect of Finkelhor's model can only be as good as the existing theoretical and research literature. Finkelhor cautions that this literature tends to have an overemphasis on psychopathology and sexually abusive behaviour as stemming from prior traumatising experiences because it is often based upon caught and convicted sexual offenders. However, these offenders may represent the extreme end of the continuum of abusers and consequently have the most extreme developmental experiences. Finkelhor suggests that his four underlying themes can be stated as questions that can also be given factor names. Finkelhor comments that applying these questions is a good starting-point for (a) understanding an individual abuser; and (b) explaining the diversity we find between abusers. He also states that the four factors allow for the incorporation of ideas from an individual psychological and a broader sociological and cultural perspective. Each of the four factors are described in more detail below.

### *Factor 1. Emotional congruence*

*Question: Why does a person find relating sexually to a child emotionally gratifying and congruent?*

The emotional congruence factor attempts to explain why an adult would find it emotionally satisfying to relate in a sexually abusive way to a child. Finkelhor outlines examples of various possible answers to this question, most of which focus on relationship rather than exclusively sexual components. They include the following. (1) Sexual abusers who victimise children are immature in their emotional development and consequently tend to wish to relate to children who appear to them to be in some way at a comparable state of emotional and psychological development. (2) Sexual abusers have poor self-esteem and a poor sense of self-efficacy in relationships. Consequently they find interactions with adults difficult. Relating to children is easier for abusers as they perceive children to be less threatening. Relationships with adults leave offenders with feelings of insecurity and inadequacy while relationships with children leave them with feelings of power and control. (3) The abuser is attempting to achieve mastery over a past traumatic experience where he was victimised, by identifying with the past perpetrator and re-enacting his own abuse through assaulting another child. (4) The abuser has a "narcissistic identification" with himself or his likeness as a child that stems from either childhood emotional deprivation or overprotection. The adult offender selects children to victimise whom he perceives to have similar characteristics to himself. In sexually assaulting them he is expressing his narcissistic self-involvement. (5) Ascendant themes in our society promote the idea that men should be powerful, dominant and the initiator in sexual relationships. Sexual abusers accept these values but perceive themselves as unable to live up to them in peer relationships. Consequently they cultivate relationships with children that allow the adoption of a dominant role.

### *Factor 2. Sexual arousal to children*

*Question: Why is a person capable of being sexually aroused by children?*

Finkelhor argues that any complete model of sexual offending must include both sexual and non-sexual motivating factors. An over-emphasis on either sexual or non-sexual factors results in an impoverished theoretical framework. However, for an individual offender sexual motivating factors may be either primary or secondary. In formulating an offender's difficulties we require a framework that allows us to understand the relative contribution made to the development and maintenance of sexually abusive behaviour that accurately reflects an individual's capacity to find children sexually arousing. Finkelhor cites various examples of theoretical and research ideas that attempt to answer the question "Why is a person capable of being sexually aroused by children?" These include: (1) A capacity to find children sexually arousing stems from critical experiences of past trauma such as sexual, physical or emotional abuse. (2) The abuser has had an experience of arousal that involved children. This experience is shaped by reinforcement (through recall, fantasy and masturbation) into a more persistent deviant pattern of sexual arousal involving children. (3) The abuser grows up in a family where children are subjected to sexual victimisation by adults. (4) The abuser misinterprets an emotional response to children as a sexual response. (5) Biological factors, such as hormonal or genetic abnormalities, predispose the development of a deviant sexual orientation towards children. (6) The abuser develops a pattern of sexual arousal towards children through exposure to child pornography, advertising that sexualises children or other culturally available influences.

### *Factor 3. Blockage*

*Question: Why is a person blocked in efforts to obtain sexual and emotional gratification from more normatively approved sources?*

The third factor outlined by Finkelhor concerns theoretical and research ideas regarding why some individuals are blocked in their ability to have their emotional and sexual needs met in adult relationships. He describes two types of blockage, developmental and situational. Developmental blockage refers "to theories like those involving Oedipal conflicts, where the person is seen as prevented from moving into the adult sexual stage of development" (p. 44). Situational blockage refers "to theories, such as those related to incest, where a person with apparent adult sexual interests is blocked from normal sexual outlets because of the loss of a relationship or some other transitory crisis" (p. 44).

### *Factor 4. Disinhibition*

*Question: Why is a person not deterred by conventional social inhibitions from having sexual relationships with children?*

Finkelhor's fourth factor clusters together theoretical and research ideas concerning how abusers are not sufficiently influenced by conventional social inhibitions to prevent them from sexually assaulting children. He cites a variety of possible explanations that appear in the literature as follows: (i) poor impulse control; (ii) senility; (iii) alcohol and other substance abuse; (iv) psychosis; (v) environmental stressors such as unemployment, loss of love relationship or bereavement; (vi) factors that may weaken familial bonds such as step-father/step-daughter relationships or significant periods of separation from children; (vii) cultural influences promoting a patriarchal society and family structure; and (viii) use of child pornography.

## *Finkelhor's four preconditions to sexual offending*

In addition to his attempt to present a framework to integrate the main ideas concerning the development of sexual offending behaviour Finkelhor presented a new formulation on the conditions that must be present for an offender to sexually abuse a child. The four preconditions model is based on Finkelhor's review of the literature on offenders, victims of child sexual abuse and their families, and societal factors that support an environment where child sexual abuse can take place. Finkelhor's four preconditions model was an attempt to integrate these previously disparate aspects of the literature. In doing so he hoped to formulate a model that did not have a bias towards placing responsibility for sexual abuse with an inability of families or children to protect themselves while at the same time acknowledging family circumstances or victim characteristics that need to be understood as part of an environment where children are sexually assaulted. Each of the four preconditions are described below.

### *Precondition 1: The motivation to sexually abuse*

The first precondition outlined in Finkelhor's model is that a potential sexual offender must be motivated in one or more ways to engage in sexually abusive behaviour directed towards children. Under this precondition motivating influences can be understood as being drawn from the first three factors of his four factor model (outlined above). That is, the offender may be partially motivated by emotional congruence factors whereby he finds some level of emotional satisfaction from directing his sexually abusive behaviour towards children; he may be partially motivated because he experiences some degree of deviant arousal from directing his sexual behaviour towards children; and he may be partly motivated through being blocked in meeting his emotional and sexual needs in a non-deviant, non-abusive manner.

### *Precondition 2: Overcoming internal inhibitions*

Conceptually Finkelhor's model allows on the one hand for individuals who may be motivated to engage in sexually abusive behaviour but do not do so because they utilize internal factors that prevent the expression of harmful behaviour, and, on the other hand, for those who overcome their internal inhibitions. As described in the "Disinhibition Factor" in the four factor model, there are many possible ways this may happen. As described earlier these range from substance misuse, to the development of distorted thinking that offenders use to justify or minimize their behaviour, to the influence of environmental stressors.

### *Precondition 3: Overcoming externally inhibiting factors*

Once a potential offender has become motivated to sexually abuse, and has overcome his internal inhibitions, the next stage within Finkelhor's framework is that he must overcome any external factors that might prevent his offence. Although some offences are opportunistic, others are carefully orchestrated through a variety of grooming and planning behaviours designed to overcome external obstacles such as lack of access to children or the presence of a protecting adult. These behaviours include forming a relationship with the parents of a child in order to gain unsupervised access to children, offering to baby-sit, seeking a job that provides access to children, or spending time in locations where children are present.

### *Precondition 4: Overcoming the resistance of the child*

The final of Finkelhor's four preconditions is that the offender must overcome the resistance of the child. Again a variety of methods may be utilised by the offender in order to achieve this. These include building and then exploiting an emotionally close relationship with a child, bribery, trickery, use of threats and use of physical force.

In summary, Finkelhor outlines a model of sexual offending that allows us to clearly express theoretical ideas about motivating influences that lead to the development of sexually abusive behaviour. In doing so we can compare one set of theoretical hypotheses with another on the same theme and set about evaluating the evidence supporting the relative merits of each. Unfortunately researchers have rarely utilized the model in this way. Finkelhor's model also allows us to consider varying influences that can be used to formulate the predisposing, precipitating and maintaining factors relevant for an individual who has engaged in sexually abusive behaviour. In doing so the model allows us to distinguish between different types of offenders who reflect different influences on their behaviour. Finkelhor's model has also been used to inform suitable intervention goals for individual offenders such as changing deviant arousal patterns, targeting and changing distorted thinking that was used to excuse or minimize offending behaviour, and identifying individual risk factors. Finally, Finkelhor's model has also been used to promote the protection of children from sexual victimisation through the provision of information on how the environments of children can be enhanced to promote their safety.

## The Marshall and Barbaree model

Barbaree, Marshall and McCormick (1998) and Marshall and Barbaree (1990) outline an important and influential model concerning the development of sexual offending behaviour. In their most recent formulation of their model they point out that although families change in how they function over time and across different settings, the majority of people who sexually abuse others have grown up in abusive rather than nurturing family environments. From this they hypothesise that children from abusive families have experiences that *for some but not all* may promote the development of sexually abusive behaviour. They argue that abusive family experiences provide children with very different lessons about how to have and maintain relationships with other people, and that these abusive family experiences (a) may prevent the growth of a range of skills and competencies for successfully negotiating interpersonal relationships and (b) may promote the primary use of a coercive interpersonal style. How this may unfold into a developmental pathway leading to sexually abusive behaviour is described below.

### *The potential limiting of the development of interpersonal skills in abusive families*

Barbaree, Marshall and McCormick argue that children from abusive families typically do not form secure attachment bonds to their parents or may experience serious disruptions in relationships with their primary attachment figures. They experience parental relationships that are of a poorer quality than children from nurturing families. They do not have the opportunity to develop interpersonal and intimacy skills within the context of a bonded relationship. They do not receive consistent and appropriate feedback on their behaviour and they develop a strategy for managing relationships with parents through the adoption of disruptive and demanding behaviour. In this relationship environment the range of successful relationship styles that a child can develop is limited.

### *The potential promotion of a coercive style of interpersonal interaction in abusive families*

According to Barbaree, Marshall and McCormick in abusive families parental control over the behaviour of other family members is often gained and maintained through coercion, intimidation and physical violence. Thus children from abusive families may not have the opportunity to learn appropriate interpersonal and intimacy skills, and develop instead a relationship template based upon inappropriate aggressive behaviour reinforced and modelled by parents. A child growing up in an abusive family may learn that intimidation, aggression and manipulation are the interpersonal strategies that are most effective in his family environment. When a child in this situation engages in interpersonal interactions outside of home, such as school, he will naturally transfer what was previously his most successful interpersonal strategy to his new relationships. Consequently this child is likely to be ill-equipped for the relationship-forming tasks he faces in contexts outside his family. The previously semi-adaptive coercive and aggressive strategy which was at least partially successful at home is maladaptive in new non-home settings. Using this interpersonal style a child is unlikely to form stable and satisfying relationships with peers, teachers and other adults who find his aggressive and coercive behaviour to be aversive. As he grows older his failure to establish and consolidate successful social relationships further impedes the development of pro-social skills and contributes to the development of a negative self-image and a reduction in the self-confidence necessary to develop a satisfying interpersonal life. From this point the child has reached what Barbaree, Marshall and McCormick call the intermediate outcome of the abusive family experience which they characterise as a "syndrome of social disability". They describe five main features of the syndrome of social disability as follows: (i) an inability to establish and maintain intimate relationships; (ii) low self-esteem; (iii) diverse anti-social and criminal attitudes and behaviours; (iv) a lack of empathy; and (v) distorted thinking that supports and justifies criminal behaviour.

While acknowledging that puberty heralds the emergence of new developmental challenges for all young people, Barbaree, Marshall and McCormick describe it as having an added significance for those whose life is characterised by the syndrome of social disability. During puberty the young person "begins to desire a more intimate and sexual quality to some relationships" (1998, p. 4). Boys from nurturing families establish successful and appropriate intimate relationships as a natural outgrowth of their history of healthy relationships. In contrast boys from abusive family backgrounds may come to have experiences of repeated failure in establishing intimate relationships based on mutual sexual attraction. Consequently, they experience themselves as powerless with regard to the establishment of healthy relationships and ultimately feel excluded and emotionally isolated. This affects their self-concept, particularly as concerned with masculinity, often leaving the young person with strong feelings of anger and resentment. For some this anger and resentment becomes directed at the object of desire, namely, intimate contact with others based upon sexual attraction. Ill-equipped to achieve intimate relationships through healthy interpersonal means the young person may apply an aggressive, manipulative and coercive strategy learnt from negotiating relationships with early attachment figures. Such a young person may seek sex either forcefully or with a younger and more vulnerable child. Such sexual experiences achieved through force, manipulation or coercion establish memories of sexual contact that may be elaborated into inappropriate sexual fantasies which are subsequently reinforced through masturbation. Repeated recall of such fantasies may promote an urge to act them out in reality. Barbaree, Marshall and McCormick argue that this process establishes and consolidates a conditioned interest in deviant sexuality. Once the young person begins to sexually offend he becomes progressively more desensitised and distorted in his thinking in relation to the distress of his victims and the fear of being caught. Barbaree, Marshall and McCormick also allow for the fact that varying levels of severity may exist in both causal and outcome factors in the development of juvenile and adult sexual abusers. Generally speaking higher levels of severity of causal factors leads to more serious deficits in social functioning and more serious levels of sexual deviance.

In summary they see the following as the key but varying causal factors in the development of sexual offending. (1) Disruption in relationships with attachment figures. (2) Experiences of sexual, physical and/or emotional abuse as a child. (3) Dysfunctional family relationships including parental reinforcement of coercive, disruptive and aggressive behaviour. (4) Inherent temperamental factors that predispose impulsiveness. (5) The emergence of a syndrome of social disability. (6) A failure to achieve normal relationships in adolescence. And (7) the replacement of normal sexual contact with abusive sexual contact achieved through force, coercion and manipulation. An advantage of the Barbaree, Marshall and McCormick model is that it offers a developmental perspective on the emergence of sexually abusive behaviour. Consequently it allows us to conceptualise the development of sexually abusive behaviour in adolescents as well as adults. A limiting aspect of the model is that it is a one-size-fits-all model based largely on working backwards from observations made concerning adult men convicted of sexual crimes. Consequently, if a more deviant and more serious type of sexual offender is represented by those who are criminally convicted for their offences then this model may have a particular relevance in helping us to understand the development of a subset of the overall population of sexual offenders. As yet we do not have empirical data that allows us to determine whether or not this is the case.

## The Hall and Hirschman quadripartite model

Hall and Hirschman (1991; 1992; Hall, 1996) identified the need for a model that (a) unified theoretical ideas about sexual offenders; (b) accounted for multiple aetiological factors in the development of offending behaviour; and (c) reflected the observed heterogeneity among those who engage in sexually abusive behaviour. Initially, Hall and Hirschman developed their model specifically in relation to adults who perpetrate sexual crimes against adult women but subsequently extended their ideas to adults who sexually offend against children. Essentially there are four components in the Hall and Hirschman model that are designed to explain sexually abusive behaviour. These are described below.

### *Component 1. The influence of physiological sexual arousal*

Physiological sexual arousal factors are conceptualised by Hall and Hirschman as a motivating influence that prompts people to engage in sexual behaviour. In adults who offend against children their sexual arousal deviates from normal patterns and their behaviour is harmfully directed against children. In those who offend against adults their sexual interests may not necessarily be deviant as they are directed towards other adults. However, relatively normative sexual drives are harmfully expressed when they disregard the consent and well-being of other adults. For some of those who offend against children or adults other non-normative features such as aggression and violence may be part of the expression of a deviant sexual arousal.

### *Component 2. The influence of cognitive distortions*

Like other theorists Hall and Hirschman identify distorted cognitions as an important feature of sexual offending. They indicate that while physiological arousal may motivate sexual offending behaviour, such drives are usually evaluated cognitively by individuals before they are acted upon. People who engage in sexually abusive behaviour may utilise a variety of distorted ways to think about their arousal that promotes the likelihood that it will be translated into action. Consequently an offender may develop distorted ideas about women or children such as "some women are just asking for it" or "children know more about sex than most people think". Alternatively, they may have cognitions that allow them to ignore the impact of their behaviour such as "this person really wants me to do this" or promote a belief that they will not be detected for their crime such as "no-one will know it was me". Often cognitive distortions that offenders use to justify their behaviour reflect aspects of distorted ideas about relationships, sexuality and gender that are part of broader messages found in our culture.

### *Component 3. The influence of affective dyscontrol*

Strong affective states such as depression, anger and hostility are regarded as important features in psychological functioning that may also facilitate sexual offending behaviour. Hall and Hirschman comment that often these types of negative affective states precede sequences of distorted thinking that culminate in sexual offending behaviour. According to their model sexually abusive behaviour occurs when such affective states are felt deeply and in such a strongly compelling way that they overcome normal emotional inhibitions that should prevent sexually abusive behaviour such as guilt, moral conviction, anxiety and victim empathy.

### *Component 4. Chronic personality difficulties that have their origin in difficult early life experiences*

The three preceding factors of physiological arousal, cognitive distortions and affective dyscontrol are features of the Hall and Hirschman model that are transitory aspects of psychological functioning that have a role in motivating sexual offenders. They are not enduring states. Within the Hall and Hirschman model their importance is acknowledged but on their own they are regarded as probably insufficient to explain the occurrence of sexually abusive behaviour. Hall and Hirschman theorise that these transitory states are usually combined with more enduring traits, such as difficulties that are reflective of harsh early life experiences. A range of early life experiences are suggested that may be of aetiological significance in the development of lasting personality difficulties that promote the likelihood of sexually abusive behaviour. Interestingly, Hall and Hirschman include aspects of development that may be experienced by many who do not engage in abusive behaviour, such as parental divorce, large family of origin, parental or sibling criminal behaviour, neglect, physical, emotional and sexual abuse, and poor socialization experiences. These are suggested as having the potential to promote the development of lasting personality problems such as selfishness, remorselessness, a tendency towards the exploitation of others, and an unstable antisocial lifestyle. Such personality difficulties, depending on their severity, could account for the chronicity of sexually offending behaviour.

It is important to note a number of features which Hall and Hirschman have deliberately included in their model. Firstly, the model focuses on psychological and interpersonal factors that they regard as having an important aetiological role in the development of sexual offending. While they acknowledge the influence of environmental factors that may inhibit (criminal sanctions, unavailability of potential victims) or promote (alcohol misuse, contact with a deviant peer group) offending behaviour they deliberately underemphasise their role in the development of sexual offending. Secondly, four subtypes of sexual offender are suggested by the model where one of the four factors is relatively more potent than the other three. Hall and Hirschman propose that this feature of their model allows it to be used as a descriptive framework accounting for the heterogeneity of sexual offenders. Consequently individual offenders can be understood as belonging to one of four categories depending on whether they were primarily motivated by (a) deviant sexual arousal; (b) cognitive factors; (c) affective factors; or (d) personality difficulties. For each subtype all four factors are present to varying degrees but one factor is regarded as dominant. Hall and Hirschman acknowledge that various factor combinations could be utilized to delineate other subtypes of offender but this would go beyond their stated intention to develop a parsimonious model. They regard the four factor based subtypes as offering sufficient complexity to provide a useful description of most offenders. Thirdly, the quadripartite model has implications for clinical work as different types of offender will require approaches to assessment and intervention tailored to reflect their primary motivational influence. Finally, the model is meant as a middle ground between single-factor and complex multi-factor models of sexually offending behaviour. It does not presume that all offenders are the same and at the same time does not presume that they are all extremely different.

## Ward and Siegert's pathways model

Ward and Siegert (2002) outline a model of the development of individuals who sexually abuse others that attempts to integrate what they regard as the best elements of the Finkelhor, Marshall and Barbaree, and Hall and Hirschman models. Their aim in doing so is to outline a comprehensive theory. Ward and Siegert refer to their work as a pathways model as it outlines five potential pathways that can lead to sexually abusive behaviour. Four of the five pathways reflect a primary causal "mechanism" that significantly influences the development of sexually abusive behaviour. However, Ward and Siegert stress that although in each pathway one "mechanism" is described as taking a leading causal role, each of the other mechanisms outlined in the model make an important contribution in all pathways. The fifth pathway is characterised as a paedophilic sexual orientation combined with major difficulties in all other areas described in the model.

Ward and Siegert begin the description of the pathways model by clarifying what they mean in their use of the term mechanism. They state,

> a mechanism is what makes things work or function and a dysfunctional mechanism is one that fails to work as intended or designed. Examples of dysfunctional mechanisms include impaired cognitive or behavioural skills and mental states such as maladaptive beliefs and desires. Psychological mechanisms generating child sexual abuse constitute *vulnerability* factors.
>
> (2002, p. 332).

It is important to note that this definition usefully clarifies that Ward and Siegert clearly mean that faulty mechanisms cause vulnerabilities to sexual offending. However, when they refer to mechanisms that fail "to work as intended or designed" they make no reference to who the designer or intender is. One possibility is that they mean a design reflective of evolution by natural selection. If this is the case then a key part of testing this aspect of their model concerns the viability of the various mechanisms as the products of the evolutionary process.

### *Pathway 1: Intimacy and social skills deficits*

The first pathway described by Ward and Siegert reflects the development of sexually abusive behaviour as an outcome of a dysfunctional intimacy and social skills mechanism. In this pathway sexual offending has its developmental roots in childhood experiences of abuse and neglect combined with insecure attachment relationships with significant care-givers. This results in an unhealthy or distorted internal working model organizing relationship behaviour that inhibits the development of good and open relationships. Poor quality relationships, and attachment styles reflective of insecurity, promote the development of poor quality relationship skills, low self-esteem, emotional loneliness and isolation. Consequently, a person who sexually offends as an outcome of pathway 1 does so in a manner that primarily reflects their intimacy and relationship related deficits. Pathway 1 offenders typically begin their sexually abusive behaviour in adulthood replacing children for adults as relationship partners. Sexually abusive behaviour often follows an experience of rejection by adult partners (or potential partners), or periods of relationship isolation. The offender treats the child he victimises as a "pseudo-adult" or "surrogate partner" and develops distorted thinking that is supportive of this view. This includes distorted thoughts that the child is accepting of the adult offender's sexual needs.

### *Pathway 2: Deviant sexual scripts*

In pathway 2 the development of sexual offending is described as primarily an outcome of a deviant sexual script. Ward and Siegert apply the notion of sexual scripts offered by Gagon (1990) and Money (1986). Sexual scripts are mental representations acquired by an individual during his life that reflect relevant past experience. They subsequently organise and guide thoughts, feelings and behaviour related to sexuality. Of overall relevance to Ward and Siegert's model, the experience of childhood sexual abuse may adversely affect the development of healthy sexual scripts in a number of ways. However, in pathway 2 Ward and Siegert have a particular sexual script distortion in mind. This pathway does not reflect a sexual script that promotes an inappropriate partner (such as a child) or inappropriate behaviour (such as a deviant act). In pathway 2, Ward and Siegert state, the major sexual script mechanism dysfunction concerns what they refer to as the "context" in which sexual behaviour is seen as acceptable. This contextual sexual script dysfunction equates sexual behaviour with the expression of interpersonal closeness. Interpersonal emotions such as loneliness are misinterpreted as signalling sexual needs. In adult relationships a person with this type of sexual script dysfunction is unlikely to establish lasting close interpersonal relationships, and is likely to find sexual intimacy with others to be impersonal and unsatisfying. Given the "interpersonal closeness and sexual behaviour are the same thing" confusion, any behaviours that a child may display to a pathway 2 offender that may reflect the child's feelings of closeness are distorted by the adult as a sexual expression. Similarly, any sexual behaviour by the adult is internally misconstrued by the offender as an expression of interpersonal closeness according to his dysfunctional sexual script.

Ward and Siegert state that a person on pathway 2 with its associated sexual script dysfunction, will experience four areas of difficulty which are commonly found among those who sexually abuse others. These are deviant patterns of sexual arousal, intimacy deficits, inappropriate emotional experiences and inappropriate cognitive distortions. On pathway 2, sexual offending typically begins in adulthood and is more likely to be episodic rather than continuous. Sexual offending will be associated with emotional loneliness and relationship rejection. Self-esteem among this group of offenders is likely to be low, reflecting experiences of interpersonal rejection. Children become the targets of sexual behaviour for this group of offenders as an outcome of opportunistic situational factors combined with the emotional and sexual demands of the offender, rather than as an outcome of a dominating deviant sexual orientation.

#### *Pathway 3: Emotional dysregulation*

The third pathway that leads to the development of sexually abusive behaviour according to Ward and Siegert is characterised by emotional dysregulation. Emotional regulation is described as the ability of an individual to control affective states in order to meet personal goals. A range of emotional regulation difficulties are outlined by Ward and Siegert as having the potential to significantly influence the development of sexually abusive behaviour. These include problems with the ability to recognise emotions, an inability to adjust emotional states when they are experienced, anger management problems, the experience of strong negative affective states such as low mood or high anxiety, and an inability to utilise appropriate social supports during times of emotional difficulty. Pathway 3 offenders respond in one of two ways to their emotional dysregulation. They either become overwhelmed and sexually uninhibited by their emotional state, or they use sexual behaviour as an inappropriate soothing strategy to allay their emotional dysregulation. In light of this Ward and Siegert describe pathway 3 offenders as tending to prefer sexual activity with age appropriate partners but shifting to sexual activity with children at times of severe emotional dysregulation. Difficulties with the regulation of emotions may be experienced in adolescence as well as adulthood. Consequently, those on pathway 3 may begin their offending behaviour during their teenage years. When they are not experiencing high levels of stress this group will exhibit normal sexual interests and behaviours. Pathway 3 offenders are unlikely to attempt to groom a "close" relationship with a child prior to sexual assault. The self-esteem of this group may be low or high depending on the individual concerned and the area of self-esteem in question.

### *Pathway 4: Anti-social cognitions*

Pathway 4 in the Ward and Siegert model concerns a subgroup of offenders whose sexually abusive behaviour is part of a wider pattern of more general criminal behaviour. This subgroup holds a range of beliefs and cognitions that support anti-social behaviour. The sexual abuse of children is one of many anti-social acts, such as substance abuse, theft and violence, in which this group engage. Pathway 4 offenders are likely to have difficulties with impulsivity and often engage in behaviours consistent with conduct disorder from childhood. More specifically their sexual offending behaviour is usually reflective of their general anti-social outlook on life combined with poorly controlled sexual impulses and opportunistic situational factors. Consequently their offending behaviour may not reflect a persistent deviant sexual preference directed towards children. Given that their abusive behaviour is part of a broader pattern of long-standing criminal and anti-social behaviour they may begin to engage in sexually abusive behaviour from a relatively early age.

### *Pathway 5: Multiple dysfunctional mechanisms*

Although those on pathway 5 of the Ward and Siegert model are referred to as having multiple-dysfunctional mechanisms they are clearly described as having a particular sexual script dysfunction that promotes child–adult sexual activity in combination with pronounced difficulties in all of the other pathway mechanisms. The inappropriately preferred sexual relationship of adults in this category is with children. Consequently, Ward and Siegert refer to them as "pure" paedophiles. They state that the development of a paedophilic sexual script among this group will usually reflect childhood experiences of sexual victimisation, or exposure to sexual behaviour and material, at a young age. Pathway 5 offenders often begin to sexually abuse others before they reach adulthood. Ward and Siegert hypothesise that a feature of this group is that they fantasise about sexual contact with children prior to committing their first offence, reflecting their underlying paedophilic sexual orientation. Ward and Siegert characterise pathway 5 offenders as (i) having an early onset of sexually abusive behaviour; (ii) having ingrained cognitive distortions regarding sexual activity with children; (iii) having deviant patterns of sexual arousal in response to children; and (iv) experiencing positive affect in response to their offending behaviour. Given their underlying sexual orientation towards children they are unlikely to develop intimate and mature relationships with other adults. They are also likely to have high self-esteem as they believe their sexually offending behaviour is justified.

In summary, Ward and Siegert propose a model of the development of sexually abusive behaviour with the aim of re-describing and incorporating what they regard as the best elements of the ideas outlined by other theorists such as Finkelhor, Marshall and Barbaree, and Hall and Hirschman. In doing so they outline five pathways that lead to the development of sexually abusive behaviour. In each pathway there is a distinct psychological mechanism that represents the primary dysfunction guiding the development of sexually abusive behaviour. However, elements of each mechanism are found on all pathways. In essence, Ward and Siegert offer a model that suggests five subtypes of sexual offender, some of whom may begin to sexually abuse others before they reach adulthood. Although Ward and Siegert outline a number of the features they regard as characteristic of those on each of the five pathways, substantial work is required to empirically evaluate the merits of this model and its value in guiding assessment and intervention.

## Lane's sexual abuse cycle

Lane (1997) has outlined a model termed the sexual abuse cycle that has found widespread use in intervention programmes for young people with sexually abusive behaviour. Essentially it consists of a description of sexually abusive behaviour as part of a maladaptive response to stressors in a young person's life. This maladaptive response is characterized by misinterpretations of the meaning of events; misinterpretations of the meaning of other people's behaviour; distorted ideas developed by young people concerning themselves, power, and interpersonal interactions; compensatory responses that include sexually abusive behaviour; transitory feelings of guilt; and cognitive distortions that promote repetition of the abuse cycle. Lane's model is based on her observation of the similarities in the build-up, commission and response to sexually abusive behaviour across different youths attending for assessment and intervention. The model attempts to extract what is common in the triggering events, feelings, cognitions and behaviours. It is Lane's observation that when the cycle is personalised, the situations, thoughts, feelings and behaviours are given a meaningful personal context for a young person who has abused. However, the underlying blue-print is the same, with each factor interacting in a way that builds a process leading to, and following on from, sexually abusive behaviour. In its application this model can help a young person to understand the pattern underlying their behaviour as a progressive interaction between situations, thoughts, feelings and behaviours rather than something that emerges without build-up or warning. It is hoped that this insight can be used to help young people deal with those aspects of their life experience that have been a part of their offence cycle and take steps to ensure that in the future they manage precursors to harmful behaviour in a preventative manner. Importantly, the cycle is a descriptive model and is not meant as a representation of causal factors leading to sexually abusive behaviour.

Lane outlines a number of concepts which are central to understanding and applying her model. These can be described as follows: (1) *Sexual abuse* is any act of sexual behaviour that occurs in the absence of consent and may involve exploitation, manipulation, coercion or force. It is characterized by some pre-thought on the part of the perpetrator and is in part an unhealthy expression of non-sexual needs. (2) *Control-seeking and dominance* are two important organizing aspects of the behaviour of young people who engage in abusive behaviour. Much of the cycle behaviour (both sexual and non-sexual) can be understood as an attempt by the young person to manage his environment and other people by controlling or dominating them. In doing so the young person is believed to be attempting to enhance his sense of self-adequacy in interpersonal and environmental interactions. (3) *The compensatory aspects of behaviour* provide another key to understanding the abuse cycle. Many of the behaviours of the cycle, including control-seeking and dominance, will, in part, be motivated by damaging attempts by the young person to compensate for powerful feelings of anxiety, helplessness, vulnerability, lack of control and sense of loss. (4) *Sexual arousal and anticipation* are part of the young person's experience during the abuse cycle. Both provide strong psychological and physiological reinforcement of behaviour. In addition sexual arousal, sexual fantasy and sexual anticipation may be part of a process that provides the young person with some degree of self-soothing in response to the feelings of anxiety, vulnerability and lack of control. (5) *Cognitive distortions* are features of the young person's psychological functioning throughout the abuse cycle. The origin of many of these distorted ways of thinking can usually be traced back to important aspects of the young person's developmental experiences in the world, particularly those that promote a view of the world as a harsh place or of individuals as worthless. Cognitions with various themes are apparent at different stages of the abuse cycle. Their differing themes function to promote progression through the cycle. Typical themes found in distorted thinking at different points in the cycle include negative self-perceptions; thoughts about complete rejection or disrespect from others; cognitions that justify or rationalize criminal or antisocial behaviour; thoughts that misrepresent the experience of those victimised by sexual abuse; and cognitions that allow the young person to negate and set aside any feelings of guilt they may experience in relation to their abusive behaviour. (6) *An addictive and compulsive quality* is apparent in some aspects of cycle behaviour. Lane acknowledges that while cycle behaviour is not truly addictive in the sense of alcohol or substance addiction, some aspects have an addictive quality. In particular, the experience of compulsions and impulsive urges to engage in abusive behaviour; the need to increase the intensity of feelings of excitement and danger as abusive behaviour becomes more habitual; the relief of unpleasant internal states such as anxiety; and the eventual narrowing of the repertoire of coping skills to maladaptive strategies such as abusive behaviour directed towards others.

Lane suggests that it is useful to think of the abuse cycle as consisting of three main phases. *A precipitating phase* where the young person perceives an event or personal interaction as problematic. This elicits feelings of dread, rejection and hopelessness. The young person responds with avoidance behaviours. *A compensatory phase* where the young person attempts to compensate for his feelings and actions through sexual and non-sexual abusive and power-based thoughts, feelings and behaviours. *An integration phase* where the young person attempts to assimilate his abusive behaviour without further undermining his sense of self. Typically this involves a process of suppression where the young person denies to himself (a) that his abusive behaviour was problematic or (b) that he may be unable stop himself from repeating it in the future. Lane describes each phase in detail as follows.

### *The precipitating phase of the abuse cycle*

The precipitating phase begins with an event that elicits a maladaptive response from a young person that reflects core distorted beliefs about himself, his abilities and the world. In response to such an event the young person thinks that he is being treated unfairly, and that this treatment reflects the fact that there is something wrong with him, and he imagines an outcome where it is inevitable that he will continue to be treated in a similar fashion in the future. He responds with an attempt to escape the imagined future outcome and his current thoughts and feelings, through suppressing or avoiding them. Lane points out two key processes that need to be understood in the precipitating phase. Firstly, we need to understand the potential origin of these core beliefs. Secondly, we need to understand the more superficial events that trigger these core beliefs. The core beliefs are established by events which place the young person in a situation where he feels helpless, lacking in control and abandoned. Lane gives an example of a young child who witnesses his father being physically violent towards his mother. This child is likely to feel afraid and vulnerable and may try to intervene. The child's intervention if attempted will be ineffective. Regardless of whether or not the child tried to stop the violence he is likely to have thoughts and feelings such as "I should have been able to help my mum"; "I'm useless because I can't stop dad from hurting mum"; "I am no good because I won't be able to stop dad from hitting mum in the future". Lane reports that in her experience the most commonly reported historical events that contribute to the development of core beliefs related to the precipitating phase of the cycle are family violence, family dysfunction, parental divorce, death of a significant other, death of a pet, change in environment, sexual, physical or emotional abuse, awareness of family members' involvement in deviant sexual behaviour, and experiences of humiliation. In contrast the more superficial proximal events that may trigger the abuse cycle's core beliefs are varied but often less dramatic. Lane cites the following as some examples; feeling put down or challenged, poor school grades, rejection by peers or others, changing school, lacking skills, conflict in relationships, conflict with authority figures, losing a game, losing a friend, and embarrassing situations.

In summary, during the precipitating phase the young person's distorted thinking reflects ideas such as: I am unfairly victimised in this situation ("Poor me"); I am alone and uncared for ("No one cares about me"); and generalisations that the situation is always going to be repeated ("Its always the same"). Feelings include hopelessness, powerlessness, fear, embarrassment and humiliation. Behaviour has an avoidance aspect to it such as avoiding contact with friends or family, retreating to one's room, engaging in solitary activities, playing computer games alone, substance misuse, excessive daydreaming or excessive sleeping.

### *The compensatory phase of sexual abuse cycle*

In the compensatory phase of the abuse cycle the young person begins to move from a victim stance combined with an avoidance strategy to a position that allows an improved self-perception. Typically this is achieved by the young person shifting their perception of who is responsible for the triggering event from an internal to an external attribution of blame. That is, they begin to become angry towards other people they perceive to be involved in the event and blame them for the situation. The young person may express their anger through a variety of behaviours that are initially non-sexual. Consequently the young person may bully or pick on others, or refuse to do as they are asked by parents, teachers or others in positions of authority. Part of a young person's compensatory response may be fantasies where he adopts a role of being powerful and in control. He may imagine himself responding in a different and more powerful way to the cycle-triggering event, or refusing to do as expected by others, or bullying people perceived to be weaker, or gaining revenge on those perceived to be stronger. Fantasies with these themes provide the young person with an enhanced sense of self and may to some extent be acted out in reality. In addition some compensatory power-based fantasies have a sexual content. A young person may imagine himself having sexual contact with someone who is very popular, or very attractive, or perhaps someone famous. Sexual fantasies may incorporate coercive or abusive behaviours or sexual contact with someone younger or more vulnerable. These types of sexual fantasies, and more specifically their coercive and abusive content, may become reinforced for a young person when coupled with masturbatory behaviour. Initially a young person may be inhibited from acting out abusive sexual fantasies because it violates their code of acceptable behaviour or out of fear of getting caught. However, over time this inhibitory effect lessens and the young person may move from fantasy to real behaviour. In doing so a young person may begin to plan an offence. He may select or groom a person to victimise, evaluate the likelihood of getting caught, think of an opportunity to exploit, make a decision to engage in the abusive behaviour and take steps to minimise or prevent detection. Distorted thinking may be used by the young person to justify his behaviour to himself ("He's too young to know what's happening"), portray the potential victim as an object or in a depersonalized manner ("She's begging for it dressed like that"), or reflect what Lane terms super-optimism ("They're so stupid, no-one will be able to catch me"). The build-up to sexually abusive behaviour is usually accompanied by physiological arousal and a thrilling affect for the young person. The outcome of this phase of the abuse cycle is that the youth sexually abuses another person.

### *The integration phase*

During the final phase of the sexual abuse cycle a young person attempts to assimilate the fact that he has sexually abused another person. However, this is rarely reflective of a concern for the harm inflicted on the person victimised. After the abusive behaviour the young person may begin to lose his sense of self-adequacy and control. His initial response may be concerned with why the perpetration of the offence did not live up to the level of gratification or excitement anticipated in fantasy. This results in the first thinking distortion of the integration phase which Lane terms the "Reinforcing distortion". The young person avoids feelings of inadequacy or disappointment by congratulating himself on his behaviour ("I was great"; "I showed her"). However, he may now fear that he will be caught and that this will result in punishment from others and public humiliation. The solution to these fears for most young people is to engage in what Lane calls a "Control distortion" ("He's so scared of me he'd never tell"; "She has no clue who I am"). However, the young person is usually left with residual self-doubts about his behaviour. Some wonder if they are sick or weird. Some feel that they have lost control. Others continue to worry that they will be caught. This leads to a "Suppression distortion" where the young person denies he has a problem and tells himself that he is in control and normal ("There's no need to worry because I'll never do it again"; "I'm not weird, lots of people do it"). Despite the reassuring nature of these distortions, feelings of anxiety and self-doubt persist. The maladaptive and illusory sense of self-adequacy of the compensatory phase has been shattered and the young person is susceptible to respond in an overly-sensitive manner to events where he perceives himself slighted, rejected or inadequate, such as those that initiated the cycle. Consequently he is more vulnerable to repeat his cycle of sexually abusive behaviour.

## The Rasmussen, Burton and Christopherson trauma outcome process

Rasmussen, Burton and Christopherson (1992) outline a sophisticated model that describes sexually abusive behaviour in children as one of three possible response wheels following a traumatic experience. The three response wheels open to children according to this model are: (1) Recovery; where the child expresses and processes feelings associated with his traumatic experience and reaches a point of resolution and acceptance. (2) Self-victimisation; where the child internally suppresses his trauma-related emotions and develops personally harmful thoughts, behaviours and emotions. (3) Assault; where the child identifies with the person responsible for his traumatic experience and engages in a range of abusive behaviours directed towards others. Rasmussen *et al.* developed their model based upon their work with children aged between four and twelve years with what they term "sexually reactive behaviour". Central to their work is an attempt to distinguish why some children respond to trauma by victimising others while other children with similarly traumatic experiences do not. Their model incorporates elements of the work of other theorists such as Lane, and Finkelhor. It also has a relevance for adolescent and adult abusers.

The starting-point of the Rasmussen *et al.* model is that a child has a traumatic experience. This may take the form of sexual victimisation or another kind of trauma such as emotional or physical abuse. Rasmussen *et al.* point out that the impact on a child of these types of experiences can be diverse and are well documented in the literature. However, from the point of view of their model, particular emphasis is given to two factors that influence the impact on a child of being abused. These are: (a) the way a victimised child may be confused by, or adopt as his own cognitions, the distorted messages regarding the abuse expressed by the perpetrator. These echoes of the cognitive distortions of the offender are referred to as "trauma echoes". And (b) triggering events, defined as any situation provoking strong feelings in the victim that are reminiscent of the original trauma. These feelings demand release or expression. Rasmussen *et al.* argue that even children must make some level of choice about how to respond to the surfacing emotions aroused by triggering events. The outcome of a child's choice of response is in essence one of the model's three wheels of potential response: recovery, self-victimisation or assault. Embarking on a particular wheel does not preclude an individual from following a different wheel at another time or context, for example a child who responds to trauma in a self-victimising manner may at times engage in healthy recovery, or under certain conditions engage in abusive behaviour towards others. A description of each of the three response wheels is given below.

### *The recovery wheel*

Rasmussen, Burton and Christopherson's recovery response to trauma consists of a number of steps. Children begin their journey towards recovery by working through feelings of denial and anger. At a developmentally appropriate level they acknowledge the losses their experience has brought to them, such as loss of innocence, trust, self-esteem. They reject the trauma echoes that resonate from the distorted cognitions expressed by the abuser. They place responsibility for the abusive behaviour with the perpetrator and accept responsibility for their own recovery. They find a means of healthy expression for the array of feelings they have in response to their experience (e.g. sadness, hurt, fear, anger, shame, embarrassment, betrayal, guilt). In time they come to view their victimisation as an unfortunate part of their life experience and continue their development free from the potentially unhealthy influence of that aspect of their past.

### *The self-victimisation wheel*

In contrast to the recovery wheel some children may respond to traumatic experience by engaging in a process that leads to self-victimisation. Again this process is made up of a number of steps. The child responds to triggering events by repressing his emotions. This leads to what Rasmussen *et al.* refer to as a constriction of affect where the normal range of a child's emotional expression becomes limited. However, the child's bottled-up feelings ultimately find uncontrolled and sublimated release in a manner that is personally harmful. A child in this situation may develop low self-esteem, and develop cognitive distortions about himself, the world and the future that incorporate the distorted ideas expressed by the abuser. In short, trauma echoes become internalised and elaborated. Ultimately this may lead to anxiety, depression and self-destructive behaviours such as self-harm, suicide or substance misuse.

### *The assault wheel*

Alternatively a child may respond to triggering events that elicit emotions related to trauma by engaging in abusive behaviour directed towards others. In the self-victimisation wheel trauma echoes become internalised and directed against the self. In the assault wheel they are externalised and used to justify abusive behaviour towards others. These thinking errors promote fantasies of getting back at people. This can lead to the planning and execution of abusive behaviour. The abusive behaviour produces a mixture of emotional responses for the child, including the release of pent-up feelings regarding personal victimisation, plus a sense of empowerment, shame, fear and disgust.

An important question that the Rasmussen *et al.* model attempts to answer is why some children respond to experiences of victimisation by being abusive towards others while other children respond to essentially similar trauma with either healthy recovery or self-victimisation. Rasmussen and colleagues attempted to explain this with reference to what they observed to be important differences in the characteristics of children who develop an assault wheel response. They outline five characteristics that make children more vulnerable to engage in sexually abusive behaviour in response to trauma. These are (i) prior traumatisation; (ii) inadequate social skills; (iii) experiencing a lack of social intimacy; (iv) impulsiveness; and (v) a general lack of accountability for their behaviour. They term these the "five precursors that lead to vulnerability to offend sexually" (1992, p. 35). Each of the five precursors are described below in more detail and the authors suggest that they should be added to Finkelhor's four preconditions to sexually abusive behaviour (as outlined earlier in this chapter) for a fuller understanding of children who engage in sexually harmful activity towards others.

### *Precursor 1. Prior traumatisation*

Rasmussen and colleagues emphasise the significance of prior traumatic experience, particularly sexual victimisation, in the emergence of sexually abusive behaviour in children. However, they acknowledge that sexual victimisation is not the only form of traumatic experience that may lead to sexually abusive behaviour. Other forms of trauma such as physical or emotional abuse may also open up a developmental pathway leading to sexually abusive behaviour if paired with other experiences that promote a sexualisation of behaviour. These other experiences might include witnessing the sexual behaviour of others, exposure to sexually explicit material, or attachment behaviour being assuaged by sexualised contact. In fact some authors emphasise the relative contribution to the emergence of sexually abusive behaviour in children made by experiences of prior physical rather than sexual victimisation (Cavanagh Johnson, 1999).

### *Precursor 2. Inadequate social skills*

Good social skills help to provide a child with good social support. Children with inadequate social skills are less likely to have well developed networks of friends and care-givers to support them in their development and help them cope with stressful experiences. This lower level of social support generally makes them more vulnerable to the development of sexually abusive behaviour in response to traumatic experiences.

### *Precursor 3. Lack of social intimacy*

A lack of social intimacy is to some degree related to whether or not a child has adequate social skills. However, Rasmussen and colleagues make the distinction that even if a child lacks social skills this does not preclude them from developing appropriately intimate relationships with important people in their lives, usually their parents. Rasmussen *et al.* define social intimacy as "a relationship in which both parties are allowed a sense of self while engaging in mutually satisfactory interactions" (1992, p. 36). A good experience of social intimacy helps a child develop a healthy sense of self and defines boundaries and relationships between self and others. According to the trauma outcome model children who do not have good social intimacy experiences and their associated protective influence on self/other boundaries are more likely to respond to personal trauma by being abusive towards others.

### *Precursor 4. Impulsiveness*

A fourth precursor to the development of sexually abusive behaviour in children outlined in this model is impulsiveness. Rasmussen *et al.* acknowledge that compared to adults, children are generally more impulsive. However, they argue that children who develop sexually abusive behaviour tend to have generalised impulse control problems in comparison with the average levels found among their peers. Impulsiveness is not only an important part of their problematic sexualised behaviour but is also frequently a feature of other difficulties such as attention deficit problems, anger management difficulties, and oppositional or conduct disordered behaviour. Impulsive children at risk of engaging in sexually harmful behaviour towards others are at a disadvantage because they are less likely to respond to internal inhibitors that may otherwise prevent its emergence.

### *Precursor 5. Lack of accountability*

Children who have developed a general sense of accountability regarding their behaviour and its potential impact on others are less likely to respond to personal trauma by engaging in abusive behaviour towards others. Children who generally lack accountability for their behaviour are at increased risk of responding to trauma by victimising others.

The Rasmussen, Burton and Christopherson model has a number of strengths. In particular it delineates three responses to trauma in children ranging from healthy recovery, to dysfunctional adjustment, to the sexual victimisation of others. It also attempts to increase our understanding of vital differences that contribute to some children responding to traumatic experiences by embarking on a developmental pathway that leads to recovery or self-victimisation from those small portion of children who respond by developing abusive behaviour towards others. It provides a number of hypotheses that can be tested empirically. Finally it has contributed to the development of ideas on assessment, formulation and intervention with children who present with sexually abusive behaviour towards others. Limitations of the Rasmussen, Burton and Christopherson model are that it may over-emphasise the role of choice on the part of children in response to their traumatic experiences. While it identifies characteristics that make some children more vulnerable to developing abusive behaviour towards others it does not describe the differentiating characteristics of those children who are more likely to respond with healthy recovery or self-victimisation.

## Conclusions

In this chapter we have outlined the main theoretical models that describe the development and maintenance of sexually abusive behaviour in children, adolescents and adults. They reflect the experience of thoughtful practitioners and researchers who have been at the forefront of developing a body of knowledge in the field of sexual offending. These models have become increasingly complex in the number of typologies they offer and make a useful contribution in helping practitioners make sense of clients who engage in abusive behaviours towards others. They have also been used to guide assessment and intervention techniques. However, the challenge that faces us at present is to subject these models to stringent empirical research that helps us to ensure their further development and appropriate application in clinical work that effectively allows us to intervene to reduce the risk of further sexual harm within the community.

## References

Barbaree, H. E., Marshall, W. L., and McCormick, J. (1998). The development of sexually deviant behaviour among adolescents and its implications for prevention and treatment. *Understanding, Assessing, and Treating Juvenile and Adult Sex Offenders. A Special Issue of the Irish Journal of Psychology, 19(1)*, 1–31.

Cavanagh Johnson, T. (1999). *Understanding Your Child's Sexual Behavior: What's Natural and Healthy*. California: New Harbinger.

Finkelhor, D. (1984). *Child Sexual Abuse: New Theory and Research*. New York: Free Press.

Gagon, J. H. (1990). The explicit and implicit use of the scripting perspective in sex research. *Annual Review of Sex Research, 1*, 1–43.

Hall, G. C. N. (1996). *Theory Based Assessment, Treatment and Prevention of Sexual Aggression*. New York: Oxford University Press.

Hall, G. C. N., and Hirschman, R. (1991). Towards a theory of sexual aggression: A quadripartite model. *Journal of Consulting and Clinical Psychology, 59(5)*, 662–669.

Hall, G. C. N., and Hirschman, R. (1992). Sexual aggression against children: A conceptual perspective on etiology. *Criminal Justice and Behaviour, 19*, 8–23.

Lane, S. (1997). The sexual abuse cycle. In G. Ryan and S. Lane (eds), *Juvenile Sexual Offending: Causes, Consequences, and Corrections*, 2nd edn. San Francisco: Jossey-Bass.

Marshall, W. L., and Barbaree, H. E. (1990). An integrated theory of the etiology of sexual offending. In W. L. Marshall, D. R. Laws and H. E. Barbaree (eds), *Handbook of Sexual Assault: Issues, Theories, and Treatment of the Offender*. New York: Plenum.

Money, J. (1986). *Lovemaps: Clinical Concepts of Sexual/Erotic Health and Pathology,*

*Paraphilia, and Gender Transposition in Childhood, Adolescence and Maturity.* Buffalo, NJ: Prometheus Books.

Rasmussen, L. A., Burton, J. E., and Christopherson, B. J. (1992). Precursors to offending and the trauma outcome process in sexually reactive children. *Journal of Child Sexual Abuse, 1(1)*, 33–48.

Ward, T., and Siegert, R. J. (2002). Towards a comprehensive theory of child sexual abuse: A theory knitting perspective. *Psychology, Crime and Law, 8*, 319–351.

Chapter 3

# A review of the research literature on young people who sexually abuse

*Kevin Epps and Dawn Fisher*

## Introduction

This chapter provides an overview of the empirical research literature on sexual offending by young people. Whilst information is lacking about the factors associated with sexual offending in undetected juvenile sexual offenders, studies into juveniles whose sexual offences do come to light often reveal the presence of a variety of psycho-social problems. Empirical studies provide evidence about the nature and extent of these problems, the degree to which they vary according to type of sexual offence, and the extent to which they are unique to sex offenders.

As one can only know about the cases which have been identified it must be acknowledged that they are likely to represent a somewhat biased sample. It is also important to acknowledge that sex offenders are not a homogenous group and thus different patterns of characteristics are likely to be associated with different typologies of offender. A number of studies do not consider these typologies separately but rather as a whole group which can mask important differences. These factors must be borne in mind when considering the findings of the various studies.

The majority of adolescent sexual offenders are male, accounting for 85 per cent of the known sample (Faller, 1990; Kelly *et al.*, 1991). To date there are few published studies of female adolescent sexual offenders and so unless specified all the studies reviewed focus on males. Females will be considered in a brief section in this chapter.

## Literature review

### *Antisocial behaviour and delinquency*

Several authors have suggested that sexual offending may have more in common with other coercive behaviours, such as bullying, than with sexual gratification (Metzner, 1987; Palmer, 1988; Ryan *et al.*, 1987). Antisocial tendencies (Malamuth, 1986), nonconformity (Rapaport and Burkhart, 1987), impulsivity (Calhoun, 1990), low socialization and low responsibility (Rapaport and Burkhart, 1984), have all been linked to sexual aggression. It is well known that the problems of conduct disorder and delinquency in young people are associated with a variety of psychosocial problems (Herbert, 1987; Johnson, 1979), some of which are also found in those who sexually offend (Jacobs *et al.*, 1997). France and Hudson (1993) suggested that "theoretical and treatment formulations for non-sexual disturbances of conduct may have useful explanatory power for at least some types of juvenile sexual offending" (p. 225).

Individual characteristics that have been linked to delinquent behaviour include deficits in: cognitive functioning, associated with low IQ (Quay, 1987); moral reasoning (Arbuthnot *et al.*, 1987; Blasi, 1980); social skills (Freedman *et al.*, 1978); social problem-solving skills (Kennedy, 1984); self-esteem (Gold, 1978; Kaplan, 1980); impulse control (Reppucci and Clingempeel, 1978); and the capacity for affective empathy and cognitive role-taking (Kaplan and Arbuthnot, 1985; Goldstein and Glick, 1987). Further research is needed to clarify which types of problem are common to both sexual and non-sexual offending, and the extent to which these vary according to type of sexual offence.

A number of studies have reported high levels of conduct disorder and delinquency in adolescent sexual offenders. Becker, Cunningham-Rathner and Kaplan (1986), for example, found that 50 per cent of their sample of juvenile male incest perpetrators had a record of previous non-sexual arrests, and that 63 per cent of those available for psychiatric assessment could be diagnosed as conduct disordered. Several other studies have reported similar findings (Awad and Saunders, 1989; Awad *et al.*, 1984; Carpenter *et al.*, 1995; Fehrenbach *et al.*, 1986; Hawkes *et al.*, 1997; James and Neil, 1996; Kavoussi *et al.*, 1988; Moody *et al.*, 1994; Pierce and Pierce, 1987; Richardson, Graham *et al.*, 1995; Saunders *et al.*, 1986). In one of the few comparative studies, Awad *et al.* (1984) compared twenty-four male juvenile sexual offenders with a group of other matched delinquents and found that the similarities in associated factors outweighed the differences between the groups. The two groups were more alike than not on measures of the prevalence of psychiatric disturbance and psychiatric history, violence and sexual deviance among their parents, disruptions in parent–child relationships, inadequate parenting, a chronic history of school problems, and past delinquencies. The differences comprised a higher prevalence of middle-class boys, lower intellectual functioning, and less truancy, alcohol abuse and temper tantrums among the sexual offenders. However, the findings of this study are limited by the small sample size and the failure to distinguish between the various kinds of juvenile sexual offender. It seems likely that the nature and extent of differences found between sexual offenders and non-sexual offenders will depend on the type of sexual offender included in the study.

Evidence that this may be the case comes from another controlled study, by

Blaske *et al.* (1989). They found significant differences between the two groups, casting doubt on the suggestion that sexual and non-sexual disturbances of conduct share a common aetiology. Blaske *et al.* compared a group of aggressive "hands-on" juvenile sexual offenders with assaultive offenders, non-violent offenders and non-delinquent adolescents, with a particular focus on emotional and interpersonal deficits. They found that the sexual offenders displayed more evidence of disturbed emotional functioning and peer relationship difficulties, whereas their family functioning was more similar to that of non-delinquents. The authors concluded that sexual offenders did not fit contemporary models of juvenile delinquency, which place particular emphasis on differential affective ties to conventional and deviant socialization agents. This study, however, did not distinguish between sexual offenders whose offences had been restricted to child molestation and those who had assaulted female peers or women.

There is in fact considerable variation in the reported rates of non-sexual offending among juvenile sexual offenders. Lewis *et al.* (1979) found that all of the male adolescent sexual offenders in their study had a history of non-sexual offending. In contrast, O'Callaghan and Print (1994), in one of the few British studies, described the juvenile sexual offenders referred to their community treatment programme in Greater Manchester (known as G-MAP) as being less delinquent than other groups of young offenders. Compared to twenty-eight male juveniles with a history of non-sexual offending, the fifty male sexual offenders engaged in less substance abuse, theft, criminal damage, car crime and violence. Bladon (2000) in another UK-based study reported on a sample of 166 young people referred to a service for abusive sexual behaviour. She reported the rates of various anti-social behaviour as follows: aggressive behaviour (70%), bullying (44%), vandalism (38%), fire-setting (26%), cruelty to animals (20%), shoplifting (20%), drug abuse (15%) and alcohol abuse (10%). The differences in these two studies highlights the effect of considering different samples.

It seems likely that the range of rates of non-sexual offending is partly explained by the type of sexual offending, which varies between studies but is not always made explicit (Davis and Leitenberg, 1987). The sexual offenders in the study by O'Callaghan and Print (1994), for example, were all child molesters, whose offending had not been especially physically violent. There is evidence that more serious and physically aggressive hands-on sexual offending is associated with higher rates of non-sexual offending (Kavoussi *et al.*, 1988; Lewis *et al.*, 1979; Smith, 1988) and with sexual offending against female peers and women (sexual assaulters), where greater force is required to overpower the victim (Richardson, Graham *et al.*, 1995). Further, sexual assaulters are twice as likely to be diagnosed as conduct disordered, or to have committed other acts of violence than are other adolescent sexual offenders (Kavoussi *et al.*, 1988; Van Ness, 1984). In addition, Calhoun *et al.* (1997) found that delinquency was the strongest predictor of both coercive sexual behaviour and attraction to sexual aggression toward women in a sample of sixty-five non-offending young men from a rural community. Failure to adequately control for type of sexual offending, especially according to victim age and degree of violence, may help to explain the varying rates of delinquency found in samples of juvenile sexual offenders. In a recent British study, Epps (2000) controlled for type of offence. He compared four groups of twenty-seven male juvenile offenders, in which two of the groups comprised boys who had sexually assaulted children only (child molesters), and boys who had sexually assaulted women and female peers only (sexual assaulters). The remaining two groups had committed either violent non-sexual offences, or property offences only. Although some of the child molesters did have an extensive history of delinquency, compared to the three other groups this group had significantly fewer recorded criminal offences, fewer criminal convictions, lower levels of self-reported delinquency, and lower levels of alcohol and substance abuse. The finding that child molesters are, on the whole, less delinquent, suggests that the development of sexual offending behaviour against children is less influenced by factors commonly associated with the development of delinquency. For example, Epps found that whilst both sexual offender groups had peer relationship difficulties, these were characterized by social isolation and victimization through bullying in the child molester group. In contrast, the difficulties in the sexual assaulter group resulted from violence and aggression toward peers and association with other, like-minded, delinquent peers, sometimes as part of a gang. Overall, they were more likely to have friends and to function as part of a peer group.

Much of the research into juvenile sexual offending has looked at adolescent sexual offenders in offence-specific community treatment programmes, which tend to focus on child molesters and are unlikely to accept boys who have been particularly physically violent or delinquent. This is acknowledged by Manocha and Mezey (1998), who describe the background characteristics of fifty-one adolescents referred to a British community assessment and treatment facility for young sexual abusers. They note that their sample "is more likely to represent those at the less abusive and delinquent end of the spectrum" (p. 600). It seems likely that the most violent, delinquent adolescent sexual offenders are less often referred to community treatment programmes. Rather, they are more frequently subject to the full force of the criminal justice system, and sentenced in similar ways to other young offenders. Some may find themselves placed in the penal system, and form part of a group of violent, delinquent adolescent sexual offenders about whom relatively little is known. Evidence for this comes from a study by Puri *et al.* (1996). They found that, of the young offenders detained in a Young Offender Institution (YOI) under a sentence reserved for the most serious kinds of juvenile offending, 26 per cent had index offences involving serious sexual crime (rape, attempted rape, indecent assault).

Whatever the case, it seems that adolescent sexual offenders with an extensive history of conduct disorder and delinquency are likely to require more intensive treatment, often in a residential treatment setting (Hagan and Cho, 1996). Some time ago, Rutter and Giller (1983) observed that the management and treatment of sexual assaulters is a particularly daunting task because all the well-known difficulties in dealing with juvenile delinquents apply to them, as well as the issue of how to manage their sexual aggressiveness. In looking at the reconviction rates among fifty adolescent sexual offenders two years after leaving a state juvenile correctional facility, Hagan *et al.* (1994) found that only 8 per cent reoffended sexually, whilst 46 per cent committed some other type of criminal offence. It is now widely reported that adolescent sexual offenders may be more at risk of committing new non-sexual offences than of reoffending sexually (Weinrott, 1996). Schram *et al.* (1991) reported that 10 per cent of their sample of 194 adolescent sexual offenders reoffended sexually within six years compared to 48 per cent who reoffended non-sexually. Kahn and Chambers (1991) also reported very similar results with a sample of 221 adolescent sexual offenders, 7 per cent re-offending sexually and 37 per cent non-sexually within twenty months of their discharge. These findings suggest that it would be a mistake for treatment programmes for delinquent juvenile sexual offenders to be so sexual-offence specific that they fail to address the broader psychosocial problems associated more generally with criminal behaviour. Given the stability of antisocial and aggressive behaviour (Loeber, 1982; Moffitt, 1993), the violent sexual offenders may also have a higher risk of re-offending against others. Indeed, Henderson *et al.* (1988) reported that about one-half of the adolescents in their treatment programme who had victim-related criminal histories prior to the sexual offence continued to exhibit sexually aggressive behaviours afterwards. However, Hagan *et al.* (2001) in an eight-year comparative study and follow-up of incarcerated juveniles reported that delinquency was a risk factor for future sexual offending; there were no differences in level of risk of sexual offending between those who offended against adults or children (Hagan *et al.*, 2001). The re-offending rates for the different groups were as follows: child sexual offenders (20%), rapists (16%) and non-sexual offending delinquents (10%). Consideration of delinquency obviously has important implications for the clinical assessment of risk of re-offending in juvenile sexual offenders and the development of management strategies to reduce risk to others (Epps, 1997).

### *Educational and academic problems*

It appears that most juvenile sexual offenders have problems in school, and underachieve academically, one of the few consistent findings in the research literature (Awad *et al.*, 1984; Bagley, 1992; Dolan *et al.*, 1996; Epps, 1991; Fehrenbach *et al.*, 1986; Gomes-Schwartz, 1984; James and Neil, 1996; Lewis *et al.*, 1979; Lonczynski, 1991; Manocha and Mezey, 1998; Pierce and Pierce,

1987; Richardson, Graham *et al.*, 1995; Saunders and Awad, 1988). Over 80 per cent of the sexual offenders described by Awad *et al.* (1984) had experienced learning and/or behavioural difficulties during some part of their school career, with a high proportion receiving remedial education (71%). Similarly, Fehrenbach *et al.* (1986) found that only 57 per cent had attained their appropriate or superior grade placement; 56.2 per cent of the sample described by Dolan *et al.* (1996) required special schooling, with 44 per cent truanting on a regular basis; and only 41.9 per cent of the offenders described by James and Neil (1996) attended secondary school on a regular basis. Ryan *et al.* (1996) reported that 60 per cent of adolescent sexual offenders had a history of truancy, learning disabilities and learning problems at school. Monck and New (1996) found that 33 per cent of their sample had statements of special educational needs, which was significantly higher than would be found in the non-psychiatric adolescent population.

However, educational and academic problems are not unique to juvenile sexual offenders. The association between educational failure and juvenile delinquency has been recognized for many years (West and Farrington, 1977) and the evidence suggests that there are few, if any, discernible differences between juvenile sexual offenders and non-sexual offenders in this area (Fehrenbach *et al.*, 1986; Lewis *et al.*, 1979; Tarter *et al.*, 1983). However, Awad and Saunders (1989) did find evidence of more serious chronic learning problems in a sample of court-referred adolescent child molesters, compared to other male delinquents matched for age, socio-economic status and time of referral. Similarly Epps (2000) found that child molesters were significantly more likely than other types of offenders to have mild or specific learning difficulties.

### *Intellectual and neurological problems*

Several studies have found lower levels of intellectual functioning in juvenile sexual offenders (Atcheson and Williams, 1954; Awad, *et al.*, 1984; Lewis *et al.*, 1981; Sauceda, 1978). There is also evidence suggesting that the proportion with an IQ of less than 80 may be greater than that found in delinquents with a history of non-sexual offending (Awad *et al.*, 1984; Sauceda, 1978). However, the results of other studies dispute this finding (Lewis *et al.*, 1979; Tarter *et al.*, 1983), again suggesting that sample selection is an important factor in determining the findings of these studies. Tarter *et al.*, for example, found no apparent differences between adolescent sexual offenders and juvenile delinquents with no history of sexual offending on a comprehensive cognitive and neuropsychological battery. Epps (2000), however, found that child molesters were significantly more likely to have a lower IQ compared to other types of offenders, by a factor of around 10 points. Bladon (2000) reported that in her UK sample of 166 young abusers, 39 per cent had moderate learning disabilities and the UK-based project, G-MAP, report that approximately half of their referrals have learning disabilities, where this was defined as an IQ of 69 and below associated with developmentally impaired intellectual and social functioning.

It appears that some juvenile sexual offenders also exhibit soft signs of neurological impairments (Bagley, 1992; Lewis *et al.*, 1981). Bagley (1992), for example, found that adolescent sexual offenders were more likely to have a history of neurological conditions such as fits and hemiplegia than non-sexual offenders. There was also more evidence of hyperactivity and restlessness in the sexual offenders. Lewis *et al.* (1981) suggested that juvenile sexual offenders are characterized by a cluster of symptoms consisting of signs of organic impairment, an IQ below 80, and an increased incidence of aggressive behaviour, both sexual and non-sexual. However, they found similar characteristics in delinquents with a history of violent, non-sexual offending, but not in those who had committed non-sexual, non-violent offences. This suggests that the cognitive and organic impairments may be more associated with violence in general rather than with sexual violence in particular, a view shared by Knight and Prentky (1993), who proposed that impairments of this kind may be restricted to the more violent sexual offenders.

France and Hudson (1993) suggested that intellectual functioning is of aetiological significance only for a subgroup of low IQ juvenile sexual offenders who differ from most juvenile sexual offenders on other dimensions as well (Awad *et al.*, 1984). Indeed, in one of the few studies looking at sexual offending among developmentally delayed adolescents, Gilby *et al.* (1989) found that 23 per cent of those in treatment had engaged in sexually abusive behaviour. It has been suggested that the prevalence of sexual offending is at least as common, if not more common, in the intellectually disabled population (Griffiths *et al.*, 1985).

### *Psychiatric and personality problems*

A psychiatric history is frequently found in the juvenile sexual offender (Barbaree, Hudson and Seto, 1993). James and Neil (1996), for example, found that nearly half of the thirty-four sexually abusive juveniles in their study were known to mental health services, either for assessment or for treatment. This finding certainly lends support to the idea that some adolescents are vulnerable in many different ways, and that sexual offending is one consequence of that vulnerability. Of course, as noted earlier, little is known about the histories of those adolescents whose sexual offending is never detected. However, research into non-clinical samples of students who self-report a history of sexual offending suggests that they exhibit lower levels of psychopathology compared to known perpetrators (Finkelhor and Lewis, 1988; Fromuth *et al.*, 1991). It is possible, nevertheless, that the sexual offences of adolescents who are already known to the various agencies as a result of their psychosocial problems are simply more likely to be detected and to face criminal prosecution.

It is also important to note that the presence of a history of psychiatric or mental health problems does not necessarily imply that the young person has suffered from some form of mental illness. A positive psychiatric history is often recorded for adolescents who have simply been referred for psychiatric assessment, many of whom will attract a diagnosis on the basis that they have sexually offended. In describing their study into 100 British sexually abusive adolescents, Richardson, Graham *et al.* (1995) noted that "our impression is that once identified as an abuser at this age, referral for a psychiatric/psychological assessment was routine" (p. 191). Kavoussi *et al.* (1988) found that the most common diagnosis is indeed "conduct disorder" (48%), with sexual assaulters (75%) being more likely than child molesters (38%) to receive this diagnosis. They suggested that the high incidence of conduct disorder indicates that many sexual offences committed by adolescents are part of a pattern of poor impulse control and antisocial behaviours, especially in the case of the sexual assaulters.

With the above considerations in mind, psychiatric problems have been found in 37 per cent to 87 per cent of juvenile sexual offenders (Awad and Saunders, 1989; Awad *et al.*, 1984; Lewis *et al.*, 1979; Manocha and Mezey, 1998). Next to conduct disorder, emotional problems such as mild depression and anxiety (Becker, Kaplan *et al.*, 1991; Blaske *et al.*, 1989; Deisher *et al.*, 1982; Groth, 1977; James and Neil, 1996; Shoor *et al.*, 1966; Van Ness, 1984) and substance abuse problems (Kavoussi *et al.*, 1988) are frequently found. It seems that the presence of mental illness is rare. Thus, in the fifty-eight juvenile sexual offenders described by Kavoussi *et al.* (1988), none met the full DSM-III criteria for Major Affective Disorder, Dysthymia, or Psychotic Disorder. Indeed, contrary to expectation, they found less evidence of psychopathology than that found in other samples of delinquents convicted of serious offences (McManus *et al.*, 1984). However, the authors note that this may be because those with more serious psychiatric problems are not referred for the type of outpatient assessment and treatment offered in their programme. Rather, they are placed in hospital or residential settings.

Nevertheless, Oliver *et al.* (1993) reported similar findings when they compared fifty juvenile sexual offenders with two non-sexual offender control groups, fifty of whom had committed violent offences and fifty non-violent offences. The sexual offenders were found to display the "least deviant personality and background characteristics among the offender groups examined" (p. 367). Among other findings, they were less likely than the other groups of offenders to have had previous contact with mental health services. Oliver *et al.* suggested that there may be a subgroup of juvenile sexual offenders who are better adjusted than other types of juvenile offenders. Unfortunately, this particular study did not distinguish between the various types of sexual offender, such as child molesters and sexual assaulters, making it difficult to draw conclusions about the nature of this proposed subgroup.

Kempton and Forehand (1992) similarly found that the juvenile sexual offenders in their study were generally perceived as having fewer broad-based behavioural and emotional difficulties than other incarcerated delinquents. Fortunately, their data also allowed for a comparison of the child molesters and the sexual assaulters (those convicted for rape or sodomy). Although they found no differences between these groups, the authors recognize that the study was severely limited in size and scope. Of the eighty-three juvenile delinquents included in the research, only fifteen were sexual offenders. In addition, data collection was restricted to administration to one teacher of the Teacher Report Form of the Child Behaviour Checklist (CBCL, Achenbach and Edelbrock, 1986). Finally, it seems that the classification of the sexual offenders may have been flawed: offenders were grouped according to their index offence, and some of those convicted of rape and sodomy might have had a history of sexual offending against children.

Three recent British studies have also found low levels of mental illness in juvenile sexual offenders (Dolan *et al.*, 1996; Epps, 2000; Manocha and Mezey, 1998; Richardson, Graham *et al.*, 1995). The study by Dolan *et al.* is especially significant because they looked at the psychosocial characteristics of 121 juvenile sexual offenders referred to an adolescent forensic psychiatric service over a seven-year period. Whilst previous psychiatric contact was documented in many of the cases (39.6%), only one adolescent had a diagnosis of mental illness (obsessive-compulsive disorder). Again, conduct disorder or mixed emotional conduct disorder was the most common diagnosis (91.7%), and only ten were left undiagnosed. Similar findings were reported in the study by Richardson, Graham *et al.* (1995). They found that none of their sample of 100 sexually abusive adolescents had been previously or currently diagnosed as suffering from a major psychiatric illness, and there was no evidence to suggest that any were mentally disordered at the time they perpetrated their sexually abusive acts. Again, the presence of conduct disorders was common, with 68 per cent meeting DSM-III-R criteria for conduct disorder. Seventy-two per cent had severe childhood behavioural problems, 69 per cent were physically aggressive, 38 per cent had a history of running away from home, and 30 per cent were known to have set fires.

### *Problems arising from sexual abuse*

It is generally accepted that sexual abuse in childhood is a damaging experience, frequently resulting in adverse psychological sequelae (Becker, Kaplan *et al.*, 1991; Finkelhor and Browne, 1985; Porter, 1986; Watkins and Bentovim, 1992), some of which may have long-lasting effects (Aber *et al.*, 1989; Widom and Ames, 1994). It has been hypothesized that the sexual aggression of at least some juveniles and adults may be due in part to the recapitulation of their own sexual victimization (Breer, 1987; Burgess *et al.*, 1987; Finkelhor, 1986; Friedrich *et al.*, 1988; Fromuth, *et al.*, 1991; Garbarino and Platz, 1984; Gray, 1988; Groth, 1979b; Muster, 1992; Rogers and Terry, 1984). Several mechanisms have been proposed to explain why some boys who have been sexually abused go on to repeat the abuse they suffered, a phenomenon termed the "cycle-of-abuse" (Woods, 1997). These explanations include simple re-enactment of the abuse, through social-learning and modelling (Laws and Marshall, 1990; Longo, 1982; McCormack *et al.*, 1992); that abusive acts are an attempt to achieve mastery over conflicts about sexuality resulting from negative sexual experiences (Bentovim *et al.*, 1991; Breer, 1987; Groth, 1977; Lanyado *et al.*, 1995; Watkins and Bentovim, 1992); and that sexual arousal becomes conditioned to sexually abusive fantasies as a result of past abusive experiences which, in turn, lead to sexually abusive behaviour (Becker and Stein, 1991).

Unfortunately, obtaining valid information about the prevalence of sexual abuse in young offenders has been problematic. The experience of having been sexually abused is one that many young people find difficult to verbalize, and disclosure in and of itself can be traumatic (Finkelhor, 1988). Awad *et al.* (1984) suggest that this may explain why none of their sample of twenty-four juvenile sexual offenders and matched delinquents reported prior sexual abuse. Similarly, Becker (1988b) and Kahn and Lafond (1988) proposed that the rates reported by juvenile sexual offenders probably underestimate the prevalence of sexual victimization in research samples because the reporting of sexual abuse often emerges only after the adolescent has been in therapy and formed a trusting relationship with a therapist. The research literature provides some support for this suggestion. Pooling data from a number of studies, Worling (1995b) found that the mean frequency of sexual abuse reported by researchers using pre-treatment data was 22 per cent (256 out of 1,180), whereas the frequency reported by investigators using post-treatment information was significantly higher at 52 per cent (46 out of 88). However, in contrast, it has also been suggested that some offenders may over-report sexual abuse as a factor mitigating their own unacceptable behaviour (Hanson and Slater, 1988).

It also seems reasonable to suggest that many of the adolescents who find themselves placed in residential or custodial settings are those who have experienced multiple and accumulative psychosocial problems, including sexual abuse (Boswell, 1997; Browne *et al.*, 1995; Falshaw and Browne, 1997). As such, the reported rates of sexual abuse may also vary according to the setting in which the young person is seen and may be highest in secure settings.

It is not surprising, therefore, that there is tremendous variability in the reported frequency of sexual abuse in the research literature, with rates ranging from 4 per cent to about 60 per cent (Awad and Saunders, 1989; Becker, Cunningham-Rathner and Kaplan, 1986; Becker, Kaplan *et al.*, 1986;

Benoit and Kennedy, 1992; Cooper *et al.*, 1996; Epps, 2000; Fagan and Wexler, 1988; Fehrenbach *et al.*, 1986; Ford and Linney, 1995; Hawkes *et al.*, 1997; James and Neil, 1996; Johnson, 1988; Kahn and Lafond, 1988; Katz, 1990; Longo, 1982; Manocha and Mezey, 1998; O'Brien, 1991; Pierce and Pierce, 1987; Richardson, Kelly *et al.*, 1995; Sefarbi, 1990; Truscott, 1993; Watkins and Bentovim, 1992). These figures range from a level equal to that found in delinquents and the general male population (Awad and Saunders, 1989; Baker and Duncan, 1985; Benoit and Kennedy, 1992; Finkelhor, 1979; Peters *et al.*, 1986), to considerably more than that found in these populations. Truscott (1993) found that more than twice as many adolescent sexual offenders as violent or property offenders reported a history of sexual abuse, suggesting that sexual abuse is a particularly salient feature in the lives of juvenile sexual offenders. There is some evidence that the rate may be highest among male adolescents who abuse children (Davis and Leitenberg, 1987; Epps, 2000; O'Brien, 1991; Richardson, Kelly *et al.*, 1995; Robertson, 1990; Worling, 1995a), especially younger boys (Worling, 1995b), and lowest among rapists (Awad and Saunders, 1989; 1991; Epps, 2000). Worling (1995b) collected data about the sexual abuse histories of eighty-seven adolescent male sexual offenders following an average of thirteen months of clinical interventions. He found that 75 per cent of those who had sexually molested male children reported a history of sexual abuse, compared to 25 per cent of those who had assaulted female children, peers or adults. He suggests that sexual victimization may be especially important for understanding the sexual offending behaviour of adolescent males who abuse male children. In addition, in one of the few British comparative studies, Richardson, Kelly *et al.* (1995) found that the juvenile sexual offenders with a history of sexual victimization began offending sexually at an earlier age compared to those without such a history.

In another study, Worling (1995c) compared twenty-nine male adolescent sexual offenders who had molested female children with twenty-seven sexual assaulters who had offended against female peers or adults. Although the majority (74%) of the sexual assaulters in the study did not report a history of sexual abuse, five of the seven who did report abuse said that they were abused by an older female. Worling suggests that these boys may have offended against women to somehow seek revenge for their own victimization.

However, Benoit and Kennedy (1992), reporting on the characteristics of 100 adolescent males incarcerated in a secure residential training school in Florida, found there was no relationship between type of offence, sexual or otherwise, and history of sexual victimization. Thus, juveniles with no history of sexual offending reported levels of sexual abuse equal to that of the sexual offenders, and there were offenders in all groups who had been repeatedly victimized sexually and physically. They suggest that high-frequency sexual victimization does not appear to be a sufficient condition for the victim to repeat these acts against another child. As noted earlier, this pattern of findings may be attributable to the higher levels of abuse and psychopathology generally found in incarcerated samples of delinquents.

It is possible that the experience of sexual abuse, although damaging in itself, is also compounded by other familial factors which are associated with sexual abuse. In one of the few British studies, Dolan *et al.* (1996) compared juvenile sexual offenders who had been sexually victimized with those who had not. The abused group were found to have come from dysfunctional families characterized by more frequent changes of carer, greater incidence of physical and sexual abuse of the offender's siblings, and maternal histories of psychiatric illness. In addition, they had higher rates of special education, secure care, substance abuse, and charges of buggery offences. In most other respects the two groups were very similar.

Clearly, the role of sexual abuse in the aetiology of juvenile sexual offending, and in non-sexual offending, is far from clear. Further research is needed to examine the possible pathways from sexual victimization to offending.

### Problems arising from physical abuse

High levels of physical abuse have also been reported among samples of juvenile sexual offenders. Truscott (1993) found that almost 83 per cent of the twenty-three adolescent sexual offenders in his study reported a history of physical abuse. In their British study, Richardson, Graham *et al.* (1995) found that 55 per cent of their sample of 100 juvenile sexual offenders had suffered physical abuse at the hands of their parents, and that 22 per cent were placed on social services child protection registers. Similarly, Benoit and Kennedy (1992) found that 40 per cent of the incarcerated child molesters in their study had been physically victimized. High levels of bullying by peers has also been reported by some juvenile sexual offenders (Hawkes *et al.*, 1997). There is some evidence that sexual assaulters report a higher incidence of physical abuse and parental physical discipline than child molesters (Epps, 2000; Worling, 1995c).

It has frequently been hypothesized that being physically abused or observing family violence may play an important role in the development of sexual violence in adolescence (Boone-Hamilton, 1991; Fehrenbach *et al.*, 1986; Gomes-Schwartz, 1984). However, the pathways by which the experience of physical abuse leads to sexual aggression are not clear (Widom, 1989). Abuse and neglect is reported by a significant proportion of delinquent adolescents, and is not specific to sexual offenders (Benoit and Kennedy, 1992; Lewis *et al.*, 1981; Truscott, 1993; Van Ness, 1984). Several studies have compared physical abuse in juvenile sexual offenders to other groups of delinquents. Van Ness (1984) found that 41 per cent of juvenile sexual offenders reported histories of physical abuse or neglect, compared to only 15 per cent of a matched sample of delinquents with no history of sexual offending. Lewis *et al.* (1981) found that while 75 per cent of a sample of incarcerated violent adolescent sexual offenders had been physically abused and 79 per cent had observed intra-family violence, only 29 per cent of non-violent delinquents had a similar history. However, delinquents with a history of non-sexual violent offending had experienced similar levels of physical abuse to the violent sexual offenders, suggesting that childhood physical abuse is associated with violent behaviour more generally. Similarly, although Benoit and Kennedy (1992) found that 40 per cent of the incarcerated child molesters in their study had been physically victimized, this figure was not significantly different to that found in the young offenders with no history of sexual offending. Likewise, Truscott (1993) found no difference in the physical abuse histories of twenty-three sexual, fifty-one violent, and seventy-nine property offenders.

Hodges *et al.* (1996) used clinical case material obtained in brief psychotherapy to examine the kinds of risk factors that may be associated with the development of sexually abusive behaviour in boys who have themselves been physically abused. They speculated that the experience of early emotional deprivation, combined with traumatization and a preoccupation with violence resulting from being physically abused, places some boys at particular risk.

### *Social competence and peer relationship problems*

Peer relationships are considered to be essential to healthy childhood and adolescent sexual development (Billy and Udry, 1985a, b; Bukowski *et al.*, 1993). Appropriate peer relationships in adolescence are especially important in the development of sexual attitudes and beliefs (Davis and Harris, 1982; Moore and Rosenthal, 1993; Thornburg, 1981). Adolescent boys who experience poor peer relationships may also be denied the opportunity of appropriate social and sexual contact with peer-age girls, and fail to learn the necessary social and conversational skills for initiating and maintaining intimate relationships (Graves, 1993). Recent research has found deficits in intimacy and social competence in sexually aggressive men (Davidson, 1983; Lisak and Ivan, 1995; Marshall, 1989), and social competence plays an important role as a differentiator among subtypes of adult sexual offenders (Fisher *et al.*, 1999; Knight, 1992; Knight and Prentky, 1990).

It is therefore not surprising to find that the role of peer relationships, and associated social and sexual difficulties, has attracted considerable attention in the literature on adolescent sexual offending. In one of the few controlled studies into adolescent sexual offending, Blaske *et al.* (1989) compared four groups of thirteen- to seventeen-year-old boys on measures of individual functioning and family and peer relationships. The sample included sexual offenders, assault offenders, non-violent offenders, and non-delinquent boys. Among other findings, Blaske *et al.* report that the sexual offenders were less emotionally bonded to peers and felt more estranged in their relationships with others. Similarly, Fagan and Wexler (1988) found that, compared to violent delinquents, the sexual offenders in their study were more socially and sexually isolated, less likely to belong to a gang, less often had girlfriends, had less sexual experiences, and expressed less interest in sex. Further, Graves (1993) found that about 75 per cent of the juvenile child molesters in his study were rated as lacking heterosocial ("dating") confidence, experience and skills. However, it seems likely that the role of peers and peer relationships in juvenile sexual offending is particularly complex. There is considerable evidence that this is one area in which there may be important differences between child molesters and sexual assaulters (Epps, 2000).

To begin with, the role of peers at the time of offending appears to vary according to type of offence. Adolescent child molesters rarely offend with other boys. Rather, they tend to offend alone. This is not surprising given the social stigma attached to sexual contact with children, and the secretive nature of child abuse. In contrast, there is evidence that sexual assaulters do offend with others, sometimes in groups ("gang rape"). In their review of the literature on adolescent sexual offenders, Davis and Leitenberg (1987) found a vast difference in the reported proportion of lone offenders, ranging from 93 per cent (Groth, 1977) to 14 per cent (Amir, 1971). However, whilst most of the studies reviewed focused on child molesters, others looked at sexual assaulters, or mixed groups, which may help to explain the wide variation. Studies looking only at sexual assaulters show lower rates of lone offending (Amir, 1971; McDermott, 1979).

Although the developmental pathways leading to sexual offending are likely to be complex and involve a multitude of variables, it seems likely that social competence and the quality of peer-relationships may be especially important in helping to shape the type and nature of sexual offending behaviour. In his four-factor model of adult sexual offending, Finkelhor (1984; 1986) suggests that sexual activity with children is more likely to occur when alternative sources of sexual gratification are blocked or inhibited in some way, termed "blockage". It seems plausible, therefore, that adolescents who are socially isolated from peers may be at greater risk of sexual contact with children, as an alternative to peer-aged sexual relationships. Evidence of blockage has been reported by O'Callaghan and Print (1994). They found that only 50 per cent of the child molesters in the G-MAP treatment programme, Manchester, England, had a number of girlfriends, compared to 81 per cent of the non-sexual offenders. Further, only 26 per cent of the sexual offenders reported having experienced non-abusive sexual intercourse with a peer, compared to 59 per cent of the non-sexual offenders. More of the sex offenders (32%) also believed they were "less successful" with girls than the non-sex offenders (19%).

There is research to support the notion that some adult child molesters perceive children as less threatening than adults (Groth *et al.*, 1982; Howells, 1979). Adult child molesters have also been found lacking in heterosocial and heterosexual skills (Overholser and Beck, 1986; Segal and Marshall, 1985). Similar deficits in social competence have also been found in adolescent child molesters, including a lack of assertiveness in social interaction (Becker and Abel, 1985), deficiencies in intimacy skills (Groth, 1977; Marshall, 1989), and shyness and timidity (DeNatale, 1989). Social isolation in adolescent child molesters seems to be a particular problem, with many finding it difficult to establish and maintain peer relationships, a view supported both by research findings and by clinical observation (Awad and Saunders, 1989; Awad *et al.*, 1984; Becker and Abel, 1985; Blaske *et al.*, 1989; Chewning, 1991; Epps, 2000; Fagan and Wexler, 1988; Fehrenbach *et al.*, 1986; Figia *et al.*, 1987; Graves, 1993; Groth, 1977; Katz, 1990; Lonczynski, 1991; Manocha and Mezey, 1998; O'Callaghan and Print, 1994; Saunders *et al.*, 1986; Shoor *et al.*, 1966; Tingle *et al.*, 1986). For example, Saunders *et al.* (1986) found that, while 60 per cent of the exhibitionists and 72 per cent of the child molesters had no close friends, only 32 per cent of the rapists were similarly isolated. O'Callaghan and Print (1994) noted that all the young abusers with whom they have worked reported feeling isolated within their own family, although it is not clear whether the experience of isolation was significantly different from that reported by adolescents with no history of sexual offending.

Perhaps allied to the social isolation described above is the finding that a significant number of sexual offenders have a low level of self-esteem (Fisher *et al.*, 1999). This is particularly true of child molesters. Most of the studies reporting on self-esteem have been examined and adult samples and studies are needed which compare adolescent sexual offenders with a control group. O'Reilly *et al.* (1998) reported that their sample of adolescent sexual offenders differed significantly from a control group of non-offending peers on general and total self-esteem scores, scoring lower than the controls. They did not differ significantly on social and personal self-esteem. It has been suggested that low self-esteem in sexual offenders is a result of poor parental attachments (Marshall *et al.*, 1993) and this is a subject for future research.

The idea that the typical adolescent sexual offender is some kind of unusual, lonely, social misfit has gained popularity. Although this is undoubtedly true in some instances, especially in child molesters, this view may have gained particular credence because it helped to distance sexual offenders from "normal" delinquents, most of whom offend with others and have extensive peer relationships, usually with other delinquents who share similar delinquent attitudes and beliefs (West and Farrington, 1977). Some years ago Cohen and Boucher (1972) noted that many popular perceptions of adult sexual offenders seem to serve the function of differentiating them from "normal" people. Thus, they are variously referred to as "loners", "monsters", "perverts", or "animals".

However, the idea that adolescent sexual offenders are socially isolated, inept individuals takes little account of the large number of socially competent adolescents, delinquent and non-delinquent, who sexually offend against women and female peers (Koss, 1988; 1992). It seems that sexual coercion and aggression toward women and female peers is seen as acceptable in some male social groups, certainly more so than sexual contact with children. Katchadourian (1990) argues that the use of sexual coercion and the various justifications for this unacceptable behaviour appear to be already established among many young men by the time of adolescence. According to the integrated theory of delinquency developed by Elliott *et al.* (1985), association with deviant peers, combined with low social bonding to family and school, is considered to be a primary determinant of delinquent behaviour. Further, Ageton (1983) found that delinquent peer group association was the single best predictor of sexual assault. Peer group endorsement of sexual intercourse and forced sexual behaviour were predictors of sexual aggression, as was engagement in various other delinquent behaviours. There is also research suggesting that a growing number of young males are forcing their girlfriends to have intercourse or perform other sexual acts against their will, often with the use of physical force (Carlson, 1987; Levine and Kanin, 1987; White and Koss, 1993).

Research into sexual aggression among male college students by Sanday (1979, 1990) and Koss and her colleagues (Koss and Dinero, 1988; White and Koss, 1993) has also implicated the role of peers. White and Koss (1993) suggested that there may be individual differences in attitudes, personality, motives for sex and domination, and opportunities for sexual aggression that explain why young men in similar circumstances differ in the likelihood of committing a sexually aggressive act. More recently, Schwartz and DeKeseredy (1997) have proposed a male peer-support model to explain the high levels of sexual aggression on North American college campuses. They argue that the college campus provides fertile ground for young men who share "rape-supportive" attitudes to congregate and to support and maintain sexually coercive behaviour toward women. The belief that masculine biological urges are so strong that they must be satisfied at any cost, together with the corresponding belief that those who do not exhibit such "strong sexual drives" are not "real men", puts pressure on adolescent males to display their sexual prowess (Hollway, 1984). It certainly seems that undergraduate rapists in North America are rarely punished for their crimes (Bernstein, 1996) and that there is a widespread tendency of college administrators to ignore or cover up reports of sexual crime (Sanday, 1990; Warshaw, 1988).

There is an important subgroup of adolescent sexual assaulters, however, who seem to be less socially skilled and who lack peer relationships, and may be more similar to child molesters in this respect (Amir, 1971; Epps, 1991). It is possible that this group of adolescent sexual assaulters were also unpopular as children, and may continue to experience social difficulties into adulthood, with an increased risk that they will continue their pattern of sexual offending behaviour. Indeed, Tingle *et al.* (1986) reported that 86 per cent of their adult rapists had few or no friends. In addition, Worling (1995c) found no differences in interpersonal functioning and self-perception between child molesters and sexual assaulters, suggesting that Finkelhor's (1984) notion of blockage may apply equally well to at least some sexual assaulters. Thus, whilst women and peer-aged girls remain the focus of sexual arousal and fantasy, they seem inaccessible, perhaps leading to feelings of frustration, anger and resentment toward women. Adolescent rapists who have been seen in clinical settings have occasionally been described as angry, insecure, manipulative and inadequate, with a strong need to control situations and people, especially women (Fehrenbach *et al.*, 1986; Groth, 1977).

These feelings may be exaggerated in boys who hold negative, stereotypical views of women, views which are commonplace in society (Epps *et al.*, 1993; Segal and Stermac, 1984; Stermac and Quinsey, 1986). The role of anger and aggression is central to the typology of rape proposed by Groth and his colleagues (Groth, 1979a; Groth and Burgess, 1977; Groth *et al.*, 1977). According to this hypothesis rape is a "pseudo-sexual" act dominated by either power needs or anger needs. For example, in "anger rape" it is proposed that the offender seeks to express rage, contempt and hate for women, perhaps to retaliate for perceived wrongdoings or rejections he has suffered at the hands of women. Sex is viewed as a weapon and, not surprisingly, anger rapists not only use excessive force whilst perpetrating rape but are often physically assaultive toward women in other contexts. Interestingly, Van Ness (1984) found problems in controlling anger to be more than twice as common in a sample of incarcerated adolescent rapists than in a non-sexual offender sample.

### *Self-image, identity problems and attitudes*

The presence of a distorted self-image is generally considered to be associated with sexual offending in adolescence (Davis and Leitenberg, 1987). Various facets of self-image have received attention in the research literature. The presence of low self-esteem, confused masculine identity, gender-identity confusion, and traditional sex-role attitudes have all been linked to sexual offending by juveniles (Davis and Leitenberg, 1987), although most of the empirical evidence comes from studies of adult sexual offenders.

Several studies have demonstrated a relationship between sexual aggression in adult males and the presence of "cognitive distortions" or "thinking errors", characterized by the endorsement of rape myths and negative, hostile attitudes toward women (Calhoun *et al.*, 1997; Hersh and Gray-Little, 1998; Lisak and Roth, 1988; Malamuth, 1986; Mosher and Anderson, 1986; Rapaport and Burkhart, 1984). It seems that sexually aggressive men generally describe themselves in more "traditional" terms than do sexually non-aggressive men (Koss and Dinero, 1988; Tieger, 1981; White and Humphrey, 1990). Research into convicted adult sexual offenders has often produced mixed results. Whilst Scott and Tetreault (1986) found support for the view that rapists have more traditional and conservative attitudes toward women than non-sexual offenders, other studies contradict this finding (Hall *et al.*, 1986; Marshall *et al.*, 1979; Overholser and Beck, 1986; Stermac and Quinsey, 1986), suggesting that negative and stereotypical attitudes toward women are commonplace among men and are not specific to sexual offenders. Similar findings have been found in adolescents (Epps *et al.*, 1993). Using the Attitudes Toward Women Scale (AWS) (Spence *et al.*, 1973) and the Burt Rape Myth Acceptance Scale (BRMAS), Epps *et al.* (1993) compared attitudes toward women and rape among thirty-one male adolescents convicted of sexual crimes and twenty-seven convicted of non-sexual violent crimes. The results showed no significant difference between the groups on either measure. In addition, a more traditional, conservative attitude toward women, as measured on the AWS, did not significantly correlate with the endorsement of rape myths as measured on the BRMAS. However, this study did not distinguish between sexual assaulters and child molesters. Nevertheless, Worling (1995c), contrary to expectations, found few differences between child molesters and sexual assaulters in the extent to which they endorsed rape-supportive attitudes. However, all the child molesters in his study had abused female children, raising the possibility that rape-supportive attitudes are associated with sexual and non-sexual violence toward all females, regardless of age. It is not known whether adolescent child molesters who sexually victimize only male children share similar views.

Related to cognitive distortions about offending is the issue of empathy. Although much has now been published on the subject of victim empathy in adult offenders this has not been specifically researched with adolescents in the same way. The adult data shows that few sexual offenders have general empathy deficits but rather lack empathy for their own victims (Fisher, 1998; Marshall, Anderson and Fernandez, 1999). One of the difficulties has been effectively measuring empathy. Until the last few years most studies relied on a measure of general empathy, the Interpersonal Reactivity Index (Davis, 1980) and measures specific to empathy for the perpetrator's own victim were not developed until the 1990s (e.g. the Victim Empathy Scale, Beckett and Fisher, 1994; the Child Molester Empathy Measure, Fernandez *et al.*, 1999). Both these measures can be used with adolescents but lack clinical norms. It is likely, however, that they are measuring the offender's distorted thinking about the victim rather than empathy per se (Fisher, 1998).

With regard to how adolescents may come to develop a particular identity and set of attitudes, Lisak (1991; 1994) and colleagues (Lisak and Ivan, 1995; Lisak and Roth, 1990) have suggested that a particularly unhelpful form of masculine identity, termed "defensive masculinity" (Chodorow, 1978), may be exacerbated when the male does not experience an adequate relationship with his father. They suggest that the presence of a father figure eases the process of "masculinization" by supplying a vivid model of "masculinity" for the son to follow. Without such a model, some boys may exaggerate what they perceive to be masculine attitudes and behaviours and reject characteristics they perceive to be "feminine", including the experience and expression of emotional states important in establishing intimate relationships. Father-absent adolescents are over-represented in sexual offender and non-sexual offender delinquent samples (Fehrenbach *et al.*, 1986; Rutter and Giller, 1983). Interestingly, in their study of 100 British adolescent sexual offenders, Richardson, Graham *et al.* (1995) found that 50 per cent had no contact with their natural father and came from families where parents had separated with a history of parental violence toward the children. There is evidence that self-esteem in male adolescents and adults is especially closely linked to the development of sexual identity and sense of masculinity (Feather, 1985), and that some types of sexual identity may be less adaptive than others (Antill and Cunningham, 1980). Specifically, that an overly masculine sexual identity may be less suited to the formation and development of intimate relationships. As noted earlier, Marshall (1989) has suggested that failure to develop intimate relationships may have important aetiological significance for the development of sexual offending.

Some empirical support for the role of the father in the development of defensive masculinity comes from cross-cultural research into child-rearing practices. For example, Coltrane's (1988; 1992) analysis of ninety pre-industrial societies demonstrated a relationship between father-distant child rearing and relatively high levels of institutionalized misogyny and the dis-empowerment of women. Men were less prone to exaggerated masculine ("hyper-masculine") behaviour and women were less likely to be socially dis-empowered in societies in which fathers participated more in child rearing. Similarly, Whiting (1965), in an analysis of six societies, suggested that father-distant child rearing is associated with "protest masculinity" which, in turn, is associated with male-perpetrated interpersonal violence.

Further support for the "gender-socialization" theory of male sexual aggression comes from studies looking at masculine identity in sexually aggressive males. Several studies have found that they are more likely than non-aggressive males to have experienced negative relationships with their fathers (Epps, 2000; Hazelwood and Warren, 1989; Lisak, 1994; Lisak and Roth, 1990; McCabe, 1989). They also score higher on a variety of psychometric measures, including measures of "hostile masculinity" (Malamuth *et al.*, 1991), hostility toward women and the need to dominate women (Lisak and Roth, 1990; Malamuth, 1986), hyper-masculinity (Gold *et al.*, 1992; Mosher and Anderson, 1986; Mosher and Sirkin, 1984), and gender role stress and emotional disconnection (Lisak *et al.*, 1995; Lisak and Roth, 1990). In addition, two studies have found that sexually aggressive men also score lower on measures of femininity (Lisak *et al.*, 1995; Lisak and Roth, 1990).

### *Substance abuse problems*

Alcohol and drugs have frequently been implicated in sexual offending among adult men (Amir, 1967; 1971; Johnson *et al.*, 1978; Rada, 1975). Substance use and abuse is also highly prevalent in delinquent young people (Elliott and Huizinga, 1984; Elliott and Morse, 1989; Hartstone and Hansen, 1984), and in some juvenile sexual offenders (Bagley, 1992; Fagan and Wexler, 1988; Hawkins *et al.*, 1987; Hsu and Starzynski, 1990; Mio *et al.*, 1986; Tinklenberg and Woodrow, 1974; Van Ness, 1984; Vinogradov *et al.*, 1988).

Ageton (1983) and Humphrey and White (1992) found correlations between reports of sexual aggression and delinquent behaviours, including alcohol and drug use at levels significantly beyond those of sexually non-aggressive adolescents. It is likely that the use of alcohol and drugs before and during offending may serve multiple functions: as a disinhibitor for the perpetrator, as an excuse after the fact, and as a strategy to reduce victim resistance. It seems that intoxication at the time of the offence is uncommon. Thus, Groth (1977) reported that 11 per cent of juvenile sexual offenders were intoxicated, Wasserman and Kappel (1985) 10 per cent, and Fehrenbach *et al.* (1986) found only 6 per cent. However, use of alcohol without intoxication may be more common in some types of sexual offending. It appears that between one-third and two-thirds of rapists and many rape victims have consumed alcohol prior to the rape (Lott *et al.*, 1982; Wolfe and Baker, 1980). In a study of sixty-three adolescent rapists (some of whom were actually child molesters, having raped children) Vinogradov *et al.* (1988) found that the large majority reported "regular" (not defined) use of alcohol and other drugs. In forty-eight of sixty-seven rape episodes, the offender described himself as under the influence of one or more psychoactive drugs at the time of the offence, and 15 per cent reported taking a drug less than fifteen minutes before the rape.

Many juvenile sexual assaulters also feel that forced sex is more justifiable if the victim is drunk or "stoned" (Goodchilds *et al.*, 1988). It is generally agreed that programmes aimed at the treatment of alcohol and drug abuse in high-risk adolescent populations would be important in the primary prevention of rape as well as other violent crimes (Lightfoot and Barbaree, 1993; Vinogradov *et al.*, 1988).

However, there is little agreement in the literature as to the extent of alcohol and drug involvement in juvenile sexual offences. In their review of the literature on adolescent sexual offenders, Davis and Leitenberg (1987) concluded that "there are no data to indicate whether adolescents who commit sexual offences are more likely than other adolescents to have a history of alcohol or drug abusing problems, or whether there is a higher incidence of adolescent sexual offenders in the drug or alcohol abusing population of adolescents than in the general population of adolescents" (p. 420). Several typologies of substance-abusing adult offenders have been proposed (Hodgins and Lightfoot, 1988; Lightfoot and Hodgins, 1988), including one for rapists which distinguished between alcoholic and non-alcoholic rapists (Rada, 1975). There is insufficient knowledge about substance abuse in juvenile sexual offenders to allow for the development of typologies. However, it seems reasonable to speculate that substance abuse may be more common in those with a more extensive history of non-sexual offending and involvement with delinquent peers. It is not surprising, therefore, that substance abuse seems to be more common among adolescent rapists (Vinogradov *et al.*, 1988). Lightfoot and Barbaree (1993) suggest that, for those who are chronic users, their high frequency of substance abuse may impair the development of appropriate heterosexual behaviours and problem-solving abilities, thus increasing the risk of sexual offending.

### *Sexual problems*

Several factors have been posited to be related to either the development or maintenance of deviant sexual acts in juvenile sexual offenders, including prior maltreatment experiences (Becker, Hunter *et al.*, 1989), exposure to sexually explicit materials and substance abuse (Becker and Stein, 1991), and exposure to aggressive role models (Ryan *et al.*, 1987). There is also evidence to suggest that some adult sexual offenders have experienced some form of prior sexual dysfunction, most often impotence or premature ejaculation (Longo, 1982). It seems reasonable to hypothesize that these kinds of sexual difficulties may occur more often in those juvenile sexual offenders who themselves have been subject to sexual abuse. However, compared to adult sexual offenders, the presence of sexual problems and sexual deviancy in juvenile sexual offenders has received scant attention. Instead, emphasis has been placed on the developmental, psychological, educational and family problems, which Barbaree *et al.* (1993) refer to as the "child and family perspective".

There are several possible explanations for this difference in emphasis, including the unfamiliarity of child and family professionals with sexual issues; the conceptualization of juvenile sexual offending as an expression of "normal", albeit misled and inappropriate, sexual curiosity and experimentation rather than the manifestation of deviant sexual preferences; and the ethical problems associated with exploring sexual attitudes and behaviour in children and adolescents. Ethical concerns about the use of phallometric plethysmography (PPG) with adolescents in a clinical context has been expressed by a number of researchers and clinicians, such that very few adolescent sexual offender programmes employ this procedure. Laws and Marshall (1990), for example, note that many adolescent sexual offenders have themselves been sexually abused and suggest that it seems unwise to show them visual material depicting the abuse and exploitation of children, some of which may be used to elaborate their own deviant sexual fantasies.

However, Knight and Prentky (1993) suggest that this bias in emphasis is worrying and should be rectified. They note that deviant sexual arousal patterns in adult offenders have been identified as one of the most consistent discriminators of the propensity to engage in sexually coercive behaviour (Prentky and Knight, 1991). There are only a handful of published studies into sexual arousal and the treatment of sexual deviancy in adolescent sexual offenders, most of which are by Becker and her colleagues (Becker, Hunter *et al.*, 1992; Becker *et al.*, 1989; Becker, Kaplan and Tenke, 1992; Becker, Stein *et al.*, 1992; Hunter and Goodwin, 1992; Kaemingk *et al.*, 1995; Weinrott *et al.*, 1997). This is despite the fact that 168 juvenile sexual offender treatment programmes in the United States reported using phallometric assessment (Knopp et al., 1992). Unfortunately, controlled studies of the patterns of sexual arousal and of sexual fantasies of adolescent sexual offenders have thus far been neglected.

Becker (1988b) proposed that there may be a distinction between juvenile sexual offenders with deviant, recurrent fantasies and a preference for deviant activity, and those for whom sexual aggression is simply a part of their impulsive behaviour. Most of the studies have focused on child molesters. A study by Weinrott *et al.* (1997), for example, used a treatment technique called vicarious sensitization (VS) with sixty-nine juvenile sexual offenders, all of whom were child molesters. Treatment outcome was evaluated using phallometric data (PPG) and self-report measures, and was successful in reducing sexual arousal to prepubescent children. Virtually nothing is known about the sexual arousal patterns in adolescent sexual assaulters. Research into the sexual arousal patterns of incarcerated adult rapists indicates that there may be important subtypes (Barbaree *et al.*, 1994). In this study sixty incarcerated adult rapists were subtyped according to the Massachusetts Treatment Center Rapist Typology as either "opportunistic" or "vindictive" "non-sexual" offenders, or "non-sadistic" or "sadistic" "sexual" offenders. Barbaree *et al.* (1994) found that the index offences committed by the non-sexual subtypes were more likely to be impulsive, violent and to result in greater harm to the victim. The men in the sexual subtypes showed more evidence of offence-planning, were more socially isolated at the time of the offence, and showed greater arousal to rape descriptions when assessed using the PPG. The authors speculate that the rapes perpetrated by each subtype are associated with distinctly different psychological processes, requiring a different approach to treatment. Thus, the sexual subtypes are more likely to need interventions directed at the sexual fantasies and behaviours which support their offending behaviour. The non-sexual subtypes, in contrast, are more likely to require help to reduce their level of aggression and interpersonal conflict, and substance abuse.

The limited research that has been carried out into juvenile sexual offenders supports findings from the adult literature suggesting that deviant sexual arousal is especially significant in sexual offending against children, and has an early onset in male paedophilia (Hunter and Becker, 1994). This finding is not particularly surprising. One of the pre-conditions for the sexual abuse of children outlined by Finkelhor (1984; 1986) in his four-factor model is that males who sexually offend against children must find children, or at least some children, sexually arousing. The extent to which male adults and juveniles who have sexually assaulted women share similar patterns of sexual arousal is not clear. Investigations into the sexual arousal patterns of adult rapists have focused on sexual arousal to violence. Whilst some studies have found significant differences between rapists and non-rapists in their PPG responses to consenting and forced sex (Lalumiere and Quinsey 1994; Quinsey *et al.*, 1984), others have not (Baxter *et al.*, 1986).

Whatever the case, it seems safe to assume that sexual arousal to children is a necessary, although not sufficient, explanation of why some adolescents sexually abuse children. In at least some cases it seems reasonable to speculate that the experience of having been sexually abused in childhood or early adolescence may have contributed to the development of sexual arousal to children (Watkins and Bentovim, 1992). The factors responsible for the development of sexual arousal to violence, which may be a significant feature in some adolescent child molesters and sexual assaulters, are even less clear.

### *Use of pornography*

Comparatively little has been written on the subject of use of pornography by adolescent sexual offenders. A number of authors have suggested that exposure to pornography may have played a part in the development of deviant interests or stimulated sexual interest. Kaufman *et al.* (1998) compared the use of pornography in adult and adolescent offenders and reported that adults had a narrower focus. They stated that being interested in pornography represents a normative developmental experience for a large number of adolescents and is a significant source of information about sexuality. Malamuth (1993) investigated the impact of pornography on male adolescents. He reported that exposure to pornography typically occurred by secondary school stage and that 45 per cent had seen an obscene film. Malamuth pointed out that if the portrayal of sex was intertwined with violence, hatred, coercion and humiliation of women then the individual could have the experience of becoming sexually aroused to such material. Malamuth found that the type of message conveyed was crucial to the impact of the material and that sexual explicitness itself does not have harmful effects. He further suggested that those individuals who already have some risk of being attracted to sexual aggression are most likely to be influenced by such material.

O' Reilly *et al.* (1998) compared the use of pornography in a group of sexually abusive adolescents with a group of non-offending peers. They found no differences in the reported usage between the two groups in their use of magazines, films and sex lines. They further found no differences between those abusers considered still to be at high risk of offending following treatment and those considered low risk.

Becker and Stein (1991) reported that magazines were the most frequently used source of sexually explicit material (35%) followed by videos (26%). Only 11 per cent of their sample reported not using explicit material and 74 per cent reported that it increased their sexual arousal. They found no relationship between the number of victims relative to the different types of explicit material or between the use of pornography and self-reported sexual arousal. Emerick and Dutton (1993) carried out polygraph research with a group of high risk adolescents and reported that almost 80 per cent acknowledged the use of pornography for stimulation. In contrast to the Becker and Stein study they reported that the mean number of female child victims increased progressively with the severity of pornography used as a stimulus for masturbation. Ford and Linney (1995) found that 42 per cent of sexual offenders reported exposure to hard core magazines compared to 29 per cent of violent offenders. The sexual offenders were also exposed to pornography at earlier ages (5–8 years).

### *Sexual knowledge*

As with the use of pornography little has been published on whether adolescent sexual offenders are more deficient in their sexual knowledge than non-offenders. Kraft (1993) studied the sexual knowledge of a large sample of young people in Norway and found considerable gaps in their knowledge. However, as there are no norms for the sexual knowledge of non-offending adolescents it is difficult to know if the Norwegian study is representative or not. Sex education is regarded as a necessary component of treatment programmes for adolescent sexual offenders as it seems reasonable to expect them to benefit from the provision of information that helps them to better understand their sexuality, clarify their personal values and make better and less risky decisions about their sexual behaviour (Klein and Gordon, 1992).

### *Denial*

It is a common feature of sexual offenders to employ some form of denial or minimization of their offending (Salter, 1988). Denial fulfils a number of functions ranging from attempting to avoid the consequences of one's actions through to self-protection by trying to excuse, justify or minimize the behaviour. Salter (1988) has described denial as being on a continuum from total denial of the behaviour through to minimization and justification. Chaffin (1997) makes the distinction between denial and lying, seeing denial as a psychological defence mechanism motivated by the need to maintain a favourable self-image. He sees lying as a social behaviour motivated by fear of consequences.

Many studies of adolescent sexual offenders report the presence of denial and minimization (Becker, 1988a; Hunter and Figueredo, 1999; Will, 1994). While the reduction of denial is a valid treatment aim as it is necessary for the individual to take responsibility for his behaviour before he will be motivated to change his offending behaviour, it is important to note that the reduction of denial is not related to reduction in risk. Kahn and Chambers (1991) reported that those adolescents who denied their offences did not re-offend when compared to a group of admitters. This finding has also been replicated with adults by Hanson and Bussiere (1998) and Beech, Fisher and Beckett (1999) who found that reductions in denial did not equate to changes in other treatment areas.

### *Distinctions based on offence characteristics*

In research into adult sexual offenders, victim age appears to be an important discriminator, producing rapist/child molester groups of offenders who differ on several dimensions (Bard *et al.*, 1987; Knight, 1988; Panton, 1978; Quinsey *et al.*, 1993). Bard *et al.* (1987) compared the developmental, clinical and criminal characteristics of 184 adult child molesters and rapists. Only men whose sexual assaults were on victims over sixteen years old were classified as rapists, whilst those whose victims were under sixteen years old were classified as child molesters. This system of classification has now been adopted in most of the research into adult sexual offending and has informed the development of the taxonomic system developed by Knight and Prentky and colleagues (Knight, 1988; 1992; Knight and Prentky, 1990; Prentky and Knight, 1991).

Bard *et al.* (1987) found that, compared to rapists, adult child molesters are less likely to have been conduct disordered during childhood and adolescence, to have a history of victim-involved crime, to have a history of drug and alcohol abuse, and to use aggression and violence during their sexual offences, although child molesters show greater variance in sexual aggression. The authors suggest that this may be due to the presence of different types of child molesters with radically different levels of aggression. In contrast, child molesters are more likely to show a pattern of social withdrawal and avoidance, to have been raised in an intact family, to have experienced more medical problems, to have a slightly lower IQ score, to score lower on psychometric measures of aggression and narcissism, to present symptoms of psychoticism, passive sexuality and psychosexual disturbance, and to have been a victim of sexual abuse. Overall, they found more variability in the characteristics of child molesters. In addition to the greater variance found in the level of sexual aggression, there was more variability in educational attainment and intellectual functioning, especially at the lower end of the scale. Thus, they found that 27.9 per cent of the sixty-eight child molesters, but only 10.6 per cent of the 107 rapists in their study had IQ scores below 85.

Bard *et al.* concluded that their data "suggest major modal differences in interpersonal style, social, intellectual, and physical competence, and symptomatology between the two groups, and support the discriminant validity of victim age" (p. 217). There is evidence of a similar pattern of differences between juvenile child molesters and sexual assaulters (Epps, 2000). Nevertheless, it is likely that there may be other clinical phenomena that are more important than the victim-age distinction in understanding certain sexual offenders.

## Conclusions

The above review suggests that many young offenders share similar characteristics, experiencing a variety of psychosocial problems. However, it also identifies areas in which there seem to be important differences between juvenile sexual offenders and non-sexual offenders, and between child molesters and sexual assaulters. Barbaree *et al.* (1993) may well have been correct when they proposed that the population of juvenile sexual offenders is every bit as heterogeneous as the population of adult sexual offenders. There is some evidence that offence and victim characteristics are associated with particular kinds of offender characteristics. Offence characteristics that seem to be particularly important are the use of force and violence (aggressive hands-on, versus non-aggressive hands-off), the degree of violence, the age of the victim (child versus adult), the gender of the victim, the relationship to the offender (relative, stranger, or acquaintance), and whether the victim was a family member (intra-familial versus extra-familial). Unfortunately, much of the research on juvenile sexual offenders has confounded these variables.

Future research into sexual offending in young people should aim to group offenders according to offence and offender characteristics. There is now considerable evidence that different clusters of psychosocial problems are associated with different types of sexual offending which, in turn, follow different developmental pathways. Identification of these pathways will have important implications for prevention, through early intervention, and for treatment. With respect to child molesters, for example, both the research and clinical literature point to the significance of unpopularity and social isolation from the peer group, often from an early age, yet little is known about the social, psychological and behavioural variables that give rise to this problem or the ways in which these variables interact with other factors, such as being a victim of sexual abuse. It seems reasonable to suggest that early interventions, such as those aimed at improving peer relationships and social functioning in at-risk children, may have long-term benefits in offsetting the development of patterns of thinking and behaviour that result in sexual offending against children.

## References

Aber, J. L., Allen, J. P., Carlson, V., and Cicchetti, D. (1989). The effects of maltreatment on development during early childhood: Recent studies and their theoretical, clinical, and policy implications. In D. Cicchetti and V. Carlson (eds), *Child Maltreatment: Theory and Research on the Causes and Consequences of Child Abuse and Neglect*. Cambridge: Cambridge University Press.

Achenbach, T. M., and Edelbrock, C. (1986). *Manual for the TRF and Teacher Version of the Child Behavior Profile*. Burlington, VT: Department of Psychiatry, University of Vermont.

Ageton, S. S. (1983). *Sexual Assault Among Adolescents*. Lexington, MA: Lexington Books.

American Psychiatric Association (1987). *Diagnostic and Statistical Manual of Mental Disorders*, 3rd edn, revised (DSM-III). Washington, DC: American Psychiatric Association.

Amir, M. (1967). Alcohol and forcible rape. *British Journal of Addictions, 62*, 219–232.

Amir, M. (1971). *Patterns in Forcible Rape*. Chicago: University of Chicago Press.

Antill, J., and Cunningham, J. (1980). The relationship of masculinity, femininity, and androgeny to self-esteem. *Australian Journal of Psychology, 32*, 195–207.

Arbuthnot, J., Gordon, D. A., and Jurkovic, G. J. (1987). Personality. In H. C. Quay (ed.), *Handbook of Juvenile Delinquency*. New York: John Wiley (pp. 139–182).

Atcheson, J. D., and Williams, D. C. (1954). A study of juvenile sexual offenders. *American Journal of Psychiatry, 111*, 366–370.

Awad, G. A., and Saunders, E. B. (1989). Adolescent child molesters: Clinical observations. *Child Psychiatry and Human Development, 19*, 195–206.

Awad, G. A., and Saunders, E. B. (1991). Male adolescent sexual assaulters: Clinical observations. *Journal of Interpersonal Violence, 6*, 446–460.

Awad, G. A., Saunders, E. B., and Levene, J. A. (1984). A clinical study of male adolescent sexual offenders. *International Journal of Offender Therapy and Comparative Criminology, 28*, 105–116.

Bagley, C. (1992). Characteristics of 60 children and adolescents with a history of sexual assaults against others: Evidence from a comparative study. *Journal of Forensic Psychiatry, 3*, 299–309.

Bagley, C., and Shewchuk-Dann, D. (1991). Characteristics of 60 children and adolescents who have a history of sexual assault against others: Evidence from a controlled study. *Journal of Child and Youth Care, 6*, 43–52.

Baker, A. W., and Duncan, S. P. (1985). Child sexual abuse: A study of prevalence in Great Britain. *Child Abuse and Neglect, 9*, 457–467.

Barbaree, H. E., Hudson, S. M., and Seto, M. C. (1993). Sexual assault in society: The role of the juvenile offender. In H. E. Barbaree, W. L. Marshall and S. M. Hudson (eds), *The Juvenile Sex Offender*. London: Guilford Press.

Barbaree, H. E., Marshall, W. L., and Hudson, S. M. (eds) (1993). *The Juvenile Sex Offender*. London: Guilford Press.

Barbaree, H. E., Seto, M. C., Serin, R. C., Amos, N. L., and Preston, D. L. (1994). Comparisons between sexual and nonsexual rapist subtypes: Sexual arousal to rape, offense precursors, and offense characteristics. *Criminal Justice and Behavior, 21*, 95–114.

Bard, L. A., Carter, D. L., Cerce, D. D., Knight, R. A., Rosenberg, R., and Schneider, B.

(1987). A descriptive study of rapists and child molesters: Developmental, clinical and criminal characteristics. *Behavioural Sciences and the Law, 5*, 203–220.

Baxter, D. J., Barbaree, H. E., and Marshall, W. L. (1986). Sexual responses to consenting and forced sex in a large sample of rapists and non-rapists. *Behaviour Research and Therapy, 24*, 513–520.

Becker, J. V. (1988a). Adolescent sex offenders. *Behaviour Therapist, 11*, 185–187.

Becker, J. V. (1988b). The effects of child sexual abuse on adolescent sexual offenders. In G. E. Wyatt and E. J. Powell (eds), *Lasting Effects of Sexual Abuse*. Beverly Hills, CA: Sage.

Becker, J. V., and Abel, G. G. (1985). Methodological and ethical issues in evaluating and treating adolescent sexual offenders. In E. M. Otey and G. D. Ryan (eds), *Adolescent Sex Offenders: Issues in Research and Treatment*. Rockville, MD: US Department of Health and Human Services.

Becker, J., and Stein, R. M. (1991). Is sexual erotica associated with sexual deviance in adolescent males? *International Journal of Law and Psychiatry, 14*, 85–95.

Becker, J. V., Cunningham-Rathner, J., and Kaplan, M. S. (1986). Adolescent sexual offenders: Demographics, criminal and sexual histories, and recommendations for reducing future offenses. *Journal of Interpersonal Violence, 1*, 431–445.

Becker, J. V., Hunter, J. A., Goodwin, D. W., Kaplan, M. S., and Martinez, D. (1992). Test–retest reliability of audio-taped phallometric stimuli with adolescent sexual offenders. *Annals of Sex Research, 5*, 45–51.

Becker, J. V., Kaplan, M. S., Cunningham-Rathner, J., and Kavoussi, R. (1986). Characteristics of adolescent incest sexual perpetrators: Preliminary findings. *Journal of Family Violence, 1*, 85–97.

Becker, J. V., Kaplan, M. S., and Tenke, C. E. (1992). The relationship of abuse history, denial and erectile response profiles of adolescent sexual perpetrators. *Behaviour Therapy, 23*, 87–97.

Becker, J. V., Stein, R. M., Kaplan, M. S., and Cunningham-Rathner, J. (1992). Erection response characteristics of adolescent sex offenders. *Annals of Sex Research, 5*, 81–86.

Becker, J. V., Hunter, J., Stein, R., and Kaplan, M. (1989). Factors associated with erection in adolescent sex offenders. *Journal of Psychopathology and Behavioural Assessment, 11*, 353–362.

Becker, J. V., Kaplan, M. S., Tenke, C. E., and Tartaglini, A. (1991). The incidence of depressive symptomatology in juvenile sex offenders with a history of abuse. *Child Abuse and Neglect, 15*, 531–536.

Beckett, R., Fisher, D. (1994) The victim empathy scale. *Unpublished Adult sexual Offender Assessment Park*. Oxford Forensic Psychology Service.

Beech, A. R., Fisher, D., Beckett, R. C. (1998). *STEP 3: An Evaluation of the Prison Sex Offender Treatment Programme*. London: Home Office.

Beech, A., Fisher, D., Beckett, R. (1999). *STEP 3: An Evaluation of the Prison Sex Offender Treatment Programme*. London: Stationery Office.

Benoit, J. L., and Kennedy, W. A. (1992). The abuse history of male adolescent sex offenders. *Journal of Interpersonal Violence, 7*, 543–548.

Bentovim, A., Vizard, E., and Hollows, A. (1991). *Children and Young People as Abusers*. London: National Children's Bureau.

Bernstein, N. (1996). Behind some fraternity walls, brothers in crime. *New York Times*, 6 May, pp. A1, B8.

Billy, J. O., and Udry, J. (1985a). The influence of male and female best friends on adolescent sexual behaviour. *Adolescence, 20*, 21–32.

Billy, J. O., and Udry, J. (1985b). Patterns of adolescent friendship and effects on sexual behaviour. *Social Psychology Quarterly, 48*, 27–41.

Bladon, E. M. M. (2000). "Child and Adolescent Sexual Offenders: Nature of Offending, Diagnoses and Treatment Outcome". Unpublished Ph.D. thesis, Institute of Psychiatry, London.

Blasi, A. (1980). Bridging moral cognition and moral action: a critical review of the literature, *Psychological Bulletin, 88(1)*, 1–45.

Blaske, D. M., Borduin, C. M., Henggeler, S. W., and Mann, B. J. (1989). Individual, family, and peer characteristics of adolescent sex offenders and assaultive offenders. *Developmental Psychology, 25*, 846–855.

Blues, A., Moffat, C., and Telford, P. (1999). Work with adolescent females who sexually abuse. In M. Erooga and H. Masson (eds), *Children and Young People who Sexually Abuse Others*. London: Routledge.

Boone-Hamilton, B. (1991). *A Family Psychosocial Assessment Tool: Implications for Treatment of the Adolescent Sex Offender and the Family*. Paper presented at the 62nd annual meeting of the Eastern Psychological Association, New York.

Boswell, G. (1997). The backgrounds of violent young offenders: The present picture. In V. Varma (ed.), *Violence in Children and Adolescents*. London: Jessica Kingsley.

Breer, W. (1987). *The Adolescent Molester*. Springfield, IL: Charles. C. Thomas.

Brown, S. E. (1984). Social class, child maltreatment, and delinquent behaviour. *Criminology, 22*, 259–278.

Browne, K., Falshaw, L., and Hamilton, C. (1995). The characteristics of young persons resident at the Glenthorne Centre during the first half of 1995. *Youth Treatment Service Journal, 1*, 52–71.

Bukowski, W. M., Sippola, L., and Brender, W. (1993). Where does sexuality come from?: Normative sexuality from a developmental perspective. In H. E. Barbaree, W. L. Marshall and S. M. Hudson (eds), *The Juvenile Sex Offender*. London: Guilford Press.

Burgess, A. W., Hartman, C. R., and McCormack, A. (1987). Abused to abuser: Antecedents of socially deviant behaviors. *American Journal of Psychiatry, 144*, 1431–1436.

Calhoun, K. (1990). *Lies, Sex, and Videotapes: Studies in Sexual Aggression*. Presidential address, presented at the Southeastern Psychological Association, Atlanta, USA.

Calhoun, K. S., Bernat, J. A., Clum, G. A., and Frame, C. L. (1997). Sexual coercion and attraction to sexual aggression in a community sample of young men. *Journal of Interpersonal Violence, 12*, 392–406.

Carlson, B. (1987). Dating violence: A research review. *Social Casework, 68*, 16–23.

Carpenter, D. R., Peed, S. F., and Eastman, B. (1995). Personality characteristics of adolescent sex offenders: A pilot study. *Sexual Abuse, 7*, 195–203.

Chaffin, M. (1997). *Managing Teen Offenders: Unsupportive Families and Family Reunification*. Illinois: American Professional Society on the Abuse of Children APSAC.

Chewning, M. F. (1991). A Comparison of Adolescent Male Sex Offenders with Juvenile Delinquents and Non-referred Adolescents. Unpublished Ph.D. thesis, Virginia Commonwealth University. *Dissertation Abstracts International, 51*, (7-B) 3557.

Chodorow, N. (1978). *The Reproduction of Mothering*. Berkeley: University of California Press.

Cohen, M. L., and Boucher, R. J. (1972). Misunderstandings about sex criminals. *Sexual Behaviour, 5*, 56–62.

Coltrane, S. (1988). Father–child relationships and the status of women: A cross-cultural study. *American Journal of Sociology, 93*, 1060–1095.

Coltrane, S. (1992). The micropolitics of gender in non-industrial societies. *Gender and Society, 6*, 86–107.

Cooper, C. L., Murphy, W. D., and Haynes, M. R. (1996). Characteristics of abused and non-abused adolescent sexual offenders. *Sexual Abuse: A Journal of Research and Treatment, 8(2)*, 105–119.

Davidson, A. T. (1983). Sexual exploitation of children: A call to action. *Journal of the National Medical Association, 75*, 925–927.

Davis, M. H. (1980). A multi-dimensional approach to individual differences in empathy, *Catalogue of Selected Documents in Psychology, 10*, 85.

Davis, S. M., and Harris, M. B. (1982). Sexual knowledge, sexual interests, and sources of information of rural and urban adolescents from three cultures. *Adolescence, 17*, 471–492.

Davis, G. E., and Leitenberg, H. (1987). Adolescent sex offenders. *Psychological Bulletin, 101*, 417–427.

Deisher, R. W., Wenet, G. A., Paperny, D. M., Clark, T. F., and Fehrenbach, P. A. (1982). Adolescent sexual offence behaviour: The role of the physician. *Journal of Adolescent Health Care, 2*, 279–286.

DeNatale, R. A. (1989). 'An Investigation of Demographic, Emotional and Attitudinal Indicators of Male Juvenile Sex Offenders'. Unpublished thesis. *Dissertation Abstracts International, 50*, 1103.

Dolan, M., Holloway, J., Bailey, S., and Kroll, L. (1996). The psycho-social characteristics of juvenile sexual offenders referred to an adolescent forensic service in the UK. *Medicine, Science and the Law, 36*, 343–352.

Elliott, D. S., and Huizinga, D. (1984). *The Relationship between Delinquent Behavior and Alcohol, Drug Abuse, and Mental Health Problem Behaviors*. Research report 26. Boulder, CO: Behavioral Research Institute.

Elliott, D. S., and Morse, B. J. (1989). Delinquency and drug abuse as risk factors in teenage sexual activity. *Youth and Society, 21*, 32–60.

Elliott, D. S., Huizinga, D., and Ageton, S. S. (1985). *Explaining Delinquency and Drug Use*. Beverly Hills, CA: Sage.

Emerick, R. L., and Dutton, W. A. (1993). The effect of polygraphy on the self-report of adolescent sexual offenders: Implications for risk assessment. *Annals of Sex Research, 6*, 83–103.

Epps, K. J. (1991). The residential treatment of adolescent sex offenders. In M. McMurran and C. McDougall (eds), Proceedings of the first Division of Criminological and Legal Psychology annual conference. *Issues in Criminological and Legal Psychology, 17(1)*, 58–67.

Epps, K. J. (1997). Managing risk. In M. Hoghughi, S. Bhate and F. Graham (eds), *Sexually Abusive Behaviour in Adolescence*. London: Sage.

Epps, K. J. (2000). 'The Psychosocial Characteristics of Adolescent Boys who Sexually Offend: A Comparative Study'. Unpublished thesis, University of Birmingham, England.

Epps, K. J., Haworth, R., and Swaffer, T. (1993). Attitudes toward women and rape among male adolescents convicted of sexual versus nonsexual crimes. *Journal of Psychology, 127*, 501–506.

Fagan, J., and Wexler, S. (1988). Explanations of sexual assault among violent delinquents. *Journal of Adolescent Research, 3*, 363–385.

Faller, K. C. (1990). *Understanding Child Sexual Maltreatment*. Beverly Hills, CA: Sage.

Falshaw, L., and Browne, K. (1997). Adverse childhood experiences and violent acts of young people in secure accommodation. *Journal of Mental Health, 6*, 443–455.

Feather, N. T. (1985). Masculinity, femininity, self-esteem, and subclinical depression. *Sex Roles, 12*, 491–500.

Fehrenbach, P. A., and Monastersky, C. (1988). Characteristics of female sexual offenders. *American Journal of Orthopsychiatry, 58*, 148–151.

Fehrenbach, P. A., Smith, W., Monastersky, C., and Deisher, R. W. (1986). Adolescent sexual offenders: Offender and offence characteristics. *American Journal of Orthopsychiatry, 56*, 225–233.

Fernandez, Y. M., Marshall, W. L., Lightbody, S., and O'Sullivan, C. (1999). The child molester empathy measure: description and examination of its reliability and validity. *Sexual Abuse: A Journal of Research and Treatment, 11*, 17–31.

Figia, N. A., Lang, R. A., Plutchik, R., and Holden, R. (1987). Personality differences between sex and violent offenders. *International Journal of Offender Therapy and Comparative Criminology, 31*, 211–226.

Finkelhor, D. (1979). *Sexually Victimized Children*. New York: Free Press.

Finkelhor, D. (1984). Four preconditions: A model. In D. Finkelhor (ed.), *Child Sexual Abuse: New Theory and Research*. New York: Free Press.

Finkelhor, D. (1986). *A Sourcebook on Child Sex Abuse*. Newbury Park, CA: Sage.

Finkelhor, D. (1988). The trauma of child sexual abuse. In G. E. Wyatt and G. J. Powell (eds), *Lasting Effects of Child Sexual Abuse*. Beverly Hills, CA: Sage.

Finkelhor, D., and Browne, A. (1985). The traumatic impact of child abuse: A conceptualisation. *American Journal of Orthopsychiatry, 55*, 530–541.

Finkelhor, D., and Lewis, I. S. (1988). An epidemiological approach to the study of child molestation. In R. A. Prentky and V. Quinsey (eds), *Human Sexual Aggression: Current Perspectives*, Annals of the New York Academy of Science, 528. New York: New York Academy of Sciences.

Fisher, D. (1998). 'Assessing Victim Empathy'. Unpublished Ph.D. thesis. University of Birmingham, UK.

Fisher, D., Beech, A. R., and Browne, K. D. (1999). Comparison of sex offenders to non-sex offenders on selected psychological measures. *Journal of Offender Therapy and Comparative Criminology, 43(4)*, 473–492.

Ford, M. E., and Linney, J. A. (1995). Comparative analysis of juvenile sexual offenders, violent nonsexual offenders, and status offenders. *Journal of Interpersonal Violence, 10*, 56–70.

France, K., and Hudson, S. M. (1993). The conduct disorders and the juvenile sex offender. In H. E. Barbaree, W. L. Marshall and S. M. Hudson (eds) (1993). *The Juvenile Sex Offender*. London: Guilford Press.

Freedman, B. J., Rosenthal, L., Donahoe, C. P., Schlundt, D. G., and McFall, R. M. (1978). A social-behavioural analysis of skill deficits in delinquent and nondelinquent adolescent boys. *Journal of Consulting and Clinical Psychology, 46*, 1448–1462.

Friedrich, W. N., Beilke, R. L., and Urquiza, A. J. (1988). Behaviour problems in young sexually abused boys: A comparison study. *Journal of Interpersonal Violence, 3*, 21–28.

Fromuth, M. E., Burkhart, B. R., and Jones, C. W. (1991). Hidden child molestation: An investigation of adolescent perpetrators in a nonclinical sample. *Journal of Interpersonal Violence, 6*, 376–384.

Garbarino, J., and Platz, M. (1984). Child abuse and juvenile delinquency: What are the links? In E. Gray (ed.), *Child Abuse: Prelude to Delinquency?* Final Report. Chicago: National Committee for Prevention of Child Abuse.

Gilby, R., Wolf, L., and Goldberg, B. (1989). Mentally retarded adolescent sex offenders: A survey and pilot study. *Canadian Journal of Psychiatry, 34*, 542–548.

Gold, M. (1978). Scholastic experiences, self-esteem, and delinquent behaviour: A theory for alternative schools. *Crime and Delinquency, 24*, 290–308.

Gold, S. R., Fultz, J., Burke, C. H., Prisco, A. G., and Willett, J. A. (1992). Vicarious emotional responses of macho college males. *Journal of Interpersonal Violence, 7*, 165–174.

Goldstein, A. P., and Glick, B. (1987). *Aggression Replacement Training: A Comprehensive Intervention for Aggressive Youth*. Champaign, IL: Research Press.

Gomes-Schwartz, B. (1984). Juvenile sexual offenders. In US Department of Justice, *Sexually Exploited Children: Service and Research Project*. Washington, DC: US Department of Justice.

Goodchilds, J. D., Zellman, G. L., Johnson, P. B., and Giarusso, R. (1988). Adolescents and their perception of sexual interaction. In A. W. Burgess (ed.), *Rape and Sexual Assault*, vol. 2. New York: Garland.

Graves, R. E. (1993). "Conceptualizing the Youthful Male Sex Offender: A Meta-Analytic Examination of Offender Characteristics by Offense Type". Unpublished dissertation. Utah State University, Utah.

Gray, E. (1988). The link between child abuse and juvenile delinquency: What we know and recommendations for future policy and research. In G. Hotaling, D. Finkelhor, J. T. Kirkpatrick and M. A. Straus (eds), *Family Abuse and its Consequences*. Newbury Park, CA: Sage.

Griffiths, D., Hingsburger, D., and Christian, R. (1985). Treating developmentally handicapped sexual offenders: The York Behaviour Management Services treatment program. *Psychiatric Aspects of Mental Retardation Reviews, 4*, 49–54.

Groth, A. N. (1977). The adolescent sexual offender and his prey. *Journal of Offender Therapy and Comparative Criminology, 21*, 249–254.

Groth, A. N. (1979a). *Men Who Rape: The Psychology of the Offender*. New York: Plenum Press.

Groth, A. N. (1979b). Sexual trauma in the life histories of rapists and child molesters. *Victimology, 4*, 10–16.

Groth, A. N., and Burgess, A. W. (1977). Motivational intent in the sexual assault of children. *Criminal Justice and Behaviour, 4*, 253–271.

Groth, A. N., Burgess, A. W., and Holstrom, L. L. (1977). Rape: Power, anger and sexuality. *American Journal of Psychiatry, 134*, 1239–1243.

Groth, A. N., Hobson, W. F., and Gary, T. S. (1982). The child molester: Clinical observations. In J. Conte and D. A. Shore (eds), *Social Work and Child Sexual Abuse*. New York: Haworth.

Hagan, M. P., and Cho, M. E. (1996). A comparison of treatment outcomes between adolescent rapists and child sexual offenders. *International Journal of Offender Therapy and Comparative Criminology, 40*, 113–122.

Hagan, M. P., King, R. P., and Patros, R. L. (1994). Recidivism among adolescent perpetrators of sexual assault against children. *Journal of Offender Rehabilitation, 21*, 127–137.

Hagan, M. P., Gust-Brey, K. L., Cho, M. E., and Dow, E. (2001). Eight-year comparative analyses of adolescent rapists, adolescent child molesters, other adolescent delinquents, and the general population. *International Journal of Offender Therapy and Comparative Criminology, 45*, 314–324.

Hall, E. R., Howard, J. A., and Boezio, S. L. (1986). Tolerance of rape: A sexist or antisocial attitude? *Psychology of Women Quarterly, 10*, 101–108.

Hanson, R. K., and Bussiere, M. T. (1998). Predicting relapse: A meta-analysis of sexual offender recidivism studies. *Journal of Consulting and Clinical Psychology, 66*, 348–362.

Hanson, R. K., and Slater, S. (1988). Sexual victimization in the history of sexual abusers: A review. *Annals of Sex Research, 1*, 485–499.

Hartstone, E., and Hansen, K. V. (1984). The violent juvenile offender: An empirical portrait. In R. Mathis, P. DeMuro, and R. A. Allinson (eds), *Violent Juvenile Offenders: An Anthology*. San Francisco, CA: National Council on Crime and Delinquency.

Hawkes, C., Jenkins, J. A., and Vizard, E. (1997). Roots of sexual violence in children and adolescents. In V. P. Varma (ed.), *Violence in Children and Adolescents*. London: Jessica Kingsley.

Hawkins, J. D., Lishner, D., Jenson, J., and Catalano, R. F. (1987). Delinquents and drugs: What the evidence suggests about prevention and treatment planning. In B. Brown and R. Mills (eds), *Youth at High Risk for Substance Abuse*. Rockville, MD: US Department of Health and Human Services.

Hazelwood, R. R., and Warren, J. (1989). The serial rapist: His characteristics and victims (conclusion). *FBI Law Enforcement Bulletin, 58*, 18–25.

Henderson, J. E., English, D. J., and MacKenzie, W. R. (1988). Family centered casework practice with sexually aggressive children. *Treatment of Sex Offenders in Social Work and Mental Health Settings, 7*, 89–109.

Herbert, M. (1987). *Behavioural Treatment of Children with Problems*, 2nd edn. London: Academic Press.

Hersh, K., and Gray-Little, B. (1998). Psychopathic traits and attitudes associated with self-reported sexual aggression in college men. *Journal of Interpersonal Violence, 13*, 456–471.

Hodges, J., Lanyado, M., and Andreou, C. (1996). Sexuality and violence: Preliminary clinical hypotheses from psychotherapeutic assessments in a research programme on young sexual offenders. *Journal of Child Psychotherapy, 20*, 283–308.

Hodgins, D. C., and Lightfoot, L. O. (1988). Types of male alcohol and drug abusing incarcerated offenders. *British Journal of Addictions, 83*, 1201–1213.

Hollway, W. (1984). Women's power in heterosexual sex. *Women's Studies International Forum, 7*, 66–68.

Howells, K. (1979). Some meanings of children for paedophiles. In M. Cook and G. Wilson (eds), *Love and Attraction*. Oxford: Pergamon.

Hsu, L. K. G., and Starzynski, J. (1990). Adolescent rapists and adolescent child sexual assaulters. *International Journal of Offender Therapy and Comparative Criminology, 34*, 23–30.

Humphrey, J. A., and White, J. W. (1992). *Perpetration of Sexual Assault: Social Psychological Predictors*. Paper presented at the American Society of Criminology, New Orleans, LA, USA.

Hunter, J. A., and Becker, J. V. (1994). The relationship between phallometrically measured deviant sexual arousal and clinical characteristics in juvenile sexual offenders. *Behaviour Research and Therapy, 32*, 533–538.

Hunter, J. A., and Figueredo, J. (1999). Factors associated with treatment compliance in a population of juvenile sexual offenders. *Sexual Abuse: A Journal of Research and Treatment, 11*, 49–67.

Hunter, J. A., and Goodwin, D. W. (1992). The utility of satiation therapy in the treatment of juvenile sexual offenders: Variations and efficacy. *Annals of Sex Research, 5*, 71–80.

Jacobs, W. L., Kennedy, W. A., and Meyer, J. B. (1997). Juvenile delinquents: A between-group comparison study of sexual and non-sexual offenders. *Sexual Abuse: A Journal of Research and Treatment, 9(3)*, 201–217.

James, A. C., and Neil, P. (1996). Juvenile sexual offending: One-year period prevalence study within Oxfordshire. *Child Abuse and Neglect, 20*, 477–485.

Johnson, R. E. (1979). *Juvenile Delinquency and its Origins*. New York: Cambridge University Press.

Johnson, S. D., Gibson, L., and Linden, R. (1978). Alcohol and rape in Winnipeg, 1966–1975. *Journal of Studies on Alcohol, 39*, 1887–1894.

Johnson, T. C. (1988). Child perpetrators: Children who molest other children: Preliminary findings. *Child Abuse and Neglect, 12*, 219–229.

Kaemingk, K. L., Koselka, M., Becker, J. V., and Kaplan, M. S. (1995). Age and adolescent sexual offender arousal. *Sexual Abuse, 7*, 249–257.

Kahn, T. J., and Chambers, H. J. (1991). Assessing re-offence risk with juvenile sex offenders. *Child Welfare, 70(3)*, 333–345.

Kahn, T. J., and Lafond, M. A. (1988). Treatment of the adolescent sex offender. *Child and Adolescent Social Work, 5*, 138–148.

Kanin, E. J. (1985). Date rapists: Differential sexual socialization and relative deprivation. *Archives of Sexual Behaviour, 14*, 219–231.

Kaplan, H. B. (1980). *Deviant Behavior in Defense of Self*. New York: Academic Press.

Kaplan, P., and Arbuthnot, J. (1985). Affective empathy and cognitive role-taking in delinquent and non-delinquent youth. *Adolescence, 20*, 323–333.

Kaplan, M. S., Becker, J. V., and Martinez, D. F. (1990). A comparison of mothers of adolescent incest vs non-incest perpetrators. *Journal of Family Violence, 5*, 209–214.

Katchadourian, H. (1990). Sexuality. In S. S. Feldman and G. R. Elliot (eds), *At the Threshold: The Developing Adolescent*. Cambridge, MA: Harvard University Press.

Katz, R. C. (1990). Psychosocial adjustment in adolescent child molesters. *Child Abuse and Neglect, 14*, 567–575.

Kaufman, K. L., Holmberg, J. K., Orts, K. A., McCrady, F. E., Rotzien, A. L., Daleiden, E. L., and Hilliker, D. R. (1998). Factors influencing sexual offenders modus operandi: An examination of victim–offender relatedness and age. *Child Maltreatment, 3*, 349–361.

Kavoussi, R. J., Kaplan, M., and Becker, J. V. (1988). Psychiatric diagnosis in adolescent sex offenders. *Journal of the Academy of Child and Adolescent Psychiatry, 27*, 241–243.

Kelly, L., Regan, L., and Burton, S. (1991). *An Exploratory Study of the Prevalence of Sexual Abuse in a Sample of 16–21 Year Olds*. London: Child Abuse Studies Unit, North London Polytechnic.

Kempton, T., and Forehand, R. (1992). Juvenile sex offenders: Similar to, or different from, other incarcerated delinquent offenders? *Behaviour Research and Therapy, 30*, 533–536.

Kennedy, R. E. (1984). Cognitive behavioral interventions with delinquents. In A. W. Meyers and W. E. Craighead (eds), *Cognitive Behavior Therapy with Children*. New York: Plenum Press.

Klein, M., and Gordon, S. (1992). Sex Education in C. E. Walker and M. C. Roberts (eds), *Handbook of Clinical Child Psychology* (2nd ed) Oxford: John Wiley and Sons.

Knight, R. A. (1988). A taxonomic analysis of child molesters. In R. A. Prentky and V. Quinsey (eds), *Human Sexual Aggression: Current Perspectives*. New York: New York Academy of Sciences.

Knight, R. A. (1992). The generation and corroboration of a taxonomic model for child molesters. In W. O'Donohue and J. H. Greer (eds), *The Sexual Abuse of Children: Theory, Research and Therapy*. Hillsdale, NJ: Erlbaum.

Knight, R. A., and Prentky, R. A. (1987). The developmental antecedents and adult adaptations of rapist subtypes. *Criminal Justice and Behaviour, 14*, 403–426.

Knight, R. A., and Prentky, R. A. (1990). Classifying sexual offenders: The development and corroboration of taxonomic models. In W. L. Marshall, D. R. Laws and H. E. Barbaree (eds), *Handbook of Sexual Assault: Issues, Theories, and Treatment of the Offender*. New York: Plenum Press.

Knight, R. A., and Prentky, R. A. (1993). Exploring characteristics for classifying juvenile sex offenders. In H. E. Barbaree, W. L. Marshall and S. M. Hudson (eds) (1993). *The Juvenile Sex Offender*. London: Guilford Press.

Knopp, F. H., and Lackey, L. D. (1987). *Female Sexual Abusers: A Summary of data from 44 Treatment Providers*. New York: Safer Society Press.

Knopp, F. H., Freeman-Longo, R., and Stevenson, W. F. (1992). *Nationwide Survey of Juvenile and Adult Sex Offender Treatment Programs and Models*. Orwell, VT: Safer Society Press.

Koss, M. P. (1988). Hidden rape: Sexual aggression and victimization in a national sample in higher education. In A. W. Burgess (ed.), *Rape and Sexual Assault*, vol. 2. New York: Garland.

Koss, M. P. (1992). Rape on campus: Facts and measures. *Planning for Higher Education, 20*, 21–28.

Koss, M. P., and Dinero, T. E. (1988). Predictors of sexual aggression among a national sample of male college students. In R. A. Prentky and V. L. Quinsey (eds), *Human Sexual Aggression: Current Perspectives*. New York: New York Academy of Sciences.

Kraft, P. (1993). Sexual knowledge among Norwegian adolescents. *Adolescence, 16*, 3–21.

Lalumiere, M. L., and Quinsey, V. L. (1994). The discriminability of rapists from non-sex offenders using phallometric measures: A meta-analysis. *Criminal Justice and Behaviour, 21*, 150–175.

Lanyado, M., Hodges, J., Bentovim, A., Andreou, C., and Williams, B. (1995). Understanding boys who sexually abuse other children: A clinical illustration. *Psychoanalytic Psychotherapy, 9*, 231–242.

Laws, D. R., and Marshall, W. L. (1990). A conditioning theory of the etiology and maintenance of deviant sexual preference and behavior. In W. L. Marshall, D. R. Laws, and H. E. Barbaree (eds), *Handbook of Sexual Assault: Issues, Theories, and Treatment of the Offender*. New York: Plenum Press.

Levine, E., and Kanin, E. (1987). Sexual violence among dates: Trends and implications. *Journal of Family Violence, 2*, 55–65.

Lewis, D. O., Shankok, S. S., Pincus, J. H., and Glaser, G. H. (1979). Violent juvenile delinquents: Psychiatric, neurological, psychological, and abuse factors. *Journal of the American Academy of Child Psychiatry, 18*, 307–319.

Lewis, D. O., Shankok, S. S., and Pincus, J. H. (1981). Juvenile male sexual assaulters. In D. Lewis (ed.), *Vulnerabilities to Delinquency*. Jamaica, NY: Spectrum.

Lightfoot, L. O., and Barbaree, H. E. (1993). The relationship between substance use and abuse and sexual offending in adolescents. In H. E. Barbaree, W. L. Marshall and S. M. Hudson (eds), *The Juvenile Sex Offender*. London: Guilford Press.

Lightfoot, L. O., and Hodgins, D. (1988). A survey of alcohol and drug problems in incarcerated Canadian offenders. *International Journal of the Addictions, 23*, 687–706.

Lisak, D. (1991). Sexual aggression, masculinity and fathers: Signs. *Journal of Women in Culture and Society, 16*, 238–262.

Lisak, D. (1994). Subjective assessment of relationships with parents by sexually aggressive and nonaggressive men. *Journal of Interpersonal Violence, 9*, 399–411.

Lisak, D., and Ivan, C. (1995). Deficits in intimacy and empathy in sexually aggressive men. *Journal of Interpersonal Violence, 10*, 296–308.

Lisak, D., and Roth, S. (1988). Motivational factors in non-incarcerated sexually aggressive men. *Journal of Personality and Social Psychology, 55*, 795–802.

Lisak, D., and Roth, S. (1990). Motives and psychodynamics of self-reported, unincarcerated rapists. *American Journal of Orthopsychiatry, 60*, 268–280.

Lisak, D., Hopper, J., and Song, P. (1995). Factors in the cycle of violence: Gender rigidity and emotional constriction. Cited in D. Lisak and C. Ivan (1995), Deficits in intimacy and empathy in sexually aggressive men. *Journal of Interpersonal Violence, 10*, 296–308.

Loeber, R. (1982). The stability of antisocial and delinquent child behaviour: A review. *Child Development, 53*, 1431–1446.

Lonczynski, C. M. (1991). Adolescent sexual offenders: Social isolation, social competency skills and identified problem behaviours. *Dissertation Abstracts International, 51*, 5040.

Longo, R. E. (1982). Sexual learning and experience among adolescent sexual offenders. *International Journal of Offender Therapy and Comparative Criminology, 26*, 235–241.

Lott, B., Reilly, M. E., and Howard, D. R. (1982). Sexual assault and harassment: A campus community case study. *Signs, 8*, 296–319.

Malamuth, N. M. (1986). Predictors of naturalistic sexual aggression. *Journal of Personality and Social Psychology, 50*, 953–962.

Malamuth, N. M. (1993). Pornography's impact on male adolescents. *Adolescent Medicine, 4*, 563–576.

Malamuth, N. M., Sockloskie, R. J., Koss, M. P., and Tonaka, J. S. (1991). Characteristics of aggressors against women: Testing a model using a national sample of college students. *Journal of Consulting and Clinical Psychology, 59*, 670–681.

Manocha, K. F., and Mezey, G. (1998). British adolescents who sexually abuse: A descriptive study. *Journal of Forensic Psychiatry, 9(3)*, 588–608.

Marshall, W. L. (1989). Intimacy, loneliness and sexual offenders. *Behaviour Research and Therapy, 27*, 491–503.

Marshall, W. L., and Mazzucco, A. (1995). Self-esteem and parental attachments in child molesters. *Sexual Abuse: A Journal of Research and Treatment, 7(4)*, 279–285.

Marshall, W. L., Christie, M. M., and Lanthier, R. D. (1979). Social competence, sexual experience and attitudes to sex in incarcerated rapists and paedophiles. Report to Solicitor General of Canada. In W. L. Marshall, D. R. Laws and H. E. Barbaree (eds), *Handbook of Sexual Assault: Issues, Theories and Treatment of the Offender*. London: Plenum Press.

Marshall, W. L., Seidman, B., and Check, J. V. (1991). Intimacy and loneliness in sex offenders. Unpublished data. Cited in W. L. Marshall, S. M. Hudson and S. Hodkinson (1993), The importance of attachment bonds in the development of juvenile sexual offending. In H. E. Barbaree, W. L. Marshall and S. M. Hudson (eds), *The Juvenile Sex Offender*. London: Guilford Press.

Marshall, W. L., Hudson, S. M., and Hodkinson, S. (1993). The importance of attachment bonds in the development of juvenile sexual offending. In H. E. Barbaree, W. L. Marshall and S. M. Hudson (eds), *The Juvenile Sex Offender*. London: Guilford Press.

Marshall, W. L., Anderson, D., and Champagne, F. (1996). Self-esteem and its relationship to sexual offending. *Psychology, Crime and Law, 3*, 81–106.

Marshall, W. L., Anderson, D., and Fernandez, Y. (1999). *Cognitive Behavioural Treatment of Sexual Offenders*. Chichester: Wiley.

Mathews, R., Hunter, J. A., and Vuz, J. (1997). Juvenile female sexual offenders: Clinical characteristics and treatment issues. *Sexual Abuse: A Journal of Research and Treatment, 9*, 187–199.

McCabe, M. P. (1989). The contribution of sexual attitudes and experiences during childhood and adolescence to adult sexual dysfunction. *Sexual and Marital Therapy, 4*, 133–141.

McCormack, A., Rokous, F. E., Hazelwood, R. R., and Burgess, A. W. (1992). An exploration of incest in the childhood development of serial rapists. *Journal of Family Violence, 7*, 219–228.

McDermott, M. J. (1979). *Rape Victimization in 26 American Cities*, Report No. SD-VAD-6. Washington, DC: National Criminal Justice Information and Statistics Service.

McManus, M., Alessi, N. E., Grapentime, W. L., and Brickman, A. (1984). Psychiatric disturbance in serious delinquents. *Journal of the American Academy of Child and Adolescent Psychiatry, 23*, 602–615.

Metzner, J. L. (1987). The adolescent sex offender: An overview. *The Colorado Lawyer*, October, 1847–1851.

Mio, J. S., Nanjundappa, G., Verleur, D. E., and de-Rios, M. D. (1986). Drug abuse and the adolescent sex offender: A preliminary analysis. *Journal of Psychoactive Drugs, 18*, 65–72.

Moffitt, T. E. (1993). Adolescence-limited and life course-persistent antisocial behaviour: A developmental taxonomy. *Psychological Review, 100*, 674–701.

Monck, E., and New, M. (1996). *Report of a Study of Sexually Abused Children and Adolescents and of Young Perpetrators of Sexual Abuse who were Treated in Voluntary Agency Community Facilities*. London: HMSO.

Moody, E. E., Brissie, J., and Kim, J. (1994). Personality and background characteristics of adolescent sexual offenders. *Journal of Addictions and Offender Counselling, 14*, 38–48.

Moore, S., and Rosenthal, D. (1993). *Sexuality in Adolescence*. London: Routledge.

Mosher, D. L., and Anderson, R. D. (1986). Macho personality, sexual aggression, and reactions to guided imagery of realistic rape. *Journal of Research in Personality, 20*, 77–94.

Mosher, D. L., and Sirkin, M. (1984). Measuring a macho personality constellation. *Journal of Research in Personality, 18*, 150–163.

Muster, N. J. (1992). Treating the adolescent victim-turned-offender. *Adolescence, 27*, 441–450.

O'Brien, M. J. (1991). Taking sibling incest seriously. In M. Q. Patten (ed.), *Family Sexual Abuse: Frontline Research and Evaluation*. Newbury Park, CA: Sage.

O'Callaghan, D., and Print, B. (1994). Adolescent sexual abusers: Research, assessment and treatment. In T. Morrison, M. Erooga and R. C. Beckett (eds), *Sexual Offending against Children: Assessment and Treatment of Male Abusers*. London: Routledge.

Oliver, L. I., Hall, G. C. N., and Neuhaus, S. M. (1993). A comparison of the personality and background characteristics of adolescent sex offenders and other adolescent offenders. *Criminal Justice and Behaviour, 20*, 359–370.

O' Reilly, G., Sheridan, A., Carr, A., Cherry, J., Donohoe, E., McGrath, K., Phelan, S., Tallon, M., and O'Reilly, K. (1998). A descriptive study of adolescent sexual offenders in an Irish community-based treatment programme. *Irish Journal of Psychology, 19*, 152–167.

Overholser, J. C., and Beck, S. (1986). Multimethod assessment of rapists and child molesters and three control groups on behavioural and psychological measures. *Journal of Consulting and Clinical Psychology, 54*, 682–687.

Palmer, C. T. (1988). Twelve reasons why rape is not sexually motivated: A sceptical examination. *Journal of Sex Research, 25*, 512–530.

Panton, J. H. (1978). Personality differences appearing between rapists of adults, rapists of children and nonviolent sexual molesters of female children. *Research Communications in Psychology, Psychiatry and Behaviour, 3*, 385–393.

Peters, S. D., Wyatt, G. E., and Finkelhor, D. (1986). Prevalence. In D. Finkelhor (ed.), *A Source-Book on Child Sexual Abuse*. Beverly Hills, CA: Sage.

Pierce, L. H., and Pierce, R. L. (1987). Incestuous victimization by juvenile sex offenders. *Journal of Family Violence, 2*, 351–364.

Porter, E. (1986). *Treating the Young Male Victim of Sexual Assault: Issues and Intervention Strategies*. Oregon, USA: Safer Society Press.

Prentky, R. A., and Knight, R. A. (1991). Dimensional and categorical discrimination among rapists. *Journal of Consulting and Clinical Psychology, 59*, 643–661.

Puri, B. K., Lambert, M. L., and Cordess, C. C. (1996). Characteristics of young offenders detained under Section 53(2) at a Young Offenders' Institution. *Medicine, Science and the Law, 36(1)*, 69–76.

Quay, H. C. (1987). Intelligence. In H. C. Quay (ed.), *Handbook of Juvenile Delinquency*. New York: John Wiley.

Quinsey, V. L., Chaplin, T. C., and Upfold, D. (1984). Sexual arousal to non-sexual violence and sadomasochistic themes among rapists and non-sex offenders. *Journal of Consulting and Clinical Psychology, 52*, 651–657.

Quinsey, V. L., Rice, M. E., Harris, G. T., and Reid, K. S. (1993). The phylogenetic and ontogenetic development of sexual age preferences in males: Conceptual and measurement issues. In H. E. Barbaree, W. L. Marshall and S. M. Hudson (eds), *The Juvenile Sex Offender*. London: Guilford Press.

Rada, R. T. (1975). Alcohol and rape. *Medical Aspects of Human Sexuality, 9*, 48–65.

Rapaport, K., and Burkhart, B. R. (1984). Personality and attitudinal characteristics of sexually coercive college males. *Journal of Abnormal Psychology, 93*, 216–221.

Rapaport, K., and Burkhart, B. R. (1987). *Male Aggression Symposium: Responsiveness to Rape Depictions*. Paper presented at the Society for the Scientific Study of Sex, Atlanta, USA.

Reppucci, N. D., and Clingempeel, W. G. (1978). Methodological issues in research with correctional populations. *Journal of Consulting and Clinical Psychology, 46*, 727–746.

Rich, J. (1956). Types of stealing. *Lancet*, 496.

Richardson, G., Graham, F., Bhate, S. R., and Kelly, T. P. (1995). A British sample of sexually abusive adolescents: Abuser and abuse characteristics. *Criminal Behaviour and Mental Health, 5*, 187–208.

Richardson, G., Kelly, T. P., Bhate, S. R., and Graham, F. (1995). Group differences in abuser and abuse characteristics in a British sample of sexually abusive adolescents. *Sexual Abuse: A Journal of Research and Treatment, 9*, 239–257.

Robertson, J. M. (1990). Group counselling and the high risk offender. *Federal Probation, 54*, 48–51.

Rogers, C. M., and Terry, T. (1984). Clinical intervention with boy victims of sexual abuse. In I. R. Stuart and J. G. Greer (eds), *Victims of Sexual Aggression: Men, Women and Children*. New York: Nostrand Reinhold.

Rutter, M., and Giller, H. (1983). *Juvenile Delinquency: Trends and Perspectives*. Harmondsworth: Penguin.

Ryan, G., Lane, S., Davis, J., and Isaac, C. (1987). Juvenile sex offenders: Development and correction. *Child Abuse and Neglect, 11*, 385–395.

Ryan, G., Miyoshi, T. J., Metner, J. L., Krugman, R. D., and Fryer, G. E. (1996). Trends in a national sample of sexually abusive youth. *Journal of the American Academy of Child and Adolescent Psychiatry, 33*, 17–25.

Salter, A. C. (1988). *Treating Child Sex Offenders and Victims: A Practical Guide*. Newbury Park, CA: Sage.

Sanday, P. R. (1979). *The Socio-Cultural Context of Rape*. Washington, DC: US Department of Commerce, National Technical Information Services.

Sanday, P. R. (1990). *Fraternity Gang Rape*. New York: New York University Press.

Sauceda, J. M. (1978). Juvenile sexual assaulters: A comparative study. Unpublished manuscript. Cited in G. A. Awad, E. B. Saunders and J. A. Levene (1984). A clinical study of male adolescent sexual offenders. *International Journal of Offender Therapy and Comparative Criminology, 28*, 105–116.

Saunders, E. B., and Awad, G. A. (1988). Assessment, management and treatment planning for male adolescent sexual offenders. *American Journal of Orthopsychiatry, 58*, 571–579.

Saunders, E. B., Awad, G. A., and White, G. (1986). Male adolescent sexual offenders: The offender and the offence. *Canadian Journal of Psychiatry, 31*, 542–549.

Schram, B. D., Milloy, C. D., and Rowe, W. E. (1991). *Juvenile Sex Offenders: A Follow-Up Study of Re-Offence Behavior*. Washington State Institute for Public Policy.

Schwartz, M. D., and DeKeseredy, W. S. (1997). *Sexual Assault on the College Campus: The Role of Male Peer Support*. London: Sage.

Scott, R. L., and Tetreault, L. A. (1986). Attitudes of rapists and other violent offenders towards women. *The Journal of Social Psychology, 127*, 375–380.

Sefarbi, R. (1990). Admitters and deniers among adolescent sex offenders and their families: A preliminary study. *American Journal of Orthopsychiatry, 60*, 460–465.

Segal, Z. V., and Marshall, W. L. (1985). Heterosexual social skills in a population of rapists and child molesters. *Journal of Consulting and Clinical Psychology, 53*, 55–63.

Segal, Z. V., and Stermac, L. (1984). A measure of rapists' attitudes towards women. *International Journal of Law and Psychiatry, 7*, 437–440.

Shoor, M., Speed, M. H., and Bartelt, C. (1966). Syndrome of the adolescent child molester. *American Journal of Psychiatry, 122*, 783–789.

Smith, W. R. (1988). Delinquency and abuse among juvenile sexual offenders. *Journal of Interpersonal Violence, 3*, 400–413.

Spence, J., Helmreich, R. L., and Stapp, J. (1973). A short version of the Attitudes Toward Women Scale (AWS). *Bulletin of the Psychonomic Society, 2*, 219–220.

Stermac, L. E., and Quinsey, V. L. (1986). Social competence among rapists. *Behavioural Assessment, 8*, 171–185.

Tarter, R. E., Hegedus, A. M., Alterman, A. I., and Katz-Garris, L. (1983). Cognitive capacities of juvenile, violent, nonviolent, and sexual offenders. *Journal of Nervous and Mental Disease, 171*, 564–567.

Thornburg, H. D. (1981). The amount of sex information learning obtained during early adolescence. *Journal of Early Adolescence, 1*, 171–183.

Tieger, T. (1981). Self-rated likelihood of raping and the social perception of rape. *Journal of Research in Personality, 15*, 147–158.

Tingle, D., Barnard, G. W., Robbins, L., Newman, G., and Hutchinson, D. (1986). Childhood and adolescent characteristics of pedophiles and rapists. *International Journal of Law and Psychiatry, 9*, 103–116.

Tinklenberg, J. R., and Woodrow, K. M. (1974). Drug use among youthful assaultive and sexual offenders. *Aggression, 52*, 209–224.

Truscott, D. (1993). Adolescent offenders: Comparison for sexual, violent, and property offences. *Psychological Reports, 73*, 657–658.

Van Ness, S. R. (1984). Rape as instrumental violence: A study of youth offenders. *Journal of Offender Counselling, Services, and Rehabilitation, 9*, 161–170.

Vinogradov, S., Dishotsky, N. I., Doty, A. K., and Tinklenberg, J. R. (1988). Patterns of behavior in adolescent rape. *American Journal of Orthopsychiatry, 58*, 179–187.

Warshaw, R. (1988). *I Never Called It Rape*. New York: Harper & Row.

Wasserman, J., and Kappel, S. (1985). *Adolescent Sex Offenders in Vermont*. Burlington: Vermont Department of Health.

Watkins, B., and Bentovim, A. (1992). The sexual abuse of male children and adolescents: A review of current research. *Journal of Child Psychology and Psychiatry, 33*, 197–248.

Weinrott, M. R. (1996). *Juvenile Sexual Aggression: A Critical Review*. Colorado: Institute of Behavioral Science.

Weinrott, M. R., Riggan, M., and Frothingham, S. (1997). Reducing deviant arousal in juvenile sex offenders using vicarious sensitization. *Journal of Interpersonal Violence, 12*, 704–728.

West, D. J., and Farrington, D. P. (1977). *The Delinquent Way of Life*. London: Heinemann.

White, J. W., and Humphrey, J. A. (1990). *A Theoretical Model of Sexual Assault: An Empirical Test*. Paper presented at symposium on sexual assault: Research, treatment and education, Southeastern Psychological Association meeting, Atlanta, GA, USA.

White, J. W., and Koss, M. P. (1993). Adolescent sexual aggression within heterosexual relationships: Prevalence, characteristics and causes. In H. E. Barbaree, W. L. Marshall and S. M. Hudson (eds), *The Juvenile Sex Offender*. London: Guilford Press.

Whiting, B. (1965). Sex identity conflict and physical violence: A comparative study. *American Anthropologist, 67*, 123–140.

Widom, C. S. (1989). Does violence beget violence? A critical examination of the literature. *Psychological Bulletin, 106*, 3–28.

Widom, C. S., and Ames, M. A. (1994). Criminal consequences of childhood sexual victimization. *Child Abuse and Neglect, 18*, 303–318.

Will, D. (1994). A treatment service for adolescent sexual offenders. *Psychiatric Bulletin, 18*, 742–744.

Wolfe, J., and Baker, V. (1980). Characteristics of imprisoned rapists and circumstances of the rape. In C. Warner (ed.), *Rape and Sexual Assault: Management and Intervention*. London: Aspen.

Woods, J. (1997). Breaking the cycle of abuse and abusing: Individual psychotherapy for juvenile sex offenders. *Clinical Child Psychology and Psychiatry, 2*, 379–392.

Worling, J. R. (1995a). Adolescent sibling-incest offenders: Differences in family and individual functioning when compared to adolescent nonsibling sex offenders. *Child Abuse and Neglect, 19*, 633–643.

Worling, J. R. (1995b). Sexual abuse histories of adolescent male sex offenders: Differences on the basis of the age and gender of their victims. *Journal of Abnormal Psychology, 104*, 610–613.

Worling, J. R. (1995c). Adolescent sex offenders against females: Differences based on the age of their victims. *International Journal of Offender Therapy and Comparative Criminology, 39*, 276–293.

Zgourides, G., Monto, M., and Harris, R. (1997). Correlates of adolescent male sexual offence: Prior adult sexual contact, sexual attitudes and use of sexually explicit materials. *International Journal of Offender Therapy and Comparative Criminology, 41*, 272–283.

Chapter 4

# Families of young people who sexually abuse

## Characteristics, context and considerations

*Yvonne Duane and Tony Morrison*

*Sam (details changed to protect client) was thirteen years old when he was referred to a specialist programme in the North-West of England for young people who had sexual behaviour problems. Sam admitted that he had sexually abused his two sisters and several young cousins over a period of two years. In total it was estimated that Sam had committed some thirty assaults. After a lengthy interview with Sam, his mother was seen. Barely had the discussion started before Sam's mother explained how she had first discovered Sam's sexual behaviour problem three years earlier. She had returned from shopping to discover Sam playing a clearly sexual "doctors and patient" game with his younger sister. She immediately phoned the local social services department and a social worker visited and reassured her that Sam's behaviour was experimental and that she should not worry.*

*Two years on and thirty assaults later, Sam's mother recounted with distress and bitterness how her family had been devastated by her son's behaviour, how she was being blamed by her sister for allowing Sam to play with his young cousins and how she had decided to have Sam admitted to care. As the workers sought in vain to stress the importance of her contribution to Sam's treatment work, Sam's mother angrily rejected all such efforts stating, "You told me not to worry, that it would all be alright and now he has ruined my family." In the eighteen months that followed Sam languished in a children's home, had few contacts with his family, and made minimal progress on his sexual problems, and his mother refused to engage with the programme. On his last day in the programme to the consternation of both staff and the other group members, Sam left with the parting remark that he knew that he would never pose any risks now that his brain had been sorted out.*

As a testament to the failure of services this is a salutary tale on many levels: the lack of basic training for frontline staff, the absence of information and counselling services for parents and the failure to appreciate the crisis that is generated within families when they discover a child who has sexual behaviour problems. The combination of delay, escalation of problems, removal from home, and the inability to engage the parents, probably meant that the treatment outcome for Sam, even in a long-term group programme, was largely undermined before the very first group session.

The purpose of this chapter is fourfold: firstly to discuss the critical importance of working with the families of these young people; secondly to describe, at least from an Irish/UK perspective, the current state of the art and the challenges facing staff seeking to develop service to families graphically illustrated in the case example of Sam; thirdly to present the available research on the characteristics of such families; and fourthly to identify some considerations at the start of any work with families. Our interests arise from both research and practice perspectives. This is reflected in the structure of the chapter, which locates the literature review on the characteristics of these families within a wider discussion of the realities and challenges posed in offering services to these families. It is with these practice realities that we start.

## Challenges in working with families

Before addressing the specific issues posed by family work, it may be helpful at the outset to remind ourselves that working with young people who sexually abuse others is still a very young field. There are huge gaps in research, almost no controlled treatment outcome studies and as we shall see later only a very sparse literature on the families of these young people. Indeed the number of extant specific books on this topic can be counted on the fingers of two hands. Moreover, given that the dominant practice model for work with juveniles has been handed down from models formulated for adult sex offenders, it is not surprising that family work has been so little discussed in the literature, with the exception of the chapter by Thomas (1991). Indeed it may be that one of the defining differences between the adult and adolescent fields is the fact that adolescents are still in a formative stage of development, in which parents/carers can still exercise a major influence in re-engaging the majority of children back to a normative developmental pathway. This stands in contrast to work with adults which is much more focused on self-control and long-term risk and relapse management strategies based on a view that their risk is over a lifetime not within a developmental stage (Ryan, 1999).

The reality in the UK is that family work is still largely under-recognized, under-funded, under-researched and unpublished. In other words we have not arrived at the point where family work is accepted as a core part of any service to young people who commit sexual offences. Its status is that of an optional extra which depends on the commitment, orientation and resources of individual practitioners. For those who are engaged in such work, it is largely a lone journey through uncharted waters, without compass, maps or preparation, seeking by trial and error to avoid being sucked under by the sheer size and complexity of the task, or simply to lose direction and run aground in the fog of organizational paralysis and inter-agency confusion.

In a recent conference workshop some forty practitioners gathered to identify the issues in relation to family work. Although there was unanimous agreement on its importance, the hurdles were numerous.

### *Lack of a clear mandate from agencies*

Although a growing awareness of the risk posed by young people who commit sexual assaults has resulted in an increase of offence-specific programmes in the UK, these almost all target the young person. Funding rarely includes provision for work with families, and therefore such work gets squeezed in between other priorities. In addition, there is a more widespread lack of clarity across agencies as to roles and responsibilities in this field, particularly as between criminal justice, child protection and health systems, each of which may view the nature, causes and interventions for these young people somewhat differently. For instance services provided by child mental health and some child protection professionals are more likely to emphasize family factors in their interventions than are youth justice staff who are more likely to emphasize offence-specific and personal competency interventions. Thus different agencies may define needs, causes and treatment targets very differently. They also bring different skills and training around working with families and young people.

### *Lack of practice models and training*

Again and again practitioners working with these families have reported a sense of isolation and the absence of research, or even simple descriptions of clinical work with families. This results in considerable caution and even anxiety as to whether "we are doing it right". The absence of specific family practice models means that practitioners have to try to adapt models of family work that have been applied to other adolescent and family problems, to the problem of sexually abusive behaviour. This in turn can result in skilled practitioners who have considerable experience with other very troubled youth feeling initially very de-skilled. Practitioners need training if they are to be helped to integrate prior family work skills and knowledge from other areas into this field and to date there has been minimal training to address family work.

### *Failure to respond to family crises*

As Thomas (1991) observes, "families frequently react with shock, disbelief and confusion followed by intense feelings of shame, anger guilt and depression. . . . This is exacerbated when the victim and the abuser are living within the same family" (p. 337). The capacity of agencies and workers involved with the family to firstly recognize, and secondly respond quickly to this crisis, is in our view crucial to the engagement of parents and the subsequent management of the case. A failure to engage parents at the outset can, as the opening case example illustrates, fatally undermine subsequent treatment efforts. Too often parents are left out in the cold, or are only addressed by agencies in terms of whether they are willing to act protectively in relation to the victim without any consideration of their own feelings and distress. Many parents report having identified sexual problems in their child's behaviour early on only to have it minimized, reframed or ignored until the behaviour became so serious that agencies felt compelled to act. Parents recount even then how often they are left in the waiting room whilst specialists assess their children and pay minimal attention to the parents' feelings or their need for information.

### *Definition, complexity and size of the task*

As our review of the characteristics of these families will illustrate, these are often troubled and troubling families with multiple and sometimes conflicting needs amongst their members. It is not surprising therefore that the range of demands, tasks and priorities for workers is great. Thomas (1991) states that the worker may act as "crisis manager, systems organiser, teacher, guide, advocate, resource person, as well as a supportive and confronting therapist" (p. 334). The multiple roles of the worker can be both stressful and unpredictable. Addressing these different tasks requires more than one worker as well as close co-ordination between agencies.

Thus, one of the biggest problems is to define and maintain a clear boundary around the task(s) in families in which the more one digs, the bigger the problems become. It is not uncommon for further disclosures of sexual or other forms of abuse to arise during the course of family work. Of even greater concern it is often the case that no reparative therapeutic work has been offered to the victim. Deciding for instance to what extent family work is tightly focused on areas pertinent to and supportive of the offence-specific work being done with the young person, as opposed to addressing other often pressing family issues, is a key decision, especially where sibling abuse has occurred. Without careful assessment, and multi-disciplinary planning, individual workers can easily be swamped by a multitude of tasks, and lose focus on the key issues. It is not surprising, therefore, that already over-pressed agencies are very cautious about committing time and resources if this looks like signing a blank cheque.

### *Consequences of not engaging families*

The consequences of not engaging families are considerable, as the opening case illustration showed. Although for a small minority of these young people their futures may not lie at home, or they may not wish to return home, the majority will be unconvicted young people living at home, neither subject to family court proceedings (care or supervision orders) nor placed on child protection registers. In other words their engagement and maintenance in any form of therapeutic work will hinge upon the support and endorsement of such work from those who care for them. The longer the family is left without services and support the less likely it is that they will engage with it when it is eventually offered. Even for those adolescents who are subject to court orders, at the psychological level the permission and support of parents or carers remains far more significant in their engagement in therapeutic work than such external influences. The issue from the young person's perspective is a simple one: will their parents/carers be able to accept and love them if they reveal the true nature of their sexually abusive behaviour?

Sadly in a few cases the degree of family breakdown, rejection or dysfunction may be such that it is clearly not in the interests of those adolescents to have contact at all, or, in some situations, only unsupervised contact with family members. This is particularly true where the adolescent himself has been severely abused or coerced by a parent into a sexually abusive role within or beyond the family. Fortunately such cases are rare but would indicate that contact with the family may be abusive and anti-therapeutic. In such cases the focus of family work will be partly on helping the young person address these issues in order to move on, and then to support him and his new guardians, whether foster parents or residential caregivers, in building a positive relationship. Whatever the circumstances in which such young people are living, family or caregiver issues exist and need to be addressed. Although the focus of this chapter is on working with natural parents the principles clearly apply more widely to all caregivers, as do many of the consequences of not engaging them.

Whilst some of the issues resulting from a failure to engage parents have already been identified it is worth setting down the full range of potential consequences here, although the degree to which they occur depends on the situation of the individual family and the services offered:

1 Families left isolated at the point of disclosure will be unable to process their emotional reactions, leaving individual family members isolated, fearful and unable to support each other. As the natural tendency by parents is to try to protect their other children from this crisis, siblings are often left bereft of any information or unclear why their sibling is not there any more. They may also be concerned that this is somehow their fault or that they will be next. In addition they may worry about the

parents' distress. These features are much more likely to occur where disclosure, reporting and subsequent investigation has been triggered by someone external to the family.

2 Parents may fail to offer protection within their family for their children, or may deal with the issue of protection in a way that creates further protection issues. The latter might include placing the abuser with a relative who has children, or as in one case, sending the young person to live in secret under the bed of his grandmother in an elderly persons' home.

3 There is the real danger that parental anger at the abuse, especially sibling abuse, will lead to immediate rejection of the child responsible. Peter was literally abandoned into care on the day it was discovered that he had abused his younger sister. Although it was undoubtedly necessary for him to leave the home, the manner and subsequent lack of contact with him place him in a double-bind as far as talking openly within the group programme about his abusive behaviour. He rightly calculated that this could only result in further rejection.

4 Resentment towards outside agencies is a common feature in child protection cases, especially where the report has not come from the family itself. In the case of Sam quoted at the start, his mother had unsuccessfully sought help two years earlier but was totally opposed to any engagement with any agency by the time Sam's sexually abusive behaviour had started to spiral out of control. Some parents relate how over a period of years they have tried to raise concerns with professionals about their child's sexual behaviour only to be fobbed off with false or minimizing reassurances.

5 Parental minimization or denial of the problem is an understandable response by any family in the circumstances they find themselves in. To acknowledge that one's child has sexually abused another challenges not only the parents' capacity to love and accept their child, but also their own sexual identity and parental confidence. It may bring to light many other hidden or denied aspects of the family's functioning, but even in the best-case scenarios, the questions, doubts and feelings of shame, disgust and fear of public humiliation are profound. The need for external help, support and acceptance as people, even if parental behaviour has to change, will be crucial if parents are to recover sufficient self-esteem, acceptance and competence to resume their role. One family, who had tentatively supported their fifteen-year-old son through the first six months of a group programme, withdrew him, stating that there was no longer any need for him to be thinking about these issues. This came shortly after their youngest son was attacked in their street for having a "pervert" as an older brother and a petrol bomb was forced through their front letter box.

6 The lack of family engagement affects assessment, planning and the success or otherwise of therapeutic work, in addition to its immediate

consequences for family members. Too often "assessment" is restricted simply to a focus on the level of sexual risk the young person poses in order to make immediate decisions with regard to living arrangements, placement, protection or schooling. It may also entail expensive external "expert" risk assessments. The exclusive focus on risk leads to a narrow view of these young people, a failure to locate their sexual behaviour within a developmental and family context, and too often a restricted and occasionally entirely absent account from parents. Even where parents have been seen as part of the assessment, it is not with a view to engaging them but simply to obtaining the young person's developmental history. In part this is due to the pressures of time, for instance in preparing court reports, but there is a wider context to this.

Although partnership with parents is seen as the key to effective child protection work with children who are victims, this is not the case with those identified as young offenders. As Goldson (2000) comments, "children in trouble have been increasingly regarded and thus treated as offenders first and children second" (p. 256). According to Goldson, current youth justice policies lead us to "adulterize" children in trouble and to "responsibilitize" them, "thus saving us the messiness of knowing too much about delinquents, their families, their opportunities, their backgrounds or their experiences" (p. 256). This context, combined with the fact that work with young people who sexually offend has been developed using models from adult programmes, leads to a de-emphasis on the role of family at all stages in the care-planning process. This is contrary however to emerging research on the influence of family on delinquency. In a recent review of family and peer influences on delinquency Blechman and Vryan (2000) quote Kandel (1996) in stating that influence of parents has been under-estimated and that of peers over-estimated. As the review of the characteristics of these families will show, an understanding of, and engagement with, their "messiness" is essential if work to reduce the risk of further offending is to succeed. Failure to engage parents in the assessment and care-planning processes not only underestimates the degree to which issues of attachment, loss and parental supervision and involvement are at the root of the sexual difficulties of these adolescents, but also undermines the possibility of good assessments and viable planning.

7 If parents are not engaged alongside work with the young person, the chances of treatment success are reduced and the chances of drop-outs are significantly higher. For instance Sheridan *et al.* (1998) found the following characteristics of the 27 per cent of the group members who were rated as the high-risk group on completion of treatment. They had "cooperated poorly, developed limited insight and remained reluctant or unable to identify patterns of their sexually abusive behaviour or intervene in it. The single most frequently occurring difficulty during treatment

was conflictual family relationships, which impinged on their ability to derive benefit from the therapy" (p. 177). It was also observed that their parents were less likely to be engaged with the programme.

### *Summary*

Thus far we have reviewed why family work with this population may have been slow to develop and the many adverse consequences of this. An underlying theme has been the importance of understanding sexually abusive behaviour by young people through a developmental perspective, which pays attention to the wider family and social context. This brings us to a consideration of the emerging literature and research on the characteristics of the families. To our knowledge this is the first dedicated account of the literature on family backgrounds, and as will be seen, there are many gaps and limitations in our knowledge. Nevertheless the emerging picture undoubtedly points towards family factors as central to any understanding of young people who sexually abuse others.

## Family characteristics

### *Clinical and theoretical perspectives*

Research specific to family environments and parental characteristics of young people who have sexually abused is sparse. However, clinical impressions abound and the family is said to be crucial in the development of sexually deviant behaviour (Barbaree *et al.*, 1998; Becker and Kaplan, 1988; Ryan *et al.*, 1987).

Families of adolescents who have sexually abused are often characterized in the literature as unstable and disorganized (Davis and Leitenberg, 1987). Family functioning has been described as either rigid and enmeshed or chaotic and confused (Knopp, 1982). Poor parenting is often noted, with parents described as either inconsistent or cold (Prentky *et al.*, 1989). Discipline in the home is often either too harsh or too lax with poor supervision, and this, it is theorized, leads to the development of anti-social behaviours (Barbaree *et al.*, 1998).

The main theoretical models highlight a number of family factors considered influential in the aetiology and maintenance of sexual offending behaviour (Barbaree *et al.*, 1998; Becker and Kaplan, 1988; Ryan *et al.*, 1987), some of which are supported by empirical research.

Becker and Kaplan's (1988) model suggests that a first sexual offence results from a combination of individual, family and social-environmental variables. Early developmental processes may break down, leading to poorly developed empathy skills (Ryan, 1998). It is observed that the quality of care is often poor in families of young people who have sexually abused, and relationships with parents are often disrupted, leading to the formation of inadequate attachments (Ward *et al.*, 1995). Parents who have experienced victimization in their own childhood may develop avoidant coping styles which may in turn manifest as a type of psychological absence leading to impaired parent–child relations (New *et al.*, 1999).

The Barbaree *et al.* (1998) model of the development of sexually deviant behaviour points to the importance of attachments and sees abusive family experiences as instrumental in the development of sexually deviant behaviour.

Marshall and Barbaree (1990) presented a framework outlining a number of factors they considered influential in the aetiology and maintenance of sexual offending. While Marshall and Barbaree acknowledge some minor role for biology they mainly focus on experiential, social and environmental influences. They focus specifically on childhood developmental experiences, social circumstances during pubescence and early adulthood, and current problems and stressors. Transitory environmental features (such as opportunity and internal states) are also taken into account. Marshall and Barbaree point to the relevance of sexual preferences, self-esteem, empathy and intimacy as key to understanding sexual offending. It is suggested that the majority of adult sex offenders grew up in families where there was a disruption in parent–child relations, where violence, abuse (physical, sexual or emotional) and neglect were common. From this standpoint the development of sexually deviant behaviour can be considered to be largely due to experiences in early family life.

Marshall and Barbaree distinguish between nurturing and abusive families and they describe families as existing along a continuum with likely shifts along this continuum from nurturing to abusive over time and setting. They identify a number of factors, which distinguish between the two ends of this continuum. A nurturing family environment facilitates the development of close interpersonal relationships. Within this context the individual learns interactional skills and intimacy behaviours, which enables them to satisfy their own social and intimacy needs in a way that is "mutually satisfying and respectful of the needs of others" (Barbaree *et al.*, 1998, p. 3). At the other end of the continuum in the abusive family environment where parental control has often been coercive, children fail to learn appropriate, effective interpersonal skills. It is proposed that the child in this environment, who has a disrupted attachment with primary caregivers, will adopt a maladaptive, coercive and manipulative strategy for interpersonal interactions. Within the family these interactions may be effective in stifling conflict in the home, and so are often reinforced. However, when this style of interaction is applied outside the family environment it fails. This in turn leads to failure in the development of stable, satisfying relationships, and difficulty in developing intimacy and relationship skills. This poor interpersonal development leads to the development of a negative self-image and low self-confidence which further mitigates against the establishment of a satisfying interpersonal life.

A syndrome of social disability develops, which includes an inability to establish and maintain intimate relationships, low self-esteem, diverse antisocial attitudes and behaviour, a lack of empathy, and cognitive distortions that support and justify criminal behaviour. This syndrome is an intermediate outcome of an abusive family experience (Barbaree *et al.*, 1998). Additional factors in the aetiology of deviant sexual behaviour are sexual, physical or emotional victimization.

In adolescence, a failure to establish appropriate intimate relationships leads to feelings of exclusion, powerlessness, a negative masculine self-concept and feelings of anger and resentment, often directed towards females. Sexual contact is sought through force or with a younger, more vulnerable partner. Coercive strategies that were learnt within abusive families are then employed.

Barbaree *et al.* (1998) argue that these early sexual experiences, which have been accomplished through coercive strategies, establish memories which may then be elaborated into inappropriate sexual fantasies. Repeated use of these fantasies leads to the urge to commit assaults. A sexual interest in antisocial sexual activities is then established through a process of conditioning. (Barbaree *et al.*, 1998). This model allows for varying levels of severity of sexually abusive behaviour from low to moderate to extreme.

Within this framework family experience is clearly implicated aetiologically. The development of sexually offending behaviour is considered the product of a number of causal factors, including: disruption of or inadequate attachment, childhood abuse (including physical, emotional and sexual), dysfunctional family relations, and temperamental factors. The literature notes that many adult sex offenders grew up in families where there was a disruption in parent–child relations where violence, abuse (physical, sexual or emotional) and neglect were common (Marshall and Barbaree, 1990).

Overall the conclusions drawn from clinical impressions and existing theories point to developmental trauma resulting from rejection and/or abuse leading to the development of sexually aggressive behaviour (Bentovim, 1998; Marshall, 1989). Overall the families of young people who sexually abuse have been characterized in the literature as dysfunctional and emotionally impoverished.

### *Methodology of empirical studies*

There is currently a small but growing body of empirical research available, that examines families of young people who have sexually abused. Many studies compare young abusers with other delinquent groups (Awad *et al.*, 1984; Bischof *et al.*, 1992, 1995; Fagan and Wexler, 1988; Lewis *et al.*, 1981; Rubenstein *et al.*, 1993; Stith and Bischof, 1996; Van Ness, 1984). Some studies have examined only incarcerated populations (Bagley and Shewchuk-Dann, 1991; Dolan *et al.*, 1996; Hsu and Starzynski, 1990; Lewis *et al.*, 1979, 1981; Rubenstein *et al.*, 1993; Van Ness, 1984), while others describe community based populations (Bischof *et al.*, 1992, 1995; Kaplan *et al.*, 1990; Manocha and Mezey, 1998; O'Reilly *et al.*, 1998; Stith and Bischof, 1996) and some consider both community and incarcerated populations (Richardson *et al.*, 1997). Most of the studies evaluate adolescents who have sexually abused, but some focus on preadolescent children with sexually aggressive behaviour (Gray *et al.*, 1997, 1999; Johnson, 1988). A few studies differentiate between types of abuse (Kaplan *et al.*, 1990; Hsu and Starzynski, 1990; O'Brien, 1991; Richardson *et al.*, 1997). Most studies base their information on young people's reports while a few use parent/caregiver reports (Awad *et al.*, 1984; Gray *et al.*, 1999; Kaplan *et al.*, 1988, 1990). Several studies use information gathered from retrospective reviews of case files (Bagley and Shewchuk-Dann, 1991; Dolan *et al.*, 1996; Manocha and Mezey, 1998; Richardson *et al.*, 1997).

So, there is much variability among the studies and much of the research is flawed methodologically. Many studies contain small sample sizes with no comparison groups, and non-offender comparison groups are rare. Therefore there are limitations to grouping together the findings from the various types of studies. As a consequence the findings are not generalizable to all young people who have sexually abused and their families. Nonetheless, the available research is valuable and does point to a number of interesting factors that may characterize the family environments and developmental experiences of young people who have sexually abused.

## Empirical research findings

### Prior experience of abuse

Numerous empirical studies have reported a high incidence of prior experience of abuse among young people who have sexually abused. Of note is the incidence of physical abuse and/or neglect (Awad *et al.*, 1984; Dolan *et al.*, 1996; Gray *et al.*, 1999; Hsu and Starzynski, 1990; Johnson, 1988; Lewis *et al.*, 1981; Manocha and Mezey, 1998; O' Reilly *et al.*, 1998; Van Ness, 1984). In a retrospective study that examined the age of onset in adult sex offenders, Knight and Prentky (1993), compared those with histories of sexual offending in their adolescence with those without such histories. Knight and Prentky found that physical abuse and neglect were more frequent among those with a history of sexual offending in adolescence. They also found that child molesters who began offending in adolescence had experienced sexual abuse as children more often than those molesters with an onset in adulthood. Several studies have reported a high incidence of sexual abuse (Dolan *et al.*, 1996; Gray *et al.*, 1997, 1999; Johnson, 1988; Manocha and Mezey, 1998; O' Reilly *et al.*, 1998; Richardson *et al.*, 1997) and or emotional abuse (Gray *et al.*, 1999; Manocha and Mezey, 1998; O' Reilly *et al.*, 1998) among juvenile sexual offenders. It is difficult to establish percentages because of the different types of samples and methodologies used and the fact that reported rates of abuse vary significantly. Rates of physical abuse and neglect range from 19 to 75 per cent while reported rates of sexual abuse range from 19 to 95 per cent. Reported rates of emotional abuse range from roughly 14 to 87 per cent.

Gray *et al.* (1999), in a review of studies on sexualized behaviour among sexually abused children, reported that sexual behaviours were among the most common after-effects (28% of a sample of 1,353) of childhood sexual maltreatment. In their study, Gray *et al.* (1999) noted that 56 per cent of their sample of children with sexual behaviour problems had been victims of multiple forms of abuse. Widom (1995) concluded that victimized children (whether as a result of neglect, sexual or physical abuse), were more likely than non-victims to be arrested for a sex crime. With regard to adolescents who have sexually abused, Ryan (1995) noted that studies show 40–90 per cent of sexually abusive adolescents had experienced some form of abuse.

### *Parental history of victimization*

A number of studies have looked at the incidence of prior victimization among the parents of young people who have sexually abused. Kaplan *et al.* (1988) reported that parents in their sample had experienced high levels of victimization in their own childhood. In a later study, Kaplan *et al.* (1990) reported that mothers of adolescent incest perpetrators were significantly more likely than mothers of non-incest perpetrators to report a personal history of early sexual victimization, later sexual dysfunction and to have had the experience of psychotherapy. O'Brien (1991) reported similar findings from his study, where 36 per cent of mothers and 10 per cent of fathers of adolescent incest perpetrators disclosed an experience of personal sexual victimization compared with 9 per cent of mothers and roughly 6 per cent of fathers of non-incest perpetrators. Manocha and Mezey (1998) and New *et al.* (1999) in their studies also reported high levels (25.5% and 55% respectively) of childhood sexual victimization among the mothers in their samples.

### *Intra-familial violence*

High levels of intra-familial violence have been observed in the families of sexually abusive adolescents. However, reported rates vary (Browne and Falshaw, 1998; Fagan and Wexler, 1988; Gray *et al.*, 1997, 1999; Lewis *et al.*, 1979; 1981; Manocha and Mezey, 1998; New *et al.*, 1999; Richardson *et al.*, 1997; Van Ness, 1984). Lewis *et al.* (1981) reported that 79 per cent of their sample had observed intra-familial violence compared with 20 per cent of their non-violent delinquent comparison group. In a recent study (New *et al.*, 1999), 72 per cent of the mothers of boys who had sexually abused reported domestic violence. In a retrospective case review of 100 young people who had sexually abused, Richardson *et al.* (1997) found that 47 per cent of their sample had experienced and/or witnessed intra-familial violence of some form. The British National Adolescent Perpetrator Network (NAPN) (1988), which holds information on 1,000 adolescent sex offenders, reports spouse abuse in 27 per cent of families. In relation to preadolescents with sexual behaviour problems, Gray *et al.* (1999) reported that approximately 87 per cent of the children in their sample had witnessed at least one physical altercation between their parents.

### Single-parent homes

Parental separation, single-parent homes and, in particular, absent-father homes are reported in a number of studies (Browne and Falshaw, 1998; Kaplan *et al.*, 1990; Graves *et al.*, 1996; Gray *et al.*, 1999; Hsu and Starzynski, 1990; Manocha and Mezey, 1998; O' Reilly *et al.*, 1998). Kaplan *et al.* (1990), in their comparison of mothers of adolescent incest offenders with adolescent non-incest sex offenders, found the majority of incest offenders had a mother who was not living with a partner. Sheridan and McGrath (1999) reported that parental separation was common in their sample at 41 per cent. In contrast, Bagley and Shewchuk-Dann (1991) reported that the majority of participants in his study came from intact families. However Bagley's families were considered to have a high degree of pathology.

A number of studies have reported a substantial incidence of disrupted care histories among young people who have sexually abused, with many having been in care at one time (rates range from 21.4% to 64.4%) (Dolan *et al.*, 1996; Manocha and Mezey, 1998).

### Family dynamics

Smith and Israel (1987) reported that among incestuous adolescents there were unhealthy family dynamics, such as inaccessible parents, lax parental control, the promotion of family secrets and the stimulation of a sexual climate. Similarly in a retrospective review of fifty-one cases, Manocha and Mezey (1998) reported a "lack of sexual boundaries" in approximately 26 per cent of families and the presence of sexually explicit materials in one-third of families within their sample. In 29 per cent of Manocha and Mezey's families, parents were described as "uncaring". Awad *et al.* (1984) compared parents of adolescents who had sexually offended with parents of non-sexual offending adolescents. They reported that the fathers of adolescent sexual offenders were more rejecting and twice as lax with parental control as were the other fathers. In relation to preadolescents, Pithers *et al.* (1998) identified poor parent–child relationships in the families of children with sexual behaviour problems. Relationships were characterized as negative, emotionally distant and conflictual.

### *Family functioning*

Poor family functioning has been observed in families of young people who have sexually offended. It is hypothesized that the families of these adolescents are either disengaged or enmeshed (Graves *et al.*, 1996). However, in an unpublished study Bera (1985) found no difference between the family systems of adolescent sexual offenders and a comparison group. Bischof, *et al.* (1992) found that families of adolescents who had sexually abused were described by youngsters as having greater family cohesion, compared with those of violent and non-violent delinquents. They were, however, less cohesive than the normative sample. In general adolescents who had sexually abused reported that their families were more helpful and supportive than those of their delinquent peers but not the normative sample. Bischof and colleagues, in a series of studies, examined communication patterns in families of adolescents who sexually offend and found poorer levels of communication between parents and children, compared with a normative sample (Bischof *et al.*, 1992, 1995; Stith and Bischof, 1996).

Other problems which have been found to characterize the families of adolescents who have sexually abused include; parental criminality; mental health problems; economic disadvantage; substance and alcohol abuse; and medical problems (Bagley and Shewchuk-Dann, 1991; Browne and Falshaw, 1998; Dolan *et al.*, 1996; Graves *et al.*, 1996; Gray *et al.*, 1999; Hsu and Starzynski, 1990; Manocha and Mezey, 1998; Pithers *et al.*, 1998). Two studies have noted the presence of additional individuals who have sexually abused within the extended families of preadolescents with sexual behaviour problems (Gray *et al.*, 1997; Johnson, 1988); estimates range from 62 to 92 per cent.

Many of the studies comparing adolescents who have sexually abused with other delinquent populations found the two groups had much in common, with regard to family environment, developmental experiences and histories of maltreatment. Interestingly, some of the research has found that adolescents who have sexually abused were distinguished from non-sexual offending delinquent peers. The youths who were sexually abused were distinguished by a higher incidence of exposure to family violence and by more frequent occurrence of physical and sexual abuse (Davis and Leitenberg, 1987; Ford and Linney, 1995, Lewis *et al.*, 1979, 1981; Rubenstein *et al.*, 1993; Van Ness, 1984).

### *Parent response to disclosure of abusive behaviour and intervention*

Duane *et al.* (2002) propose a conceptual model of the experiences of parents in response to the disclosure of sexually abusive behaviour by their adolescent sons. They constructed their model based on semi-structured interviews with five parents of three adolescents with sexually abusive behaviour difficulties. The parents were attending a support group that is part of the Northside Inter-Agency Project (NIAP) intervention programme for adolescents who sexually abuse. Each parent was interviewed three times; at the beginning of their attendance, midway through, and on completion of the programme. Duane *et al.* aimed to utilise this small group of parents to document changes over the course of attendance and to explore the psychological processes that underpin these changes. In doing so they intended to conduct a descriptive-explorative study that would generate hypotheses that could be subsequently evaluated in a properly controlled full-scale study. Thematic content analysis of the fifteen interviews suggested five main domains that summarized parents' concerns and reflections on their experiences. These are described below.

*Impact of disclosure* The impact of disclosure on parents and others in the family was the most frequently mentioned negative experience reported by parents. They described a range of painful emotions related to this including feelings of stress, trauma, helplessness, shock, sadness, confusion, searching, disbelief, shame, guilt and anger. Some reported an experience of feeling deskilled as a parent and thought that only "professionals" could help their sons. They also reported feelings of isolation, stigma and embarrassment. For those whose children's offending behaviour was extra-familial and known within their communities verbal abuse and threats were experienced by parents.

*Positive changes for parents* The following positive changes were reported by parents over the course of their attendance at the programme: an increase in general well-being and ability to cope, an increase in parent–child communication, and a decrease in the anger felt by parents towards their son.

*Observations of their sons* Some positive changes in their sons were observed by some parents during the course of the former's attendance at the adolescent intervention programme. These included an increase in general well-being, level of maturity and social interaction coupled with a decrease in isolation. Difficulties in communication with their sons was commonly reported, particularly in relation to offending behaviour. Two parents reported feelings of mistrust towards their sons. For parents where the abuse was intra-familial a struggle with feelings of divided loyalties was reported.

*Experiences in the parents' group* All five parents reported that they found attendance at the parents' group to be a beneficial experience where they felt a strong sense of support, and had a forum for discussion, reflection and learning. The group was described as "helpful", "comforting" and at times even "enjoyable". Two parents found their initial attendance in the group to be relatively stressful and "intrusive". However, over time they found it easier to attend. One parent commented that it felt easier to have discussions when the group leader was not present. Nevertheless, none of the parents reported things that they would change about the way the group was run and all reported considerable personal benefits from their attendance.

*Comments on the programme* When parents spoke about their reflections on their children's participation in the adolescent intervention part of the service they commented positively on the young person; having access to professional advice and guidance, the involvement of Juvenile Liaison Officers, the importance of their sons' having to admit and talk about their abusive behaviour as part of the intervention programme, the support that was available to their children within their own group, increased knowledge about sexual offending behaviour, and increased knowledge of the impact of abusive behaviour. Parents also spoke positively about their having access to professional advice and guidance, being kept informed of their child's progress, and increased awareness of child protection issues.

Based on their preliminary study Duane *et al.* proposed a conceptual model of parents' response and adjustment to the disclosure of sexually abusive behaviour (see Figure 4.1). This was informed by models of grief reactions and stages of change. Duane *et al.* observed that on disclosure of sexually abusive behaviour by adolescents "parents enter into a process in which thoughts about the disclosure trigger a range of emotions, including shock, confusion, searching and questioning, disbelief or minimization, acceptance, shame, self-blame, guilt, anger and sadness. Parents do not experience these feelings in any particular order and not all emotions are experienced by all" (2002, p. 53). Nevertheless some patterns of response appear more frequently. These include shock in response to disclosure, confusion with searching for answers and questioning as part of that confusion (for some there may be a vicious repeating cycle of confusion, searching for answers, questioning their validity, and return to confusion that can be resolved if an acceptance of the behaviour can be reached), use of denial and minimization as a defence against full acceptance of their son's abusive behaviour, and shame (at times related to a cycle of guilt, self-blame and anger). These findings and conceptual model may prove helpful for guiding research and clinical practice with parents.

## Discussion

The findings from this review point to the experience of abuse or trauma as a significant aetiological factor in the emergence of sexual behaviour problems in young people. Prior sexual victimization seems to be significant in determining the age at onset of sexual behaviour problems (Richardson *et al.*, 1997). However, prior physical abuse is also an important factor, particularly for more violent and sadistic young offenders (Bridge Child Care Development Service, 2001). With regard specifically to the families of young people who have sexually abused, the research, although limited, provides some support for family environment as a discriminating variable. Family dysfunction, abuse and neglect may be predictive in the development of sexually offending behaviour (Vizard *et al.*, 1995). However, because of the wide

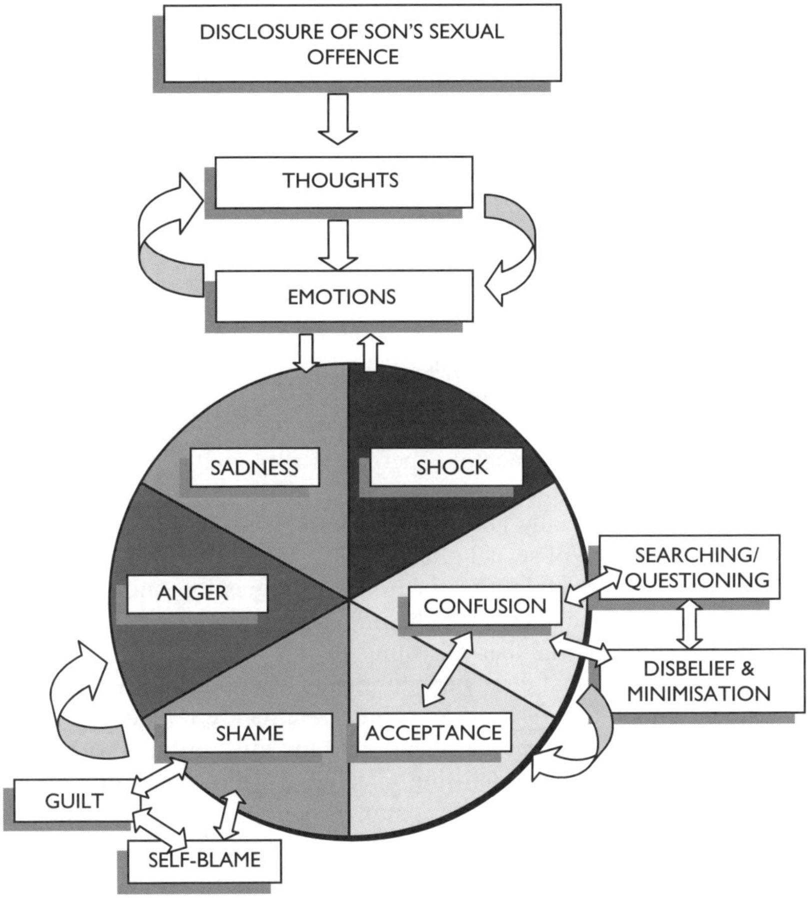


*Figure 4.1* Conceptual model of process which occurs for parents after disclosure of son's sexual offence.

Source: reproduced from Duane *et al.*, 'Experience of parents attending a programme for families of adolescent child sexual abuse perpetrators in Ireland', *Child Care in Practice*, 8, 1: 46–57, by permission of Taylor & Francis http://www.tandf.co.uk/journals/titles/13575279.html

variability in methodologies and samples, these studies are difficult to interpret. It is possible only to say that these factors may be linked to the development of sexually abusive behaviour in some young people.

Chaffin and Bonner (1998) noted that, on the basis of clinical impressions of those working within the adult sex offender population, there are many assumptions accepted as conventional wisdom within the area of young people who sexually abuse. Included amongst these is the idea that all parents and families of young people who have sexually abused are generally dysfunctional and that personal victimization is usually present in the young person's history. However, the empirical support for these is limited. The research is in its infancy and while significant progress has been made there is much ground yet to be covered. There are many gaps in the research and results need to be confirmed in well-designed larger controlled trials.

Families of young people who have sexually abused are a heterogeneous group. While the research indicates that many of these young people have grown up in dysfunctional families, there are also some who seem to have grown up in relatively well-functioning families. There is much variability in terms of developmental experiences and histories of maltreatment. The relationship between past victimization and future offending is complex and is likely to be influenced to a significant degree by the quality of care and relationships child victims experience with their parents or caregivers. The explanation is likely to be multi-causal with risk factors located in abuser histories, their personalities and their environments. Various combinations of family factors and developmental experiences may contribute to the development of disrupted attachments and inadequate empathy development, which may lead to sexually abusive behaviour in some, but not all young people. An explanation of sexual offending in adolescence involving multiple pathways with high variability in time onset, progression and desistance is probably going to fit the data best (Chaffin, 2000).

Clearly a significant number of young people who sexually abuse have grown up in dysfunctional family environments where they have experienced maltreatment and where relationships with parents are impaired. This suggests there is a need to combine offence-specific interventions with holistic interventions that focus on "defusing affective triggers, increasing developmental competence, and self efficacy, countering hopelessness, and increasing psychological safety in relationships" (Ryan, 1999, p. 427). The role of parents in helping young people address these issues and in creating a supportive family environment is crucial. Without parental support progress on both the offence-specific and the developmental issues may be frustrated at best and undermined at worst. If this alliance with parents can be forged, adolescence provides perhaps the last protected opportunity to shape relationship and problem-solving behaviours free from the burdens and responsibilities of caring for self and others.

## A continuum of services, goals and basic requirements

In this final section we consider goals and methods, as well as defining a minimum level of service for family work. The chapter concludes by highlighting some clinical issues to which practitioners must pay attention in the opening stages of any family work with this population.

### *An inter-agency framework for services to families*

Although there are many gaps in our understanding of the nature and needs of these families, it is already clear that they represent a very diverse group. Therefore a continuum of services, and not a "one size fits all" response, will be required to address the variety of situations, needs and risks presented by these different family situations. The pyramid model adapted from Ryan's (1999) ideas presented in Figure 4.2 illustrates such a continuum in which the type and intensity of service is matched to the level of the risk and the capacity and commitment of the family.

Adapting Ryan's model suggests a four-level model of service as follows:

*Level 1*: Early presentation of sexually problematic behaviour in the context of concerned parents and a reasonably positive functioning family. The intervention here would be educational and supportive in which the worker would help the parents process their feelings and then provide them with an information and home counselling pack which the parents work through with the

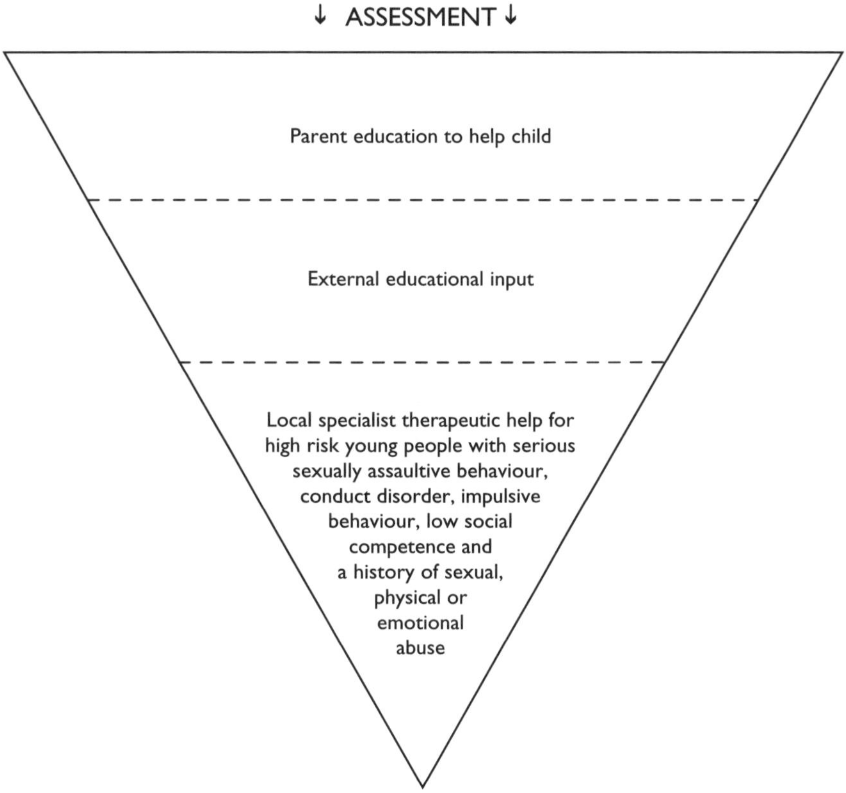


*Figure 4.2* Threshold for services (based on the ideas of Ryan, 1999).

young person, focusing on issues of consent, empathy and boundaries. One or two follow-up visits would take place to check progress.

*Level 2*: Referral to a psycho-educational group for parents where there had been further sexual behaviour problems and there is a need to bolster the parents' skills and commitment.

*Level 3*: Referral for community-based treatment programme for the young person and the parents which could be run by a mixture of specialist and generalist staff.

*Level 4*: Referral to specialist residential/secure programmes for the identified high-risk group where there are multiple problems, serious abusive behaviours and where there is a high public protection risk.

Let us take two very different sorts of family situation. Family A is a relatively well functioning, intact and cohesive family unknown to welfare or criminal justice agencies in which fourteen-year-old Stanley has committed a single indecent assault on a five-year-old child for whom he was acting as babysitter. Stanley's parents, although very distressed, responded immediately and appropriately when the victim's mother told them what had happened. They accompanied Stanley to the police station, made it clear to him that although they still loved him, what he had done was wrong, and they asked what they could do to help Stanley to ensure he did not commit any further assaults. Stanley is an only child. Family B is a family in which there are four children ranging in ages from the oldest, Brian, twelve years, to Katie, four years. There are three different fathers and currently Katie's father, Bill, is living with the family. The family are well known to welfare agencies and there have been persistent concerns about Brian's disruptive behaviour at school. One day Brian was spotted in school to have welts on his back. When asked about these he stated that Bill inflicted the marks with a leather belt. During the subsequent child protection investigation Bill told the social worker and the police that he had done this after he had caught Brian in bed with Katie getting her to play with his penis.

Plainly these two situations require different responses. Using the pyramid framework, and based upon a thorough assessment for all families where a young person has committed a sexual assault, Family A would be offered the Level 1 response whilst Family B would require a Level 3 response in addition to a requirement that Brian live outside the family at least initially.

However, such a system can only be delivered in the context of a strong inter-agency framework where there is shared commitment, some pooled resources, agreed thresholds of intervention, and a clear multi-disciplinary assessment protocol in order to identify accurately which families need what level of service.

### *Goals of family work*

It follows from the above that the goals of family work depend on the circumstances and needs of the case. The overriding objective of such family work can be defined as engaging parents/caregivers in services that enable them to care for, support and supervise young people who have committed sexual assaults, in order to reduce the risk of recidivism, protect known or potential victims, and promote the welfare of the young person. In pursuit of that overall objective some or all of the following goals may be relevant in any particular case:

- Provision of immediate crisis support for the family, especially offering or identifying sources of emotional support to reduce isolation, shame, victim blaming, withdrawal, loss of parental functioning, or emotional rejection.
- Enlisting parental agreement and engagement for both them and their child in an assessment process.
- Provision of information and educative help about normal sexual behaviour, understanding consent, abusive sexual behaviour and its effects.
- Provision of information as to how parents can most helpfully respond to both the victim and the abuser, including how to support the latter in his treatment work.
- Establishing (where viable) home safety agreements to monitor and supervise the young person and protect victims. This might include: separate sleeping arrangements; privacy rules; increased parental checks; restrictions on children being alone together behind closed doors; limits on horseplay and wrestling; monitoring TV, video and computer access; and expectations about being fully dressed (Chaffin, 2000).
- Engaging parents/caregivers in a case-planning and review process from the outset.
- Engaging parents/carers in longer-term work to increase openness and emotional expressiveness within the family; clarify, consolidate or restore appropriate parental and child roles; identify family strengths and needs; acknowledge and interrupt abusive family patterns; increase parental skills, confidence and competence in promoting accountable behaviour within the family and in handling negotiation and conflict; assist in apology or reparative work between abuser and victim; enhance their protective capacity, especially in relation to boundary-setting; assist them to positively structure the young person's time and activities in terms of peer and social activities; re-negotiate family relationships and address the transition where it is not possible for the young person to return home, in order to clarify, maintain or improve contact with the family and enable the family to be a source of continuing support and significance.

In other words the work with parents may be rehabilitative, reparative or focused on restructuring family relationships. It may be carried out through a variety of approaches: individual or couple work with parents (Burnham, *et al.*, 1999); group work with parents (McGarvey and McKeown, 1999); part or whole family work with parents and children; individual or group work with the young person.

### *Basic requirements*

Earlier in the chapter the crucial importance of engaging parents was stressed. However, resources may not stretch to address the range of tasks which have been outlined above. Nevertheless, there is a minimum level of service which would appear to be necessary without which any work with young people about their offending behaviour may become seriously compromised. These requirements are focused on two critical issues: restoring the parental functioning following the crisis of disclosure; and engaging parents in safety planning. The latter cannot be done without the former. These basic requirements are: the provision of immediate crisis support for the family; a message that parents are not there to be "blamed" or put thorough therapy; affirming the positive role they can play; agreeing a home safety plan; engaging parents in a collaborative process of assessment; early engagement of parents in the case-planning process; information as to how parents can support the offence-focused work.

For many families this basic package would represent a considerable improvement on their experiences to date. It would also act as the prerequisite for involvement in some of the more demanding work listed earlier. For young people to know that their parents were neither falling apart nor rejecting them as a result of their abusive behaviours, would restore the sense of containment and security that is vital as they seek to address their difficulties and to make changes to a more healthy and responsible lifestyle.

## Conclusion

It would be hard to describe the current state of responses and services to families of young people who commit sexual assaults in terms other than disorganized, sporadic and unpredictable. We have sought to illustrate the dire consequences that can ensue from our failure to engage parents. The research on the characteristics of these families should leave us in no doubt that family factors are central to any understanding of, or intervention in, the patterns, context and overall environment in which young people's sexually abusive behaviour exists. Indeed it is hard to see how the move to a more holistic approach to this problem will succeed unless strengthening the family environment and parental competence and confidence is a central target of our efforts. Even for the small proportion of young people who cannot return home, family remains important both for their core sense of identity and self, and at the practical level in supporting their journey into adulthood and independence. It is hoped finally that in every location those who read this chapter and who agree with its arguments will lobby vigorously at the very least for a minimum level of service for these families, even as we must build with patience a more comprehensive response.

## References

Awad, G. A., Saunders, E., and Levene, J. (1984). A clinical study of male adolescent sexual offenders. *International Journal of Offender Therapy and Comparative Criminology, 28(1)*, 105–115.

Bagley, C., and Shewchuk-Dann, D. (1991). Characteristics of 60 children and adolescents who have a history of sexual assault against others: Evidence from a controlled study. *Journal of Child & Youth Care, Special issue: Child sexual abuse*, Fall, 43–52.

Barbaree, H., Marshall, W., and McCormack, J. (1998). The development of sexually deviant behaviour among adolescents and its implications for prevention and treatment. *Irish Journal of Psychology, 19(1)*, 1–31.

Becker, J. V. and Kaplan, M. S. (1988). The assessment of adolescent sexual offenders. *Advances in Behavioural Assessment of Children and Families, 4*, 97–118.

Bentovim, A. (1998). A family systemic approach to working with young sex offenders. *Irish Journal of Psychology, 19(1)*, 119–135.

Bera, W. H. (1985). A preliminary investigation of a typology of adolescent sex offenders and their family systems. Unpublished Masters thesis, University of Minnesota.

Bischof, G., Stith, S., and Wilson, S. (1992). A comparison of the family systems of adolescent sex offenders and non-sexual offending delinquents. *Family Relations, 41*, 318–323.

Bischof, G. P., Stith, S. M., and Whitney, M. L. (1995). Family environments of adolescent sex offenders and other juvenile delinquents. *Adolescence, 30*, 117, 157–170.

Blaske, D. M., Borduin, C. M., and Henggeler, S. W. (1989). Individual, family and peer characteristics of adolescent sex offenders and assaultive offenders. *Developmental Psychology, 25(5)*, 846–855.

Blechman, E., and Vryan, P. (2000). Pro-social family therapy: A manualised prevention intervention for juvenile offenders. *Aggression and Violent Behaviour, 5(4)*, 343–378.

Bridge Child Care Development Service (2001). *Childhood Lost: Part 8 Case Review Overview Report DM*. Hay-on-Wye: Bridge Publishing.

Browne, K., and Falshaw, L. (1998). Treatment work with young people in secure care. *Irish Journal of Psychology, 19(1)*, 208–225.

Burnham, J., Moss, J., Debrelle, J., and Jamieson, R. (1999) Working with families of young sexual abusers: assessment and intervention issues. In M. Erooga and H. Masson (eds), *Children and Young People who Sexually Abuse Others*. London: Routledge.

Chaffin, M. (2000). *Family and Ecological Emphasis in Interventions: A Developmental Perspective in Working with Children, Adolescents and Adults with Sexually Abusive*

*Behaviours*. Keynote presentation at the 10th annual conference of the National Organisation for the Treatment of Abusers (NOTA), Dublin, Ireland.

Chaffin, M., and Bonner, B. (1998). Editor's introduction. *Child Maltreatment: Journal of the American Professional Society on the Abuse of Children, 3(4)*, 314–316.

Davis, G. E., and Leitenberg, H. (1987). Adolescent sex offenders. *Psychological bulletin, 101(3)*, 417–427.

Dolan, M., Holloway, J., Bailey, S., and Kroll, L. (1996). The psychosocial characteristics of juvenile sexual offenders. *Medicine, Science and the Law, 36(4)*, 343–352.

Duane, Y., Carr, A., Cherry, J., McGrath, K., and O'Shea, D. (2002). Experiences of parents attending a programme for families of adolescent child sexual abuse perpetrators in Ireland. *Child Care in Practice, 8(1)*, 46–57.

Fagan, J., and Wexler, S. (1988). Explanations of sexual assault among violent delinquents. *Journal of Adolescent Research, 3*, 363–385.

Ford, M. A., and Linney, J. A. (1995). Comparative analysis of juvenile sexual offenders, violent non-sexual offenders and status offenders. *Journal of Interpersonal Violence, 10*, 56–70.

Goldson, B. (2000), 'Children in Need' or young offenders: Hardening ideology, organisational change, and new challenges for social workers with children in trouble. *Child and Family Social Work, 5(3)*, 255–266.

Graves, R., Openshaw, D., Ascione, F., and Erickson, S. (1996). Demographic and parental characteristics of youthful sex offenders. *Individual Journal of Offender Therapy and Comparative Criminology, 40(4)*, 300–317.

Gray, A., Busconi, A., Houchens, P., and Pithers, W. D. (1997). Children with sexual behaviour problems and their caregivers: Demographics, functioning and clinical patterns. *Sexual Abuse: A Journal of Research and Treatment, 9*, 267–290.

Gray, A., Pithers, W. D., Busconi, A., and Houchens, P. (1999). Developmental and etiological characteristics of children with sexual behaviour problems: Treatment implications. *Child Abuse and Neglect, 23(6)*, 601–621.

Hsu, L. K. G., and Starzynski, J. (1990). Adolescent rapists and adolescent child sexual assaulters. *International Journal of Offender Therapy and Comparative Criminology, 34*, 23–31.

Johnson, T. C. (1988). Child perpetrators: Children who molest other children: Preliminary findings. *Child Abuse and Neglect, 12*, 219–229.

Kandel, D. (1996). Parental and peer contexts of adolescent deviance. *Journal of Drug Issues, 26*, 289–315.

Kaplan, M. S., Becker, J. V., and Cunningham-Rathner, J. (1988). Characteristics of parents of adolescent incest perpetrators: Preliminary findings. *Journal of Family Violence, 3*, 183–191.

Kaplan, M., Becker, J., and Martinez, D. (1990). A comparison of mothers of adolescent incest vs. non-incest perpetrators. *Journal of Family Violence, 5(3)*, 209–214.

Knight, R. A., and Prentky, R. A. (1993). Exploring characteristics for classifying juvenile sex offenders. In H. E. Barbaree, W. L. Marshall and S. M. Hudson (eds), *The Juvenile Sex Offender*. New York: Guilford Press, pp. 45–83.

Knopp, F. H. (1982). *Remedial Intervention in Adolescent Sex Offences: Nine Programme Descriptions*. Orwell, VT: Safer Society Press.

Lewis, D. O., Shankok, S. S., and Pincus, J. H. (1979). Juvenile sexual assaulters. *American Journal of Psychiatry, 136*, 1194–1196.

Lewis, D. O., Shankok, S. S., and Pincus, J. H. (1981) Juvenile male sexual assaulters: Psychiatric, neurological, psycho educational and abuse factors. In D. O. Lewis (ed.), *Vulnerabilities to Delinquency*. Jamaica, NY: Spectrum, pp. 29–105.

Manocha, K. F., and Mezey, G. (1998). British adolescents who sexually abuse: A descriptive study. *Journal of Forensic Psychiatry, 9(3)*, 588–608.

Marshall, W. L. (1989). Invited essay: Intimacy, loneliness and sexual offenders. *Behaviour Research and Therapy, 27*, 491–503.

Marshall, W., and Barbaree, H. E. (1990). An integrated theory of the aetiology of sexual offending. In W. L. Marshall, D. R. Laws and H. E. Barbaree (eds), *Handbook of Sexual Assault: Issues, Theories and Treatment of the Offender*. New York: Plenum Press.

McGarvey, J., and McKeown, L. (1999). Psycho-educational support for a clinically neglected population: parents and carers of young people who sexually abuse children and others. In M. Calder (ed.), *Working with Young People who Sexually Abuse: New Pieces of the Jigsaw Puzzle*. Lyme Regis: Russell House.

National Adolescent Perpetrator Network (NAPN) (1988). Preliminary report from the national task force on juvenile sexual offending. *Juvenile and Family Court Journal, 39(2)*.

New, M. J., Stevenson, J., and Skuse, D. (1999). Characteristics of mothers of boys who sexually abuse. *Child Maltreatment, 4(1)*, 21–31.

O'Brien, M. (1991). Taking sibling incest seriously. In M. Quinn-Patton (ed.), *Family Sexual Abuse: Frontline Research and Evaluation*, Beverly Hills, CA: Sage.

O' Reilly, G., Sheridan, A., Carr, A., Cherry, J., Donohoe, E., McGrath, K., Phelan, S., Tallon, M., and O'Reilly, K. (1998). A descriptive study of adolescent sexual offenders in an Irish community-based treatment programme. *Irish Journal of Psychology, 19(1)*, 152–167.

Pithers, W. D., Gray, A., Busconi, A., and Houchens, P. (1998). Caregivers of children with sexual behaviour problems: Psychological and familial functioning. *Child Abuse and Neglect, 22*, 43–55.

Prentky, R., Knight, R., Straus, H., Rokou, F., Cerce, D., and Sims-Knight, J. (1989). Developmental antecedents of sexual aggression. *Development and Psychopathology, 1*, 153–169.

Richardson, G., Kelly, T. P., Bhate, R., and Graham, F. (1997). Group differences in abuser and abuse characteristics in a British sample of sexually abusive adolescents. *Sexual Abuse: A Journal of Research and Treatment, 9(3)*, 239–257.

Rubenstein, M., Yeager, C. A., Goodstein, B. A., and Lewis, D. O. (1993). Sexually assaultive male juveniles: A follow-up. *American Journal of Psychiatry, 150*, 262–265.

Ryan, G. (1995). *Treatment of Sexually Abusive Youth: The Evolving Consensus*. Paper presented at the International Experts Conference, Utrecht, the Netherlands.

Ryan, G. (1998). The relevance of early life experience to the behaviour of sexually abusive youth. *Irish Journal of Psychology, 19(1)*, 32–48.

Ryan, G. (1999). Treatment of sexually abusive youth: The evolving consensus. *Journal of Interpersonal Violence, 14(4)*, 422–436.

Ryan, G., Lane, S., Davis, J., and Issac, C. (1987). Juvenile sex offenders: development and correction. *Child Abuse and Neglect, 11*, 385–395.

Sheridan, A., and McGrath, K. (1999). Adolescent sexual offenders: characteristics and treatment effectiveness. In M. Calder (ed.), *Working with Young People who Sexually Abuse: New Pieces of the Jigsaw Puzzle*. Lyme Regis: Russell House.

Sheridan, A., McKeown, K., Cherry, J., Donohoe, E., McGrath, C., Phelan, S., Tallon, M., and O' Reilly, K. (1998). Perspectives on treatment outcome in adolescent sexual offending: A study of community-based treatment programmes. *Irish Journal of Psychology, 19(1)*, 168–180.

Smith, H., and Israel, E. (1987). Sibling incest: A study of the dynamics of 25 cases. *Child Abuse and Neglect, 11*, 101–108.

Stith, S., and Bischof, G. (1996). Communication patterns in families of adolescent sex offenders. In D. Cahn, and S. Lloyd (eds), *Family Violence from a Communication Perspective*. London: Sage, pp. 108–126.

Thomas, J. (1991). The adolescent sex offenders family. In G. Ryan and S. Lane (eds), *Juvenile Sexual Offending: Causes, Consequences, and Corrections*. Lexington: Lexington Books.

Van Ness, S. (1984). Rape as instrumental violence: A study of youth offenders. *Journal of Offender Counselling Services and Rehabilitation, 9*, 161–170.

Vizard, E., Monck, E., and Misch, P. (1995). Child and adolescent sex abuse perpetrators: A review of the research. *Journal of Child Psychology and Psychiatry, 36(5)*, 731–756.

Ward, T., Hudson, S. M., Marshall, W. L., and Seigert, T. (1995). Attachment style and intimacy deficits in sex offenders: A theoretical framework. *Sexual Abuse: A Journal of Research and Treatment, 7*, 317–335.

Widom, C. S. (1995). *Victims of childhood sexual abuse: Later criminal consequences*. Washington, DC: National Institute of Justice.

Chapter 5

# Psychiatric disorder and adolescent sexual offending

*Declan Sheerin*

## Introduction

What value is there in identifying the types and prevalence of psychiatric disorder in adolescent sexual offenders? McElroy *et al.* (1999) suggest the following: (1) a better understanding of the relationship between sexual violence and mental illness might enable the development of more effective legal, correctional and public health policies regarding persons who commit sexual crimes; (2) psychopharmacologic treatment of appropriate psychiatric disorders in affected sexual offenders, administered in conjunction with correctional and psychosocial treatment programmes might increase the likelihood of successful rehabilitation and thereby reduce recidivism, public victimisation and the use of more costly correctional services; and (3) risk factors and preventive strategies for sexual violence might be identified and developed.

As with adult sexual offenders, psychiatric disorder appears to be common in adolescents who sexually offend. Unfortunately, it frequently goes unnoticed. Many programmes do not have the availability of a psychiatrist to assess mental state, or to ensure that co-morbid psychiatric disorders are adequately treated and programmes adjusted where necessary to meet the particular psychiatric and personality needs of each individual. To underline this lack of psychiatric involvement, it is perhaps pertinent to point out that the medical membership of NOTA (National Organisation for the Treatment of Abusers) in December 2000 was a mere twenty-seven (2.8%) of almost 1,000 members (NOTA, 2000).

This chapter covers five broad areas: (1) the specific psychiatric diagnostic categories that address some sexual behaviour problems; (2) the methodological difficulties inherent in researching psychiatric disorder in sexual offenders; (3) a review of the studies available on psychopathology in adult sexual offenders; (4) a review of the studies available on adolescent sexual offenders; and finally (5) the chapter draws conclusions from both adult and adolescent studies and provides some guidelines both for assessing psychopathology in adolescents who sexually offend and for identifying the need for a full psychiatric assessment.

## Sexual offending and psychiatric disorder

Sexual offenders have been categorised into three broad diagnostic groups (Abel *et al.*, 1986): (1) the paraphilic who habitually and compulsively only commits sexual offences; (2) the schizophrenic or psychotic individual whose sexual offences are the product of the psychosis; and (3) the antisocial personality, whose sexual offences are part of other nonsexual, sociopathic patterns. However, the picture is probably more complex than this, in that personality disorder may be the rule rather than the exception, and several other disorders may be associated with sexual offending. In addition, there is uncertainty regarding the validity of paraphilia as a diagnostic category, or whether in fact it constitutes a psychiatric disorder at all.

### *The paraphilias*

Although sexual ruminations are described as diagnostic criteria for several psychiatric disorders, sexual deviations themselves are viewed as specific psychiatric syndromes by the medical profession. These are the paraphilias and are listed as diagnostic categories in the official psychiatric nomenclatures, DSM-IV (American Psychiatric Association, 1994) and ICD-10 (WHO, 1996). In both systems, the paraphilias include disorders such as exhibitionism, fetishism, frotteurism, paedophilia, sexual masochism or sadism, transvestic fetishism, voyeurism and other disorders of sexual preference like phonecall scatologia, zoophilia, necrophilia and coprophilia. ICD-10 also includes Multiple Disorders of Sexual Preference as a diagnostic category.

Paraphilias are defined as sexual disorders characterised by recurrent, intense sexual urges, fantasies or behaviours that involve unusual objects, activities or situations, occurring over a period of at least six months (DSM-IV). The person either has acted on these fantasies or is markedly distressed by them and the fantasies and behaviours cause significant impairment in social, occupational or other important areas of functioning. Finally, for paedophilia (but not for the other paraphilias) the perpetrator must be aged sixteen or over, and the victim must be at least five years younger than the perpetrator. This means that paedophilia can be diagnosed in some adolescents (16–18 years) using DSM-IV criteria. In ICD-10 – Clinical Descriptions (WHO, 1992), there is no age stipulation for any of the paraphilias, including paedophilia. However, and rather confusingly, in the ICD-10 – Diagnostic Criteria for Research (WHO, 1993), the criteria for paedophilia include the same age stipulation as DSM-IV.

### *Definitional problems*

The development of the paraphilias as mental disorders has required some gestation and modification in the various editions of DSM and ICD. For instance, there were many difficulties in the DSM-III-R definition of paraphilia that required revision for DSM-IV, one of which was that the definition, in itself, was considered inconsistent with the definition of mental disorder in general (Gert, 1992).

A mental disorder was defined as "a clinically significant behavioural or psychological syndrome or pattern that occurs in an individual and that is associated with either present distress (a painful symptom) or disability (impairment in one or more areas of functioning) or a significant risk of suffering death, pain, disability, or loss of significant freedom" (APA, 1987, p. xxii). So, what makes a disorder a mental disorder is its symptoms, not its cause or aetiology. This is fundamental to psychiatric diagnostic practice. Also, unless the patient has a painful symptom, suffers impairment in an important area of functioning or is at significantly increased risk of suffering death, pain, etc., deviant behaviour could not of itself be defined as mental disorder – according to DSM-III-R standards. Yet the criteria for diagnosing paraphilia allowed that deviance, by itself, was sufficient to classify a behavioural syndrome as a psychiatric disorder. "The paraphilias are characterised by arousal in response to sexual objects or situations that are not part of normative arousal-activity patterns and that in varying degrees may interfere with the capacity of reciprocal, affectionate sexual activity" (APA, 1987, p. 279). Therefore, it is not essential for such arousal-activity patterns to interfere with reciprocal, affectionate sexual activity (Gert, 1992) or to involve pain, impairment or risk of suffering death, pain, disability or loss of freedom. Yet they were regarded as mental disorders. In addition, DSM-III-R states that "neither deviant behaviour, e.g., political, religious, or sexual, nor conflicts that are primarily between the individual and society are mental disorders unless deviance or conflict is a symptom of a dysfunction in the person . . ." (APA, 1987, p. xxii).

Clearly, these stipulations created a conflict within the system. To counteract this, DSM-IV added to its definition of paraphilia the phrase that the fantasies and behaviours cause significant impairment in social, occupational or other important areas of functioning. This gave a clearer rigidity to the definition of deviant sexual arousal patterns as mental disorder.

However, questions remain regarding distress consequent to deviant sexual arousal or activity. For instance, in transvestic fetishism, the distress associated with cross-dressing may, in many cases, be a consequence of the conflict between the urge to engage in deviant sexual behaviour and the anticipated or real social disapproval or shaming of that behaviour, if discovered and punished (Gert, 1992). Given that "neither deviant behaviour, e.g., political, religious, or sexual, nor conflicts that are primarily between the individual and society are mental disorders unless deviance or conflict is a symptom of a dysfunction in the person . . ." (APA, 1987, p. xxii) then the origin of the distress becomes important in deciding whether a mental disorder is present or not. Based on the same principles, if someone were engaged in politically deviant behaviour – and if the distress associated with urges to engage in this behaviour were independent of the chance of being found out and punished – then that person could be said to be suffering from a mental disorder, by DSM criteria (Gert, 1992).

In summary, serious questions remain about the validity of the paraphilias as a psychiatric construct, a construct further undermined when we compare diagnostic criteria for paraphilia with those of other disorders, particularly impulse-control disorders (IPD) and obsessive-compulsive disorders (OCD).

### *The relationship between paraphilia and other diagnostic categories*

The paraphilias do not appear to represent "stand-alone" categories. Whether these behaviours constitute an addiction, a compulsion, a form of hypersexuality, or a disorder of impulse control is controversial. ICD-10 excludes the paraphilias from Habit and Impulse Disorders (F63) "by convention", though clearly indicating that paraphilias would meet the general criteria for impulse disorders. DSM-IV makes a similar distinction in its category Impulse-Control Disorder Not Otherwise Specified (312.30), excluding paraphilias again by convention.

Pearson (1990) noted similarities between paraphilias and OCD, apparent in individuals experiencing erotic cravings and impulses with a sense of mounting tension prior to committing the act, which often was performed in a stereotypical manner. Predominantly obsessional thoughts or ruminations are defined as "ideas, images, or impulses that enter the individual's mind again and again . . . They are almost invariably distressing (because they are violent or obscene) . . . and the sufferer often tries, unsuccessfully, to resist them" (WHO, 1993, p. 142). DSM-IV makes the link with OCD very clear by stating in the diagnostic guidelines for OCD that if the content of the obsessions and compulsions is restricted to another Axis 1 disorder, for instance, preoccupation only with sexual urges or fantasies, then the obsessions and compulsions are part of a paraphilia diagnosis.

Further evidence for the link between paraphilias and OCD is provided through case reports describing the treatment of various paraphilias with medications that have proven efficacy in the treatment of OCD (Jenike, 1989; Pearson, 1990). Selective serotonin re-uptake inhibitors (SSRIs) have been shown to decrease the intensity and intrusiveness of fantasies, resulting in more conventional sexual behaviours (Bianchi, 1990; Kafka, 1991; Perilstein *et al.*, 1991). One case report describes an adolescent with multiple paraphilias, who also met criteria for OCD and bipolar disorder (Galli *et al.*, 1998). The intrusive sexual and aggressive thoughts responded to fluoxetine. The paedophilic behaviour may however have been a manifestation of a primary OCD with paedophilic, frotteuristic, sadistic, zoophilic and necrophilic obsessional thoughts and compulsive behaviours. Such reports are suggestive of improved impulse control with the use of an SSRI, though the apparent therapeutic response may partially be explained on the basis of an SSRI's effects on neuronal systems regulating behaviour or on antidepressant-induced anorgasmia (Perilstein *et al.*, 1991).

In conclusion, two key points need to be made. Firstly, preliminary phenomenological, co-morbidity, and treatment response data suggest that paraphilias may be related to other major psychiatric disorders, especially mood, obsessive-compulsive, impulse control, personality and substance use disorders (McElroy *et al.*, 1999). Therefore, when sexual offending behaviour is considered within psychiatric classification, it appears to be situated in many areas and crosses many boundaries (see Figure 5.1). This may of course indicate co-morbidity, or, it may simply underline the degree of leakage of definitional integrity between psychiatric disorders.

Secondly, classificatory criteria should be re-evaluated for paedophilia. The age restriction in DSM-IV may be quite arbitrary and worth removing to increase public awareness that paraphilias can begin at a young age (Galli *et al.*, 1998). Given the link in DSM-IV between OCD and paraphilia, and given

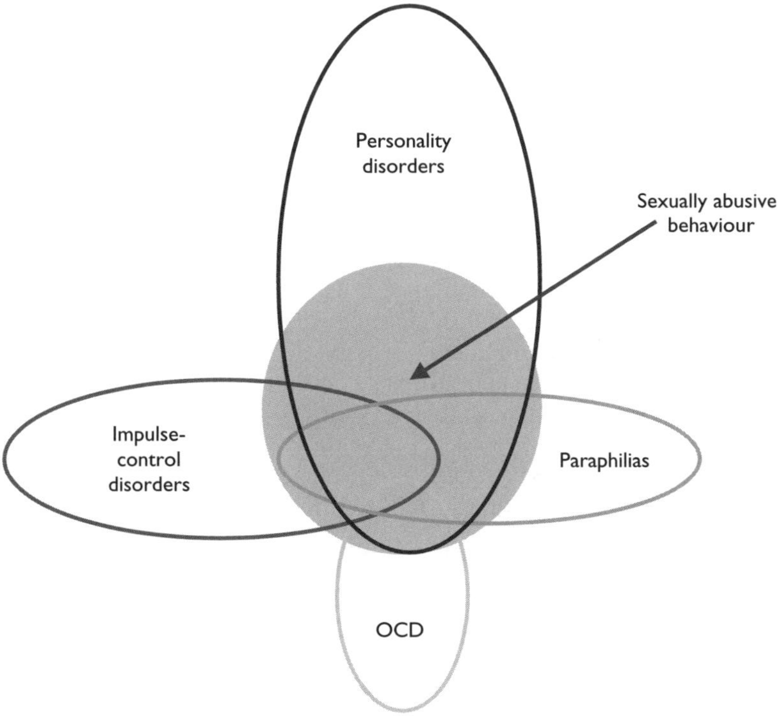


*Figure 5.1* Diagnostic overlaps and sexually offending (other psychiatric disorders like schizophrenia and bipolar disorder, which may rarely involve sexually abusive behaviour, have not been included in this figure).

that OCD can be diagnosed at any age, as can all paraphilias besides paedophilia, there seems little reason to restrict the diagnosis of paedophilia, or at least a subgroup of paedophilia with OCD-type fantasies and urges, to sixteen-year-olds and over. It should be a matter of content rather than age.

## Researching psychopathology in sexual offenders

It could be argued that researching psychopathology in sexual offenders is an impossible task. This is for two reasons. Firstly, some methodological problems are virtually intractable and a study devoid of even the most fundamental of these would be very difficult to design indeed (Problem A). Secondly, the offenders, by their very nature, are highly likely to dissimulate (Problem B). Problem A is addressed later in this chapter, alongside discussion of the studies themselves; Problem B is addressed below.

### *Problems in assessing psychopathology: denial*

Given that denial of offending behaviour is a frequent experience of those working with adolescents and adults who sexually offend, an inevitable question arises: will denial of offending behaviour extend to denial of psychopathology and associated psychological features like hostility and anger? If minimisation occurs is this likely to be linked to minimisation of psychopathology or, if the offender has admitted in part to his sexual offence, will he exaggerate psychopathology in the hope of currying sympathy, creating exonerating motives, or getting himself "off the hook"? Or will he be truthful, having admitted in part or in full his offence?

Denial or minimisation of sexual offending behaviour may be accompanied by denial or minimisation of accompanying psychopathology (Grossman and Cavanaugh, 1990). Also, denial or minimisation of paraphilia is considered common amongst sexual offenders (Grossman, 1985; Kelly and Cavanaugh, 1982). These two facts have compromised co-morbidity research into paedophilia, sexual offending and psychiatric disorders (Kafka and Prentky, 1994).

Inevitably, the context in which the evaluation occurs will influence the motivation to "come clean" or dissimulate. Grossman and Cavanaugh (1989), using the Minnesota Multiphasic Personality Inventory (MMPI), assessed two groups of men alleged to have committed sexual offences – those that admitted their offence and those that denied engaging in paraphilic behaviour. Several scales of the MMPI are believed to discriminate honest responders from experimental subjects instructed to minimise or exaggerate symptoms (Greene, 1980; Grow *et al.*, 1980). On all of these indices of the MMPI, those that denied paraphilia showed more evidence of minimising psychopathology than those who admitted to paraphilia. Analysis of the clinical scales showed that the non-admitters showed less psychopathology consistently on all ten of the standard MMPI clinical scales.

Therefore, patients that deny allegations of sexual offending when undergoing psychiatric or psychological evaluation, are prone to minimise other symptoms of psychopathology. Unfortunately, interpreting the implications of this study is difficult, given that the study itself is subject to Problem A. None of the men in the study had been found guilty – they were either pre-trial, facing no formal legal charges, or had already been found Not Guilty by Reason of Insanity. So, it was of course possible that in the group of non-admitters some did not in fact commit any sexual offence. If that were so, then the denial or minimisation on the MMPI scales might indicate a different motive, for instance, a general attitude of defensiveness and uncooperativeness. Recommending extreme alertness when evaluating sexual offenders who deny having engaged in paraphilic behaviour implies that all those alleged to have committed sexual offences but who deny the allegations are in fact sexual offenders anyway.

It is unknown to what extent denial of hostility is related to denial of psychopathology or to denial of offences (Hall, 1989; Panton, 1978). Using the MMPI and the Buss-Durkee Hostility Inventory (BDHI), eighty-two alleged child molesters were assessed (Wasyliw *et al.*, 1994). The MMPI validity scales (those shown to discriminate between exaggerators, honest responders and minimisers in a variety of clinical and forensic settings) were all significantly correlated with BDHI total scores, with minimisation associated with lower BDHI scores and exaggeration associated with higher scores. The authors concluded that (a) alleged sexual offenders who minimise psychopathology in general admit to less hostility than do those who do not minimise psychopathology; (b) alleged sexual offenders who exaggerate psychopathology also acknowledge more hostility than do those who do not exaggerate; and (c) alleged sexual offenders who deny their allegations admit to less hostility than do those who acknowledge their allegations. They noted that admitters of charges exaggerated psychopathology significantly more often than deniers.

In conclusion, a fairly complex pattern of response bias may be present. The deniers (some of whom may be innocent) have no reason to exaggerate psychological problems since they may believe that any admission of psychological disorder may place them at risk of being perceived as abnormal and therefore as being more likely to have committed deviant behaviours. For some individuals who have admitted to charges, in contrast, there may be an attempt to exaggerate other aspects of psychopathology in an attempt to blame their behaviour on mental disorder and thus disown personal responsibility (Fedoroff *et al.*, 1992; Grossman *et al.*, 1992). This finding is consistent with prior research showing that alleged sexual offenders display substantial response bias on psychological tests and that some measures used in forensic situations could be potentially misleading, given the evidence that there is substantial motivation on the part of the alleged offender to present an overly benign or malignant psychological image of themselves (Wasyliw *et al.*, 1994).

## Diagnostic studies of adult sexual offenders

The literature on psychiatric disorders in adults who sexually offend can be highly informative regarding adolescents who offend, particularly when approximately one-third of adult offenders begin offending in adolescence (Longo and Groth, 1983). While there are several studies of psychopathology in adults who have committed sexual offences, the degree of response bias and the methodological limitations that simply litter several of these studies need to be kept in mind. Studies need to be taken for what they are – an assessment of a particular group of men in particular circumstances, the results of which can not be generalised to the overall population of adults or adolescents who commit sexual offences.

### *Sexual offending and psychiatric disorder (Axis I) in adults*

There were few studies of the psychiatric diagnostic status of sexual offenders prior to the early 1980s when DSM-III (1980) was employed. Before this time data from studies were often based on file information, self-reports and non-standardised psychological assessment tools and led to results to which little weight can now be given. For example, Revitch (1965) reported that many sexual murderers were psychotic. Henn *et al.* (1976) found in a study of 239 defendants, that 38 per cent had personality disorders and 11 per cent schizophrenia or a schizoaffective disorder, though what diagnostic instrument was used is not stated.

In an early 1980s study, sixty-four men charged with at least one sexual offence were referred by the court for psychiatric evaluation (Bonheur and Rosner, 1981). Almost half of this group were aged between seventeen and twenty-one years. DSM-II (1968) criteria were used for diagnostic purposes. Schizophrenia was diagnosed in 47 per cent of cases. This was of course a biased sample as not all sexual offenders are arrested and those who are arrested are not necessarily prosecuted. Also, this was a select group singled out by the courts for psychiatric assessment and therefore with the likelihood of including more "psychiatric cases". The authors also point out that DSM-III would most likely have reclassified the schizophrenia group as having either schizophreniform disorder, atypical psychosis or a borderline, schizotypal or narcissistic personality disorder. Nevertheless, they stress that the majority of these defendants were troubled by chronic mental disorders.

A later study, using the same group of men, compared the psychiatric diagnoses of two offender groups: those charged with sexual crimes as well as larceny (SC&L) and those charged with sexual crimes (SC) only (Bonheur, 1983) In the SC&L group, 65 per cent suffered from one or another form of schizophrenic disorder in contrast to 38 per cent of the SC-only group. There is no indication of how diagnoses were made but again, if the revised edition of DSM-III had been available for the study then some men might have been reclassified. Also, the study is subject to the same sampling biases of its predecessor; the numbers are too small in one group and the distinction made between the two groups is spurious as those charged with larceny may not have committed it and those not charged with larceny may have committed offences unknown to the authorities.

Lau (1982) examined 142 sexual offenders remanded to a psychiatric observation unit in a prison; 24 per cent were regarded as schizophrenic while 66 per cent had no mental disorder. The study does not state how diagnoses were made. A further study evaluated ninety-five defendants charged with sexual offences (Packard and Rosner, 1985). Almost a third of this sample were under twenty-one years of age. One-fifth were given a diagnosis of schizophrenia, affective disorder or an atypical psychosis. Only 6 per cent of the sample were given a diagnosis of a paraphilia. Their sample was however made up primarily of minority groups (84% were either African-American or Hispanic).

In the early 1990s the quality of studies improved somewhat. Kafka and Prentky (1994) assessed DSM-III-R Axis I diagnoses of mood, anxiety, substance abuse disorders and impulse disorders not elsewhere classified (NOS) in a group of men with either paraphilias or paraphilia-related disorders (PRD). PRDs were defined as repetitive, intensely arousing sexual behaviours that endure for at least six months and are accompanied by significant distress or social impairment, but, in contrast to paraphilias, were not currently considered deviant – for instance, compulsive masturbation, dependence on pornography or phone sexual or sexual accessories such as objects (dildoes) or drugs (nitrates). Although 15 per cent of the sample reported no lifetime nonsexual Axis I co-morbid disorder, both groups reported a significant lifetime prevalence of any mood disorder (77%), especially early-onset dysthymic disorder (53%); any psychoactive substance abuse disorder (63%), especially alcohol abuse; any anxiety disorder (40%), especially social phobia; but a low prevalence of impulse disorders NOS (13.3%). They noted that no consistent diagnosis existed that distinguished males in the two groups. The concept of PRDs is open to criticism. It was originally based on the DSM-III-R classification of "nonparaphilic sexual addictions" (Sexual Disorders Not Otherwise Specified). This term was subsequently deleted for DSM-IV psychiatric diagnostic nosology, probably due to lack of empirical support.

In a study by Black *et al.* (1997) thirty-six respondents (8 female) to an advertisement for "compulsive sexual behaviour" were assessed using the National Institute for Mental Health (NIMH) Diagnostic Interview Schedule (DIS). Seventeen per cent of the sample reported no lifetime Axis I nonsexual disorder. However, lifetime prevalence was common: mood disorders (39%), especially major depression or dysthymia; anxiety disorders (50%), especially phobic disorder; and psychoactive substance abuse disorder (64%), especially alcohol abuse.

In a Swiss retrospective study of sixty-seven sexual offenders for whom a psychiatric expert report had been requested by the judicial authorities (Curtin and Niveau, 1998), psychiatric diagnoses were classified according to DSM-III and subsequent editions. Schizophrenia and other psychotic conditions were relatively rare (5%) whereas affective disorders were diagnosed in 12 to 14 per cent of all offenders. Paraphilias were identified in 24 per cent of the sexual offenders.

Firestone *et al.* (1998) assessed the DSM diagnostic status of forty-eight homicidal sexual offenders (HSO), compared to a group of incest offenders. Each offender was interviewed by a psychiatrist and given a DSM-III diagnosis. Compared to incest offenders, HSOs were more often diagnosed as suffering from psychosis (15% versus 0%), antisocial personality disorder (51% versus 4%), any paraphilia (79% versus 24%), atypical paraphilia (23% versus 2%), sexual sadism (75% versus 2%) and substance abuse (40% versus 6%). Seventy-five per cent of the HSOs had three or more diagnoses compared with 6 per cent of the incest offenders. There was also an increased rate of paraphilic co-morbidity in HSOs, which had been previously reported for rapists (Abel *et al.*, 1981) and sexual murderers (Langevin *et al.*, 1988). A limitation of this diagnostic study however was that the psychiatrists and research assistants were not blind to the group membership of the individuals under consideration so that the index offence of homicide may have influenced the DSM diagnoses.

McElroy *et al.* (1999) assessed the psychiatric features of thirty-six consecutive male sexual offenders admitted to prison, jail or probation to a residential treatment facility, using structured clinical interviews for DSM-IV Axis I and II disorders. Subjects had very high lifetime Axis I disorders (97%) with 78 per cent meeting criteria for three or more disorders. However, none had schizophrenia and only one had a schizoaffective disorder – bipolar type. Further analysis was performed on the subgroup of men with paraphilias. They were significantly younger than non-paraphilic offenders when they committed their first offence and were more likely to have co-morbid mood, anxiety and eating disorders. Like all other studies in this field, there are inherent problems in this study: small sample size, unblended psychiatric evaluators, no control group (including a non-sexual offender forensic group). The cohort may not be representative of sexual offenders in general, so that the high rates of Axis I disorders could represent recruitment bias. Also, McElroy points out the considerable definitional overlap in many diagnostic categories (i.e. bipolar mood disorders, some impulse control disorders, borderline and antisocial personality disorders) so that some participants may have been misclassified as having one or more such disorders. In addition, certain psychiatric diagnoses were not evaluated, for instance, a history of attention-deficit hyperactivity disorder which may have falsely elevated the diagnosis of bipolar disorder.

A Minneapolis study of forty-five paedophile sexual offenders engaged in residential or outpatient treatment programmes was conducted by Raymond *et al.* (1999). They used the Structured Clinical Interview for DSM-IV (SCID-P) for Axis I and II disorders and included only those who met criteria for paedophilia. Ninety-three per cent of the subjects met criteria for an Axis I disorder other than paedophilia, with 76 per cent having a current diagnosis. Fifty-six per cent of the subjects met criteria for five or more co-morbid conditions in addition to paedophilia. The lifetime prevalence of mood disorder was 67 per cent with 31 per cent currently meeting criteria. The most common diagnosis was major depression, with over half of the group reporting a history of this disorder and 20 per cent being currently depressed. Sixty-four per cent had a history of anxiety disorders with 53 per cent meeting criteria for current anxiety disorder. Sixty per cent had a history of substance abuse, 53 per cent met criteria for other paraphilia diagnoses and 34 per cent met criteria for a sexual dysfunction diagnosis.

In one of the few studies of female offenders Green and Kaplan (1994) assessed psychiatric diagnoses in eleven incarcerated female offenders using the Structured Clinical Interview for DSM-III-R (SCID). The mean number of Axis I diagnoses per offender was almost five (4.8). Sixty-four per cent experienced a past or current episode of depression; 73 per cent suffered substance abuse; 73 per cent suffered PTSD linked to previous physical or sexual abuse in childhood or adolescence.

#### *Summary*

Many adults who sexually molest children have paedophilia and other paraphilias (Abel *et al.*, 1988; Galli *et al.*, 1999). The studies above seem to indicate that paraphilia and sexual offending in adults may be associated with elevated rates of mood, substance abuse, obsessive-compulsive and impulse control disorders, and they may respond in part to agents with antidepressant or mood stabilising properties. More serious offences may be associated with increased psychopathology; however, it seems clear that as studies have improved over the years, prevalence rates for psychoses have fallen while rates for depression and anxiety have risen. Given that a substantial proportion of child molestation is perpetrated by adolescent males and that many paedophiles report that the onset of deviant sexual impulses and behaviours occurred before the age of eighteen, it is crucial to assess the presence of paedophilia (minus the age limitation), and mood and anxiety disorders in adolescents who sexually molest children.

### *Sexual offending and personality disorder (Axis II)*

Personality disorder is defined by ICD-10 as "a severe disturbance in the characterological constitution and behavioural tendencies of the individual, usually involving several areas of the personality, and nearly always associated with considerable personal and social disruption" (WHO, 1992, p. 202). It is considered unlikely that the diagnosis is appropriate before sixteen or seventeen years. Personality disorders, as defined, display "markedly disharmonious attitudes and behaviour, involving usually several areas of functioning, e.g., affectivity, arousal, impulse control, ways of perceiving and thinking, and style of relating to others" and the "abnormal behaviour pattern is enduring, of long-standing . . . [and] . . . is pervasive and clearly maladaptive to a broad range of personal and social situations" (WHO, 1992, p. 202).

The age criteria require some comment. ICD-10 states that "personality disorder tends to appear in late childhood or adolescence and continues to manifest itself into adulthood" (WHO, 1992, p. 202) and DSM-IV states that "the pattern is stable and of long duration and its onset can be traced back at least to adolescence or early adulthood" (APA, 1994, p. 633). In other words, although it may be present in a child or adolescent, one can only make the diagnosis after the age of sixteen or seventeen.

Several of the studies mentioned below have been referenced in the preceding section on Axis I disorders and the details of these studies can be found there. In Bonheur and Rosner's (1981) study of sixty-four male sexual offenders, thirty-three defendants had personality disorders (16% schizoid, 19% passive-aggressive and 16% inadequate). In Lau's (1982) study of 142 sexual offenders only 1.5 per cent had personality disorders. In Bonheur's (1983) later study, 35 per cent of the SC&L group suffered from a personality disorder in contrast to 62 per cent of the SC only group (primarily schizoid personality disorder). In the Swiss retrospective study of sixty-seven sexual offenders, a personality disorder was diagnosed in half of the offenders, borderline personality disorder (44%) and antisocial personality disorder (17%) being the most common (Curtin and Niveau, 1998).

In McElroy *et al.*'s study (1999) of thirty-six male sexual offenders, 94 per cent met DSM criteria for at least one Axis II disorder and 33 per cent met criteria for three or more. The most common displayed disorders were cluster B: 72 per cent met criteria for antisocial personality disorder, 42 per cent for borderline personality disorder and 17 per cent for narcissistic personality disorder. Also, 28 per cent met criteria for paranoid personality disorder (cluster A) and 25 per cent met criteria for obsessive-compulsive personality disorder (cluster C). There was also no difference between personality disorders in those with or without paraphilia.

In Raymond *et al.*'s (1999) study of forty-five paedophile sexual offenders' axis, 60 per cent received a diagnosis of personality disorder: cluster A (18%), cluster B (33%) and cluster C (43%). Commonest personality disorders were, obsessive-compulsive, antisocial, avoidant and narcissistic. The high incidence of personality disorder is in line with the prevalence of 43 per cent for personality disorders found in a group of New York sexual offenders (Packard and Rosner, 1985), though these were mostly either psychopathic, schizoid, schizotypal or paranoid personality disorders. Firestone *et al.* (1998)

compared the psychopathy status of forty-eight homicidal sexual offenders (HSO), all eighteen years or over, to a group of incest offenders, using the Psychopathy Checklist-Revised. The PCL-R is designed to assess antisocial behaviours (e.g. impulsivity, promiscuous sexual activity, criminal versatility, parasitic lifestyle, early behaviour problems, juvenile delinquency) and personality characteristics (e.g. glibness/superficial charm, grandiose sense of self-worth, callous/lack of empathy, shallow affect) considered fundamental to psychopathy (Hare, 1991). The HSO group were found to have significantly more psychopathic features than the incest offenders on Factor 1 (personality traits) and Factor 2 (antisocial history). The HSOs, compared with other pathological and criminal populations, show relatively greater personality disturbance than criminal behaviour.

In Green and Kaplan's (1994) study of eleven incarcerated female offenders, they also administered the SCID-II for personality disorders. The mean number of Axis II diagnoses was almost four (3.6). Avoidant, borderline and dependent personality disorders were the most frequent amongst this group.

### *Summary*

Personality disorders are likely to be present in adults who sexually offend, ranging from somewhere between 60 per cent (for those engaged in court-ordered residential or outpatient treatment programmes) to over 90 per cent (for those in prison or on probation to a residential treatment facility); antisocial, borderline, schizoid and paranoid, and obsessive-compulsive personality disorders being the most frequent. Given that personality disorders have their origins in childhood or adolescence, then it is likely that some manifestations of these disorders are identifiable in many adolescents who sexually offend, for instance, as conduct disorders, OCD symptoms, impulse control disorders or emergent borderline personality disorders. Conduct disorder is a well-accepted precursor of antisocial personality disorder in adults.

## *Schizophrenia and schizophrenic-spectrum disorders*

Although recent studies indicate very low rates of schizophrenia among sexual offenders, the frequent finding in older studies of schizophrenia or schizophrenia-spectrum disorders merits particular attention. Henderson and Kalichman (1990) suggest that a proportion of sexual offenders are characterised by signs of severe thought disorder. In their review of the literature on MMPI profiles with sexual offenders, they concluded that elevated scores on Scale 8 (Schizophrenia) and Scale 4 (Psychopathic Deviate) are frequently found in offenders who sexually assault adults or children, though the latter group appear to have higher Scale 8 scores. Elevations on the Scale 8 would indicate disturbed thoughts, interpersonal alienation and hostility. It is not however a diagnosis of schizophrenia.

Henderson and Kalichman (1990) compared MMPI profiles for 113 men found guilty of sexual offences against children with paraphilic symptoms computed from the Multiphasic Sex Inventory completed by the men. The MMPI scales indicative of obsessive-compulsive thinking (Scale 7) and disturbed thought processes (Scale 8) correlated strongly with self-reported paraphilic activity. Child sexual offenders frequently have high scores on the following MMPI scales; Scale 2 (Depression), Scale 6 (Paranoia), Scale 8 (Schizophrenia) and Scale 0 (Social Introversion) when compared with those whose sexual offending is directed against adults (Levin and Stava, 1987). One study assessed 144 men using the MMPI (Kalichman, 1991). The men were divided into three groups: those that abused prepubescent, post-pubescent or adult victims. The child offenders appeared more emotionally disturbed, immature and distressed than their adult offender counterparts who appeared more antisocial, sociopathic and defensive. Kalichman believes his results support Finkelhor and Araji's (1986) hypothesis that the personality of sexual offenders tends to be congruent with the developmental period of their victims. However, the group studied consisted of incarcerated criminal sexual offenders and the results cannot be generalized to non-convicted or forensic hospital patients.

One interpretation of these MMPI findings in the context of sexual offenders is that they may be describing a schizotypic profile, suggesting a link between sexually deviant behaviour and schizotypy (Kalichman, 1990). Based on Meehl's seminal work on schizophrenic thought disturbance (Meehl, 1962), schizotypy is seen to occur in the mid-range of a spectrum from a schizotaxic genotype in the absence of symptom expression to full phenotypic schizophrenia. Schizotypy presents with variable levels of cognitive slippage, affective disturbances, perceptual aberration, and social anhedonia, among other elements of psychopathology. Meehl's schizotypy is similar, though not identical to schizotypal and schizoid personality disorders as defined in DSM-IV and ICD-10. He described a group with chaotic sexuality, defined as either acted-out or fantasised episodes characterised by a scrambling of heterosexual, homosexual, autoerotic, voyeuristic-exhibitionistic, sado-masochistic, oral, anal and genital components (Henderson and Kalichman, 1990). Dunaif and Hoch (1955) described seven case studies of men with what would now be termed schizotypal disorder. All men had been convicted of sexual offences yet were presented in the paper to illustrate schizotypal disorder. Schizotypal disorder is considered to be part of the genetic spectrum of schizophrenia but which pursues a course more similar to that of a personality disorder. One of the criteria for the diagnosis of schizotypal personality disorder is the presence of "obsessive ruminations without inner resistance, often with dysmorphophobic, sexual or aggressive contents" (WHO, 1992, p. 96). This criterion is not included in the DSM-IV definition.

So, there appears to be a subgroup of sexual offenders who are schizotypic and present with disturbed thought processes as well as sexual deviances

(Henderson and Kalichman, 1990). Indeed, further criteria for schizotypal disorder include excessive social anxiety and lack of close friends (DSM-IV), poor rapport with others and a tendency to social withdrawal (ICD-10) – social skills deficits are frequently evident in those who sexually offend. The false beliefs, distorted perceptions and irrational justifications concerning violence against women reported from several studies of sexual offenders may be accounted for in some cases, especially those characterised as paraphilic, by a more general disturbance in thought processes. In those cases where obsessive ruminations coexist, risk of sexual offending may be substantial.

### *Mental illness and adult sexual offending: conclusions*

There is extensive research on the relationship between violent crime and mental illness, but not between sexual violence and mental illness (McElroy *et al.*, 1999). This chapter has thus far drawn together work on adult offenders from a clinical and a forensic perspective, alongside specific research on schizophrenia-spectrum disorders in sexual offenders. One tentative conclusion can be made: a substantial proportion of adult sexual offenders may suffer from a wide range of psychiatric disorders, including paraphilias, substance abuse disorders, mood and anxiety disorders, psychotic disorders, schizophrenia-spectrum disorders and personality disorders. Besides those with antisocial personality disorders, at particular risk may be those individuals with disturbances of thought, social isolation and depression, who entertain obsessive ruminations of a poorly focused sexual nature, and without inner resistance.

## Diagnostic studies of adolescent sexual offenders

Few systematic studies have been carried out on adolescents who sexually abuse other children. Galli *et al.* (1999) pointed out that although these studies generally report high rates of psychopathology, the vast majority of the studies did not use operational diagnostic criteria or structured clinical interviews to assess psychiatric disorders. Also, adolescents who commit sexual offences have been studied in various different settings and often offences of varying severity have been grouped together. However, unlike adult studies, several of the studies used comparison or control groups.

### *Sexual offending and psychiatric disorders (Axis I) in adolescents*

An early study of twenty-five juveniles referred for psychiatric examination because of what was termed “some type of sexual perversion” revealed that the “perverted sexual pattern” was inextricably linked with a pattern of general delinquency in most of the twenty-five cases (Waggoner and Boyd, 1941). Atcheson and Williams (1954) reviewed records of male and female juvenile offenders (7–16 years) in Toronto from 1939 to 1984 and compared these with a randomly selected sample of other offenders. They found a sixfold increase in "serious personality maladjustment" (based on recorded psychiatric symptomatology, previous inpatient or outpatient stay) in the male sexual offender group compared to the control nonsexual offender group.

Lewis *et al.* (1979) compared seventeen juvenile males incarcerated in a secure unit for violent sexual assaults to sixty-one boys incarcerated for violent nonsexual acts. They found that both groups had a high prevalence of psychiatric symptoms. For the sexual offenders, 75 per cent had symptoms of depression, 46 per cent had auditory hallucinations, 73 per cent had paranoid symptoms, and 70 per cent had loose, rambling, illogical thought processes. This study was based on symptom assessment, and did not use structured interviewing and did not assess for diagnostic status.

Becker *et al.* (1991) assessed depressive symptomatology using the Beck Depression Inventory (BDI) in 246 male juvenile sexual offenders. The BDI is a self-report measure for depressive symptomatology with good reliability and validity. All subjects were judged to be non-psychotic on clinical interview. The mean score for the group was found to be in the mildly depressed range (14.3) and 42 per cent attained scores above 15 putting them in the moderate to severe depression (major depression) range. Those with a history of sexual or physical abuse had significantly high scores – 49 per cent of whom had scores indicative of major depression compared with 37 per cent of the non-abused group. Becker *et al.* point out that it was impossible to tell whether the depressive symptoms predated the occurrence of sexually offending behaviour or were instead due to the disclosure of the abuse and its consequences.

Twenty-nine adolescent child molesters were assessed using a battery of tests and assessments that included a DSM-III diagnosis (Awad and Saunders, 1989). They had been caught, brought to the attention of the police and had either admitted their guilt or been found guilty in court. Forty-eight per cent had a diagnosed learning disability and one-third had been diagnosed as suffering from emotional problems prior to committing a sexual offence. Eighty-seven per cent were found to suffer from a diagnosable psychiatric disorder, though the types are not stated. Forty-five per cent showed antisocial kinds of behaviour and about half of that group had a delinquency record predating the sexual offences. A third had received outpatient psychiatric treatment prior to their referral. They concluded that there was an overlap between serious psychopathology and both antisocial and sexually deviant behaviour and that psychopathology characterised the majority of these offenders. Also, psychopathology per se (excluding conduct disorder and sexual deviance) could not be considered a cause of the offence since there was a wide range of psychopathology and the majority of male adolescents showing these disorders do not commit sexual offences (Awad and Saunders, 1989).

Twenty-eight adolescent sexual offenders (ASO) were compared with thirty-three conduct disordered adolescents (CD) and thirty-four adolescents in a control group (CA) (Hastings *et al.*, 1997). The offender group were recruited from both outpatients and inpatients and were homogeneous with regard to offence (child sexual abuse, at least five years younger and under sixteen, genital stimulation, oral sex or penetration). They were administered the Revised Behaviour Problem Checklist (RBPC) which consists of six scales (ADHD, anxiety/withdrawal, conduct disorder, socialized aggression, psychotic behaviour and motor excess). Significant group differences were found on all subscales. Socialised aggression was significantly higher for CD than ASO, and for the ASO than the CA group. For all other subscales, the CD and ASO groups scored significantly higher than the CA group but there were no other significant differences between the CD and ASO groups.

In another study, nineteen adolescent males who had made obscene phone calls or committed exhibitionism ("hands off" offences) were assessed by clinical interview (Saunders and Awad, 1991). Seventy-nine per cent of the adolescents had chronic learning difficulties; 58 per cent had a history of antisocial behaviour; 79 per cent were considered moderately to severely maladjusted. However, it is not clear what criteria were used in arriving at these conclusions. Ten of the sample had also committed "hands on" offences.

Kavoussi *et al.* (1988), in the first report using structured clinical interviews (SCID and K-SADS) to assess DSM-III disorders found, in a sample of fifty-eight outpatient adolescent male offenders, a high rate of conduct disorder (48%) but comparatively low rates of psychotic, mood and attention deficit/hyperactivity disorders. Substance abuse (marijuana or alcohol) was the only other diagnosis found in more than 10 per cent of the sample. None of the subjects met full criteria for major affective disorder, dysthymia or psychotic disturbance. Nineteen per cent of the juveniles had no psychiatric diagnosis; however, 20 per cent of the sample had some symptoms of adjustment disorder with depressed mood, usually as a result of being arrested. The low rates of psychiatric disorder could be explained by the fact that those sexual offenders with more severe psychopathology were not referred to this particular programme and were more likely to be in a hospital or residential setting. Also, the SCID (used in this study to assess affective, psychotic, anxiety disorders and substance abuse) is primarily an adult interview and its reliability with adolescents is questionable.

Twenty-six incarcerated sexual offenders (aged 9–14) were compared with a control group of conduct-disordered youth, matched for age, sex and ethnic status (Shaw *et al.*, 1993). The DSM-IV Field Trials version of the National Institute of Mental Health (NIMH) Diagnostic Interview Schedule for Children (DISC-2) was used to establish DSM-III, ICD-10 and Draft

DSM-IV criteria for a range of diagnoses, though ADHD was omitted from the study. Twenty-one adolescent sexual offenders (81%) met criteria for conduct disorder (two more just fell short of full criteria); anxiety disorder was present in 50 per cent, major depression or dysthymia (35%) and PTSD (12%). The two groups didn't differ regarding diagnoses. The authors concluded that sexual offending (which is a symptom of conduct disorder in DSM-III-R) is closely linked to the diagnosis of conduct disorder. This study has several limitations. Its sample size is small and selective in that the boys were only accepted to the unit on the basis of having admitted their offences, having an Intelligence Quotient over 70 and the absence of psychosis; and many of the boys had used considerable force and coercion in their offences. Also, very few parents of the sexual offender group were available for interview for the DISC-2.

### *ADHD, Tourette's syndrome and OCD*

Few studies have specifically looked at Attention Deficit Hyperactivity Disorder amongst adolescent sexual offenders. Kafka and Prentky followed up their 1994 adult study with a similar study that included a retrospective evaluation for the prevalence of childhood ADHD as defined by DSM-III-R (Kafka and Prentky, 1998). The study included sixty outpatient males (aged 15–59 years) seeking treatment for paraphilia (PA) or paraphilia-related disorders (PRDs). A semistructured questionnaire was used to detect DSM-III-R mood, anxiety, substance abuse, impulse NOS and attention-deficit disorders. The Wender Utah Rating Scale (WURS) was also used to assess retrospectively the symptoms of childhood-onset ADHD in adults. Subjects in both groups were diagnosed as having lifetime prevalence of any mood disorder (72%), especially dysthymic disorder (67%); any anxiety disorder (43%), especially social phobia (28%); any psychoactive substance abuse disorder (45%), especially alcohol abuse (30%); and any impulse disorder NOS (25%), especially speeding and reckless driving (17%). The only diagnosis that significantly distinguished the two groups was retrospectively diagnosed childhood ADHD, identified in 40 per cent of the total sample (50% of PA vs. 17% of PRD). They concluded that although depressive disorders were the most common diagnoses across groups, childhood ADHD was the only disorder significantly associated with paraphilias, or socially deviant and aggressive forms of sexual impulsivity. The diagnosis of childhood ADHD did not however distinguish paraphilic sexual offenders from non-offending paraphilic subjects. Although sample size in this study was sufficient for statistical comparison between the PA and PRD groups, they were not so for the offender and non-offender paedophile subgroups. The validity and reliability of the diagnostic inventories, including the lifetime assessment of ADHD, had also not been rigorously tested. Diagnostic evaluations were performed non-blind. The samples were biased because, as rightly pointed out by the authors, the men who seek treatment at a specialised treatment centre are more likely to have increased co-morbidity or increased severity of illness in comparison with a population-based sample (Kafka and Prentky, 1994).

Galli *et al.* (1999) assessed the psychiatric status of twenty-two adolescent males who had sexually molested a child at least once. All had admitted to their offence. They used structured clinical interviews for DSM-III-R Axis I disorders (including sections on ADHD and conduct disorders) and a semi-structured interview for DSM-III-R diagnosis of paedophilia. The sexual molestation behaviour of all subjects met A and B criteria for paedophilia (with the exception of the age requirement – Criterion C). All subjects described having impulses or urges to have sex with younger children. Thirty-six per cent described their sexual impulses as recurrent, intrusive and resisted. However, 64 per cent reported that they usually did not resist their impulses and acted on them whenever possible. In addition, 95 per cent reached diagnostic criteria for two or more paraphilias, 82 per cent for a mood disorder (55% for a bipolar disorder), 55 per cent for an anxiety disorder, 50 per cent for a substance abuse disorder, and 55 for an impulse-control disorder. Seventy-one per cent of seventeen subjects were diagnosed with ADHD and 94 per cent with conduct disorder. They concluded that some adolescent child molesters may have paedophilia or other paraphilias. Other disorders with impulsive features, especially conduct, attention-deficit/hyperactivity, bipolar and substance abuse disorders, may also be found in these adolescents (Galli *et al.*, 1999). The authors conclude that their findings are consistent with other findings of high rates of depressive and psychotic symptoms (Lewis *et al.*, 1979), conduct disorder (Kavoussi *et al.*, 1988), multiple paraphilias in adult male sexual offenders (Abel *et al.*, 1988), multiple deviant sexual behaviours in adolescent sexual offenders (Fehrenbach *et al.*, 1986; Awad and Saunders, 1989), and of co-morbid mood, substance abuse and anxiety disorders in adults with paedophilias (Kafka, 1995; Kruesi *et al.*, 1992). The limitations of this study are its small sample size, lack of a control group, recruitment of some subjects from psychiatric institutions, lack of validity and reliability of some of the assessment tools, and evaluation of psychiatric diagnosis by an un-blind investigator.

Further studies that included ADHD and Tourette's syndrome (TS) – a hereditary tic and disinhibition disorder – have been conducted. In a study of satiation therapy for thirty-nine juvenile sexual offenders, 59 per cent had a secondary psychiatric diagnosis of learning disability and/or ADHD (Hunter and Goodwin, 1992). No indication is given of how the authors arrived at this diagnosis. Increased frequency of exhibitionism has been reported in TS (Comings and Comings, 1982; Eldridge *et al.*, 1977; Nee *et al.*, 1980). Exhibitionism was reported in 19 per cent of severe TS subjects, in 17 per cent of TS with ADHD, and in 8 per cent of all TS subjects (Comings and Comings, 1987). When TS patients had co-morbid ADHD, the frequency of sexual disorders was consistently much higher than the TS subjects who did not have

ADHD. However, almost every sexual behaviour problem studied was more common in TS subjects without ADHD than in ADHD subjects without TS – suggesting that ADHD is only a contributory factor to the sexual behaviour problems of TS subjects. Also, when OCD is co-morbid with TS, this leads to a significant increase in aberrant sexual behaviours (Comings, 1994). Comings concluded that many of the sexual behaviour problems seen in TS are variants of OCD and are in part, genetically driven obsessive-compulsive behaviours.

The best-documented co-morbid diagnoses for Tic Disorders (including Tourette's) are OCD and ADHD (Castellanos, 1998; Comings and Comings, 1984; Knell and Comings, 1993; Pauls *et al.*, 1993), suggesting strong evidence for TS, OCD and ADHD being neuropsychiatric spectrum disorders. Interestingly, children or adolescents who manifest both TS and ADHD are qualitatively distinct from those with TS only (Schuerholz *et al.*, 1996) and OCD symptoms in patients co-morbid for TS are more likely to relate to aggressive, religious and sexual themes (Leckman *et al.*, 1994).

### *Personality typology and MMPI profiles in adolescent sexual offenders*

Carpenter *et al.* (1995) compared sixteen adolescents who sexually offended against peers with twenty who sexually offended against children, using the Millon Clinical Multiaxial Inventory. This psychometric scale yields eight DSM-III-R Axis II basic personality patterns. Adolescent child offenders appeared more schizoid, dependent and avoidant than peer offenders. There was no difference on the antisocial, histrionic or narcissistic scales, though both groups entered the clinically significant range on the antisocial personality scale, and for the peer group offenders, the degree of narcissism was clinically significant.

Smith *et al.* (1987) administered the MMPI to 262 adolescent sexual offenders (less than 1% of whom were incarcerated), representing a relatively less violent, less aggressive population. On the basis of the results, the authors provided four mean profiles, based on the descriptive narratives formulated by Marks *et al.* (1974), which were described as follows:

*Group I:* Normal range profile. Likely to be shy, over-controlled and a worrier with few friends; attempts to portray self as morally above reproach.

*Group II:* Most disturbed profile. Likely to be demanding and narcissistic, using illness (particularly physical illness) to gain attention. Argumentative, insecure, and likely to over-rely on personal fantasy to solve problems.

*Group III:* Normal range profile. Likely to be frank and realistic in describing self. Socially outgoing, normal affect and no impaired judgement. Likely to be emotionally over-controlled and given to (perhaps violent) emotional outbursts.

*Group IV:* Abnormal range profile. Likely to impulsively act-out, display poor self-control and poor judgement. Distrust and alienation likely to be prominent. Vulnerable to perceived threat; likely to strike out in anticipation. Schizoid and under-socialised.

Jacobs *et al.* (1997) assessed 156 incarcerated sexual and nonsexual juvenile offenders using the MMPI-A (adolescent version), the MMPI-2 and Hare's Psychopathy Checklist – Revised (PCL-R). There were trends of differences in Scale 6 (Paranoia), Scale 0 (Social introversion) and Scale 8 (Schizophrenia). Scores on each of these scales were higher in the sexual offender group. There were no group differences on the PCL-R scores. This study is limited by the use of the PCL-R on institutional records rather than on interview with the subject.

Losada-Paisey (1998) administered the MMPI-A to twenty-one juvenile male sexual offenders and thirty adolescents with non-sexual offences. All subjects were diagnosed as conduct-disordered by the attending psychiatrist. She found that Scale 3 (Hysteria) and Scale 7 (Psychasthenia) of the MMPI-A contributed primarily to juveniles being classified as non-sexual offenders whereas Scale 4 (Psychopathic Deviate) and Scale 8 (Schizophrenia) contributed primarily to subjects being classified as sexual offenders. In other words, antisocial personality traits and cognitive disorganisation as measured on the clinical scales of the MMPI-A can differentiate the adolescent non-sex from the adolescent sexual offender.

Herkov *et al.* (1996) administered the MMPI to sixty-one adolescent sexual offenders (divided into those accused of sexual abuse, rape or sodomy) and compared these to MMPI scores for fifteen adolescent psychiatric inpatients. The adolescent sexual offenders demonstrated significantly more psychopathology than those in the inpatient group. In general, increased psychopathology was associated with increased sexual deviancy. Analysis of MMPI two-point code types (a strategy for interpreting profiles when more than one of the clinical scales is elevated) revealed that Scale 6 (Paranoia) and Scale 8 (Schizophrenia) were frequently associated with the adolescents who had engaged in sodomy. A high incidence of Scale 8 as a two-point code was also associated with the rape group. The two-point coding of 6–8/8–6 has long been recognised as indicating serious psychopathology in teenagers and adults, social isolation, withdrawal and difficulties in thought processes (Archer, 1987; 1997). The two-point coding of 2–4/4–2 (Depression/Psychopathic Deviate) was most frequently associated with those accused of sexual abuse and with psychiatric inpatients, many of whom had a diagnosis of conduct disorder. The authors suggest that there may be a subgroup of juveniles whose sexual behaviour (sodomy, rape) represents a more ingrained deviant sexual arousal pattern associated with increased psychopathology.

The study was however limited by small sample size and differences in race and IQ between the groups.

### *Adolescents who commit sexual homicide*

A special group that deserves mention are adolescents who commit sexual homicide. In adult sexual murders, it is believed that psychopathology is common, particularly personality disorder diagnoses of the antisocial, narcissistic, borderline and sadistic types (Liebert, 1985; Myers *et al.*, 1993; Ressler *et al.*, 1988). Case reports are scattered throughout the literature of the last half-century of adolescents who commit sexual homicide. Myers (1994) reported on three cases of adolescent sexual homicide. Two of the three boys were diagnosed with conduct disorder and all three had signs of neuropsychiatric dysfunction (e.g. learning difficulties, past encephalopathic events).

More recently, Myers and Blashfield (1997) conducted a study where fourteen adolescents who had committed sexual homicide were administered the DSM-III-R Diagnostic Interview for Children and Adolescents (DICA-R), a structured diagnostic interview that covers the major psychiatric disorders of childhood; the Schedule for Nonadaptive and Adaptive Personality (SNAP), a self-report inventory that yields DSM-III-R personality disorders; and the Revised Psychopathy Checklist (PCL-R). Twelve youths (86%) manifested one or more Axis I diagnoses at the time of the crimes, conduct disorder occurring in all cases. Substance abuse (43%), ADHD (21%), anxiety disorders (21%) and dysthymia (14%) were the most frequent co-morbid conditions. None of the youths was found to have a current or past psychotic disorder – however, psychotic symptoms were found in the pasts of 11 per cent of the sample (probably explained by the personality disorder typology of the group). Sixty-two per cent met SNAP criteria for at least one personality disorder. Contrary to expectations, antisocial and borderline diagnoses did not occur frequently. In fact, the youths demonstrated more cluster "A" symptomatology (the paranoid, schizoid and schizotypal personality disorder spectrum) than cluster "B" (the antisocial, borderline, histrionic and narcissistic personality disorder spectrum). Also, 31 per cent had sadistic personality features. The mean PCL-R score for the group was indicative of moderate psychopathic disturbance.

## Conclusions

When drawing conclusions from these studies the same reservations regarding adult studies pertain: dissimulation and methodology. Also, studies of the psychological characteristics and psychopathology of sexual abusers are inevitably skewed, as only a small percentage of sexual abusers are actually caught (Harvey and Herman, 1992).

The assessment of sexual deviance in adolescents presents very complex problems. These adolescents do not meet DSM-IV criteria for paraphilia (which specifies a lower age limit of sixteen). In addition, DSM-IV does not provide a suitable alternative diagnosis that would give prominence to the sexual offending behaviours. While the diagnosis of conduct disorder can usually be made in these cases, its broad applicability to a variety of non-conforming children and adolescents limits its usefulness for research and treatment planning in cases of adolescent sexual offending. Many adult sexual offenders begin sexual offending in adolescence, and this fact indicates that, retrospectively, a diagnosis of sexual deviance in adolescence could have been made. This situation is comparable with the DSM-IV guidelines for personality disorder diagnoses which are seen as having an onset in adolescence but which, as a rule, are not applied in diagnosing adolescents. DSM definitions of paraphilic behaviour should be modified to make them applicable to adolescent sexual offenders.

With these reservations in mind, the review above appears to support and extend the view that there is a spectrum of adolescent sexual offenders that includes the true paraphiliac, those whose impulse control is compromised by concurrent conduct disorder or other psychiatric disorder and those whose social and interpersonal skills result in them turning to younger children for sexual gratification unavailable from peers. Also, sexual offending appears to be strongly linked to conduct disorder, particularly in those youths who force sex or whose sexual offending is considered more serious. For some boys who sexually offend and also have conduct disorder, their sexual offending behaviour may be as described by Shaw *et al.* (1993) but an interesting variation on a well-established matrix of antisocial and aggressive behaviour. In many cases, there will be a complicating learning disability (48–79% reported).

Given the prevalence rates for mood disorders and attention-deficit disorders indicated in some studies, a presumptive relationship between mood disorders (especially dysthymia), ADHD and paraphilic sexuality may exist and certainly merits further examination. Early-onset dysthymic disorder and ADHD during the formative developmental years could have a particularly pathoplastic effect on developing male sexuality, conducive to disregulated sexual appetite, thrill-seeking behaviour, social deviancy and impaired impulse control. This is further supported by the only study of genetic factors associated with deviant sexual behaviours in Tourette's syndrome. Those subjects with both Tourette's syndrome and ADHD had the most disinhibited forms of sexual expression (Comings, 1994). The presence of serious psychopathology (MMPI profiles) in adolescents accused of sodomy and rape and Cluster A personality types on SNAP assessments of adolescents who commit sexual homicide suggests a potentially serious influence of schizophrenic-spectrum disorders on the sexual behaviour of some adolescents. Over-anxious, ruminative and compulsive traits in unsocialised adolescents could also provide a fertile ground for deviant sexual fantasies to emerge.

### *Implications for assessment and intervention*

The evaluation of mentally ill adolescent sexual offenders is a common task facing mental health professionals and a challenging problem. Psychiatric co-morbidity is clearly more often the rule than the exception in adolescents who sexually offend (Shaw *et al.*, 1993). Major mental disorders and substance abuse disorders may adversely affect the expression of and any attempt to modify sexually deviant behaviour (Zonana and Norko, 1999). Therefore, it is crucial to evaluate the nature of the mental disorder and to clearly establish the relationship between manifestations of any mental disorder and the sexual-offending behaviour. There is evidence that adults, and perhaps adolescents, who commit sexual crimes, especially those who present with affective, anxiety or eating disorder symptoms, should be evaluated for paraphilias even if they deny such symptoms. Conversely, sexual offenders with paraphilias should be carefully evaluated for mood, anxiety and eating disorders (McElroy *et al.*, 1999).

Zonana and Norko (1999) suggest the following questions: What symptoms does the individual have and are these temporally linked to the sexual offending behaviour? Has the risk of offending behaviour increased historically in the presence of delusions, hallucinations, mania, depression, alcohol use, substance use, obsessional thoughts and so on? Affirmative answers will obviously guide treatment and monitoring and control of symptoms. Mental health interventions in these individuals should then be established as a necessary, but not sufficient means towards diminishing sexual-offending behaviour.

From studies of adult sexual offenders, and given the methodological reservations already stated, attention to the diagnosis and treatment of co-morbid psychiatric disorders is essential to the treatment of this population. Mood, anxiety, substance abuse disorders and paraphilias are the most common diagnoses and need to be assessed, since the presence of these problems may interfere with response to offence-specific work. In adolescents, in addition to these disorders, the presence of ADHD and borderline psychotic symptoms should routinely be assessed.

Since many adolescent sexual offenders have serious mental illnesses underlying their deviant sexual behaviour, offender treatment programmes, especially those dealing with the more serious offenders, would be substantially enhanced by the incorporation of a variety of treatment interventions typically used with individuals with serious psychopathology, including the exploration of possible psychotrophic medications. The adolescent sexual offender group is heterogeneous in nature and no single treatment regimen will be effective in all cases (Kavoussi *et al.*, 1988). An adolescent with psychosis or an affective disorder should be specifically treated for this (with lithium, antipsychotics, antidepressants, etc.) and then re-evaluated for sexual offending potential. Similarly, with impulse control problems related to ADHD, stimulants may be the preferential treatment.

Also, the presence of paraphilia (minus the age criterion) should be considered, as it may be amenable, in part, to pharmacological treatment. Treatment of some paraphilic sexual offenders has been promising despite the fact that long-term recidivism studies proving effectiveness are lacking (Zonana and Norko, 1999). Psychiatrists and psychiatric training programmes have generally avoided these disorders. With the finding that SSRIs – used by psychiatrists to treat depression and OCD – are useful in the treatment of paraphilias, psychiatrists may be more willing to consider providing treatment for this group.

The evidence from several studies that personality characteristics of offenders are heterogeneous, and that, for instance, peer offenders may differ in general from child offenders (Carpenter *et al.*, 1995), indicates that the design and implementation of adolescent sexual offender treatment programmes may be enhanced if these personality differences are taken into account. Social skills training may be particularly important for those adolescents who offend against younger children. As there appears to be a subgroup of offenders with schizotypal disorder, all adolescents and adults who sexually offend should be assessed for schizotypal features, especially those who commit very serious offences and when there is a family history of psychiatric disorder. Their management and intervention will need to be geared towards their wider needs and take into account additional symptoms they may display, for instance, paranoid ideation. It is unlikely that someone with schizotypal disorder will do well in a confrontative group setting; such an experience could be disintegrative or precipitate an overt schizophrenic disorder. Also, there are implications for follow-up. This group do not do well in treatment. If their distorted sexual offence-related thinking is indicative of wider disorders in thought processes then a cognitive approach aimed at distorted sexual offence-related thinking alone may be insufficient in reducing risk in the medium to long term.

Lack of progress in treatment is often attributed to poor motivation, inattentiveness, resistance and denial. It seems likely that unrecognised psychiatric conditions contribute to the difficulties that individuals face when they try to engage in the process of therapy and complete therapeutic tasks. It is important to take into account these co-morbid conditions when individualising treatment within sexual offender treatment programmes.

Many adolescent sexual offender treatment programmes have been set up on an ad hoc basis by enthusiastic health professionals with limited resources. They are often insufficiently multidisciplinary in nature and there can be considerable difficulty accessing expensive psychiatric involvement. Given the high incidence of psychiatric disorder in adolescents who sexually offend, programmes should have the availability on a regular, sessional basis, of an adolescent psychiatrist to assess mental state and to provide sufficient psychiatric input to ensure that co-morbid psychiatric disorders are assessed, treated adequately and programmes adjusted, where necessary, to meet the particular psychiatric and personality needs of each individual.

Where resources are limited and referral to an external psychiatric service is all that is available, then some screening procedures should be in place to ensure that those adolescents with psychiatric disorder are referred, rather than their psychiatric problems being lost in what is, inevitably, the glare of their sexual offending. Combining the use of the Child Behaviour Checklist (Achenbach, 1991a), The Youth Self-Report (Achenbach, 1991b), the Children's Yale-Brown Obsessive Compulsive Scale (Scahill *et al.*, 1997), the State-Trait Anxiety Inventory for Children (Speilberger *et al.*, 1973), the Childhood Depression Inventory (Kovacs and Beck, 1977) for younger adolescents or the Beck Depression Inventory II (Beck, 1996) for older adolescents, the Connors' Teacher and Parent Rating Scales – Revised (Conners, 1996) and the MMPI-A (Butcher *et al.*, 1992) may help as initial screenings for psychiatric disorders like depression, anxiety, ADHD, OCD and schizotypal disorder. However, these measures cannot be used to determine diagnosis because the items do not parallel diagnostic criteria, and onset and duration information is not requested (Hodges, 1993). Also, there is evidence that the sensitivity of the questionnaires is too low for diagnostic purposes. Nevertheless, they remain useful screening tools and their application may help treatment programmes remain vigilant to co-morbid and sometimes occult psychiatric symptomatology.

## References

Abel, G. G., Blanchard, E. B., and Barlow, D. H. (1981). Measurement of sexual arousal in several paraphilias: The effects of stimulus modality, instructional set and stimulus content on the objective. *Behaviour Research and Therapy, 19*, 25–33.

Abel, G. G., Rouleau, J., and Cunningham-Rathner, J. (1986). Sexually aggressive behavior. In W. Curren, A. L. McGarry, and S. A. Shah (eds), *Forensic Psychiatry and Psychology: Perspectives and Standards for Interdisciplinary Practice*. Philadelphia: F. A. Davis.

Abel, G. G., Becker, J. V., Cunningham-Rathner, J., Mittelman, M., and Rouleau, J. L. (1988). Multiple paraphilic diagnoses among sex offenders. *Bulletin of the American Academy of Psychiatry and Law, 16(2)*, 153–168.

Achenbach, T. (1991a). *Manual for the Child Behavior Checklistl 4–18 and 1991 Profile*. Burlington, VT: University of Vermont, Department of Psychiatry.

Achenbach, T. (1991b). *Manual for the Youth Self-Report and 1991 Profile*. Burlington, VT: University of Vermont, Department of Psychiatry.

APA (1968). *Diagnostic and Statistical Manual of Mental Diseases*, 2nd edn (DSM-II). Washington, DC: American Psychiatric Association.

APA (1980). *Diagnostic and Statistical Manual of Mental Diseases*, 3rd edn (DSM-III). Washington, DC: American Psychiatric Association.

APA (1987). *Diagnostic and Statistical Manual of Mental Diseases*, 3rd edn revised (DSM-III-R). Washington, DC: American Psychiatric Association.

APA (1994). *Diagnostic and Statistical Manual of Mental Diseases*, 4th edn (DSM-IV). Washington, DC: American Psychiatric Association.

Archer, R. P. (1987). *Using the MMPI with Adolescents*. Hillsdale, NJ: Lawrence Erlbaum.

Archer, R. P. (1997). *MMPI-A: Assessing Adolescent Psychopathology*. Mahwah, NJ: Lawrence Erlbaum.

Atcheson, J. D., and Williams, D. C. (1954). A study of juvenile sex offenders. *American Journal of Psychiatry, 111*, 366–370.

Awad, G. A., and Saunders, E. B. (1989). Adolescent child molesters: Clinical observations. *Child Psychiatry and Human Development, 19*, 195–206.

Beck, A. T. (1996). *Beck Depression Inventory – II*. San Antonio, TX: Psychological Corporation.

Becker, J. V., Kaplan, M. S., Tenke, C. E., and Tartaglini, A. (1991). The incidence of depressive symptomatology in juvenile sex offenders with a history of abuse. *Child Abuse and Neglect, 15*, 531–536.

Bianchi, M. D. (1990). Fluozetine treatment of exhibitionism. *American Journal of Psychiatry, 147*, 1089–1090.

Black, D. W., Kehrberg, L. L. D., Flumerfelt, D. L., *et al.* (1997). Characteristics of 36 subjects reporting compulsive sexual behaviour. *American Journal of Psychiatry, 154*, 243–249.

Bonheur, H. H. (1983). Psychodiagnostic testing of sex offenders: A comparative study. *Journal of Forensic Science, 28(1)*, 49–60.

Bonheur, H. H., and Rosner, R. (1981). Sex offenders: Diagnosis, organicity, and intelligence. *Journal of Forensic Science, 26(4)*, 782–792.

Butcher, J. N., Williams, C. L., Graham, J. R., Archer, R. P., Tellengen, A., Ben-Porah, Y. S., and Kaememer, B. (1992). *MMPI-A (Minnesota Multiphasic Personality Inventory): Manual for Administration, Scoring, and Interpretation*. Minneapolis: University of Minnesota Press.

Carpenter, D. R., Peed, S. F., and Eastman, B. (1995). Personality characteristics of adolescent sexual offenders: A pilot study. *Sex Abuse, 7*, 195–203.

Castellanos, F. X. (1998). Tic disorders and obsessive-compulsive disorders. In B. T. Walsh (ed.), *Child Psychopharmacology*. Washington: American Psychiatric Press.

Comings, D. (1994). Role of genetic factors in human sexual behavior based on studies of Tourette syndrome and ADHD probands and their relatives. *American Journal of Medical Genetics, 54*, 227–241.

Comings, D. E., and Comings, B. G. (1982). A case of familial exhibitionism in Tourette's syndrome successfully treated with haloperidol. *American Journal of Psychiatry, 139*, 913–915.

Comings, D. E., and Comings, B. G. (1984). Tourette's syndrome and attention deficit disorder with hyperactivity: Are they genetically related. *Journal of the American Academy of Child Psychiatry, 23*, 138–146.

Comings, D. E., and Comings, B. G. (1987). A controlled study of Tourette syndrome. IV. Obsessions, compulsions, and schizoid behaviors. *American Journal of Human Genetics, 41*, 782–803.

Conners, C. (1996). *Conners Rating Scales*. Odessa, FL: Psychological Assessment Resources.

Curtin, F., and Niveau, G. (1998). Psychosocial profile of Swiss sexual offenders. *Journal of Forensic Science, 43(4)*, 755–759.

Dunaif, S., and Hoch, P. (1955). Pseudoneurotic schizophrenia. In P. Hoch and P. Zubin (eds), *Psychiatry and the Law*. New York: Grune and Stratton.
Eldridge, R., Sweet, R., Lake, R., Ziegler, M., and Shapiro, A. K. (1977). Gilles de la Tourette's syndrome: clinical, genetic, psychologic, and biochemical aspects in 21 selected families. *Neurology, 27*, 115–124.
Fedoroff, J. P., Hanson, A., McGuire, M., Malin, H. M., and Berlin, F. S. (1992). Simulated paraphilias: a preliminary study of patients who imitate or exaggerate paraphilic symptoms and behaviors. *Journal of Forensic Sciences, 37*, 902–911.
Fehrenbach, P. A., Smith, W., Monastersky, C., and Deisher, R. W. (1986). Adolescent sexual offenders: Offender and offence characteristics. *American Journal of Orthopsychiatry, 56*, 225–233.
Finkelhor, D., and Araji, S. (1986). Explanations of pedophilia: A four factor model. *Journal of Sex Research, 22*, 145–162.
Firestone, P., Bradford, J. M., Greenberg, D. M., and Larose, M. R. (1998). Homicidal sex offenders: Psychological, phallometric, and diagnostic features. *Journal of the American Academy of Psychiatry and Law, 26(4)*, 537–552.
Galli, V. B., Raute, N. J., McConville, B. J., and McElroy, S. L. (1998). An adolescent male with multiple paraphilias successfully treated with fluoxetine. *Journal of Child and Adolescent Psychopharmacology, 8(3)*, 195–197.
Galli, V., McElroy, S. L., Soutullo, C. A., Kizer, D., Raute, N., Keck Jr., P. E., and McConvile, B. J. (1999). The psychiatric diagnoses of twenty-two adolescents who have sexually molested other children. *Comparative Psychiatry, 40(2)*, 85–88.
Gert, B. (1992). A sex caused inconsistency in DSM-III-R: the definition of mental disorder and the definition of paraphilias. *Journal of Medical Philosophy, 17(2)*, 155–171.
Green, A. H., and Kaplan, M. S. (1994). Psychiatric impairment and childhood victimization experiences in female child molesters. *Journal of the American Academy of Child and Adolescent Psychiatry, 33(7)*, 954–961.
Greene, R. L. (1980). *MMPI: An Interpretive Manual*. New York: Grune and Stratton.
Grossman, L. S. (1985). Research direction in the evaluation and treatment of sex offenders: An analysis. *Behavioral Sciences and the Law, 3*, 421–440.
Grossman, L. S., and Cavanaugh, J. L. (1989). Do sex offenders minimize psychiatric symptoms? *Journal of Forensic Science, 34(4)*, 881–886.
Grossman, L. S., and Cavanaugh, J. L. (1990). Psychopathology and denial in alleged sex offenders. *Journal of Nervous Mental Disorder, 178(12)*, 739–744.
Grossman, L. S., Haywood, T. W., and Wasyliw, O. E. (1992). The evaluation of truthfulness in alleged sex offenders' self-reports: 16PF and MMPI validity scales. *Journal of Personality Assessment, 59*, 264–275.
Grow, R., McVaugh, W., and Eno, T. D. (1980). Faking and the MMPI. *Journal of Clinical Psychology, 36*, 910–911.
Hall, G. C. N. (1989). Self-reported hostility as a function of offense characteristics and response style in a sexual offender population. *Journal of Consulting and Clinical Psychology, 57*, 306–308.
Hare, R. D. (1991). *The Hare Psychopathy Checklist Revised*. Toronto: Multi-Health Systems.
Harvey, M. R., and Herman, J. L. (1992). The trauma of sexual victimization: Feminist contributions to theory, research, and practice. *PTSD Research Quarterly, 3(3)*, 1–7.

Hastings, T., Anderson, S. J., and Hemphill, P. (1997). Comparisons of daily stress, coping, problem behaviour and cognitive distortions in adolescent sex offenders and conduct disordered youth. *Sex Abuse: A Journal of Research and Therapy, 9*, 29–42.

Henderson, M. C., and Kalichman, S. C. (1990). Sexually deviant behavior and schizotypy: A theoretical perspective with supportive data. *Psychiatry Quarterly, 61(4)*, 273–284.

Henn, F. A., Herjanic, M., and Vanderpearl, R. H. (1976). Forensic psychiatry: Diagnosis and criminal responsibility. *Journal of Nervous and Mental Disorder, 162(6)*, 423–429.

Herkov, M. J., Gynther, M. D., Thomas, S., and Myers, W. C. (1996). MMPI differences among adolescent inpatients, rapists, sodomists, and sexual abusers. *Journal of Personality Assessment, 66(1)*, 81–90.

Hodges, K. (1993). Structured interviews for assessing children. *Journal of Child Psychology and Psychiatry, 34(1)*, 49–68.

Hunter, J. A., and Goodwin, D. W. (1992). The clinical utility of satiation therapy with juvenile sex offenders: Variations and efficacy. *Annals of Sex Research, 5*, 71–80.

Jacobs, W. L., Kennedy, W. A., and Meyer, J. B. (1997). Juvenile delinquents: A between-group comparison study of sexual and nonsexual offenders. *Sex Abuse: A Journal of Research and Therapy, 9*, 201–217.

Jenike, M. A. (1989). Obsessive-compulsive and related disorders: a hidden epidemic. *New England Journal of Medicine, 321(8)*, 539–541.

Kafka, M. P. (1991). Successful treatment of paraphilic coercive disorder (a rapist) with fluoxetine hydrochloride. *British Journal of Psychiatry, 158*, 844–847.

Kafka, M. P. (1995). Sexual impulsivity. In E. Hollander and D. J. Stein (eds), *Impulsivity and Aggression*. Chichester: Wiley.

Kafka, M. P., and Prentky, R. A. (1994). Preliminary observations of DSM-III-R axis I comorbidity in men with paraphilias and paraphilia-related disorders. *Journal of Clinical Psychiatry, 55(11)*, 481–487.

Kafka, M. P., and Prentky, R. A. (1998). Attention-deficit/hyperactivity disorder in males with paraphilias and paraphilia-related disorders: a comorbidity study. *Journal of Clinical Psychiatry, 59(7)*, 388–396.

Kalichman, S. C. (1990). Affective and personality characteristics of MMPI profile subgroups of incarcerated rapists. *Archives of Sexual Behaviour, 19(5)*, 443–459.

Kalichman, S. C. (1991). Psychopathology and personality characteristics of criminal sexual offenders as a function of victim age. *Archives of Sexual Behaviour, 20(2)*, 187–197.

Kavoussi, R. J., Kaplan, M., and Becker, J. V. (1988). Psychiatric diagnoses in adolescent sex offenders. *Journal of the American Academy of Child and Adolescent Psychiatry, 27*, 241–243.

Kelly, J. R., and Cavanaugh, J. L. (1982). Treatment of the sexually dangerous patient. *Current Psychiatric Therapies, 21*, 101–109.

Knell, E., and Comings, D. E. (1993). Tourette syndrome and attention deficit hyperactivity disorder: Evidence for a genetic relationship. *Journal of Clinical Psychiatry, 54*, 331–337.

Kovacs, M., and Beck, A. (1977). An empirical approach towards definition of childhood depression. In J. Schulterbrandt *et al.* (eds), *Depression in Children*. New York: Raven.

Kruesi, M. J., Fine, S., Valladares, L., Phillips, R. A., and Rapoport, J. L. (1992). Paraphilias: A double-blind crossover comparison of clomipramine versus desipramine. *Archives of Sexual Behaviour, 21(6)*, 587–593.

Langevin, R., Ben-Aron, M. H., Wright, P., Marchese, V., and Handy, L. (1988). The sex killer. *Annals of Sexual Research, 1*, 263–301.

Lau, B. W. (1982). A profile study of sexual offenders in Hong Kong. *Medical Science and Law, 22(2)*, 126–134.

Leckman, J. F., Grice, D. E., Barr, L. C., de Vries, A. L., Martin, C., Cohen, D. J., McDougle, C. J., Goodman, W. K., and Rasmussen, S. A. (1994). Tic-related vs. non-tic-related obsessive compulsive disorder. *Anxiety, 1*, 208–215.

Levin, S. M., and Stava, L. (1987). Personality characteristics of sex offenders: A review. *Archives of Sexual Behaviour, 16(1)*, 57–79.

Lewis, D. O., Shankok, S. S., and Pincus, J. H. (1979). Juvenile male sexual assaulters. *American Journal of Psychiatry, 139*, 1194–1196.

Liebert, J. A. (1985). Contributions of psychiatric consultation in the investigation of serial murder. *International Journal of Offender Therapy and Comparative Criminology, 29*, 187–200.

Longo, R., and Groth, A. (1983). Juvenile sexual offenses in the histories of adult rapists and child molesters. *International Journal of Offender Therapy and Comparative Criminology, 27*, 150–155.

Losada-Paisey, G. (1998). Use of the MMPI-A to assess personality of juvenile male delinquents who are sex offenders and nonsex offenders. *Psychological Reports, 83(1)*, 115–122.

McElroy, S. L., Soutullo, C. A., Taylor, P., Jr, Nelson, E. B., Beckman, D. A., Brusman, L. A., Ombaba, J. M., Strakowski, S. M., and Keck, P. E., Jr (1999). Psychiatric features of 36 men convicted of sexual offenses. *Journal of Clinical Psychiatry, 60(6)*, 414–420.

Marks, P. A., Seeman, W., and Hallar, D. L. (1974). *The Actuarial Use of the MMPI with Adolescents and Adults*. Baltimore: Williams & Wilkins.

Meehl, P. E. (1962). Schizotaxia, schizotypy, schizophrenia. *American Psychologist, 17*, 827–838.

Myers, W. C., Reccoppa, L., Burton, K., and McElroy, R. (1993). Malignant sex and aggression: An overview of serial sexual homicide. *Bulletin of the American Academy of Psychiatry Law, 21*, 435–451.

Myers, W. C. (1994). Sexual homicide by adolescents. *Journal of the American Academy of Child and Adolescent Psychiatry, 33*, 962–969.

Myers, W. C., and Blashfield, R. (1997). Psychopathology and personality in juvenile sexual homicide offenders. *Journal of the American Academy of Psychiatry Law, 25(4)*, 497–508.

National Organisation for the Treatment of Abusers (NOTA) (2000). *Membership Network List*. Hull: NOTA.

Nee, L. E., Caine, E. D., Polinsky, R. J., and Ebert, M. H. (1980). Gilles de la Tourette syndrome: Clinical and family study of 50 cases. *Annals Neurologica, 7*, 41–49.

Packard, W. S., and Rosner, R. (1985). Psychiatric evaluations of sexual offenders. *Journal of Forensic Science, 30(3)*, 715–720.

Panton, J. H. (1978). Personality differences appearing between rapists of adults, rapists of children and non-violent sexual molesters of female children. *Research Communications in Psychology, Psychiatry and Behavior, 3*, 385–389.

Pauls, D., Leckman, J. F., and Cohen, D. J. (1993). Familial relationship between Gilles de la Tourette syndrome, attention deficit disorder, learning disabilities, speech disorders, and stuttering. *Journal of the American Academy of Child Psychiatry, 32*, 1044–1050.

Pearson, H. J. (1990). Paraphilias, impulse control, and serotonin. *Journal of Clinical Psychopharmacologica, 10(3)*, 233.

Perilstein, R. D., Lipper, S., and Friedman, L. J. (1991). Three cases of paraphilias responsive to fluoxetine treatment. *Journal of Clinical Psychiatry, 52(4)*, 169–170.

Raymond, N. C., Coleman, E., Ohlerking, F., Christenson, G. A., and Miner, M. (1999). Psychiatric comorbidity in pedophilic sex offenders. *American Journal of Psychiatry, 156(5)*, 786–788.

Ressler, R. K., Burgess, A. W., and Douglas, J. E. (1988). *Sexual Homicide*. Lexington, MA: Lexington Books.

Revitch, E. (1965). Sex murder and the potential sex murderer. *Disorders of the Nervous System, 26(10)*, 640–648.

Saunders, E. B., and Awad, O. A. (1991). Male adolescent sexual offenders: Exhibitionism and obscene phone calls. *Child Psychiatry and Human Development, 21*, 169–178.

Scahill, L., Riddle, M., McSwiggin-Hardin, M., Ort, S., King, R., Goodman, W., Cicchetti, D., and Leckman, J. (1997). Children's Yale Brown Obsessive Compulsive Scale: Reliability and validity. *Journal of the American Academy of Child and Adolescent Psychiatry, 36*, 675–684.

Schuerholz, L. J., Baumgardner, T. L., Singer, H. S., Reiss, A. L., and Denckla, M. B. (1996). Neuropsychological status of children with Tourette's syndrome with and without attention deficit hyperactivity disorder. *Neurology, 46(4)*, 958–965.

Shaw, J. A., Campo-Bowen, A. E., Applegate, B., *et al.* (1993). Young boys who commit serious sexual offences: Demographics, psychometrics, and phenomenology. *Bulletin of the American Academy of Psychiatry and Law, 21*, 399–408.

Smith, W. R., Monastersky, C., and Deisher, R. M. (1987). MMPI-based personality types among juvenile sex offenders. *Journal of Clinical Psychology, 43*, 422–430.

Speilberger, C., Edwards, C., Lushene, S., Monturi, J., and Platzek, D. (1973). *Manual for the State Trait Anxiety Inventory for Children*. Palo Alto, CA: Consulting Psychologists.

Waggoner, R. W., and Boyd, D. A. (1941). Juvenile aberrant sexual behaviour. *American Journal of Orthopsychiatry, 11*, 275–291.

Wasyliw, O. E., Grossman, L. S., and Haywood, T. W. (1994). Denial of hostility and psychopathology in the evaluation of child molestation. *Journal of Personality Assessment, 63(1)*, 185–190.

WHO (1992). *The ICD-10 Classification of Mental and Behavioural Disorders: Clinical Descriptions and Diagnostic Guidelines*. Geneva: World Health Organization.

WHO (1993). *The ICD-10 Classification of Mental and Behavioural Disorders: Diagnostic Criteria for Research*. Geneva: World Health Organization.

WHO (1996). *Multi-Axial Classification of Mental and Behavioural Disorders in Children and Adolescents*. Cambridge: Cambridge University Press.

Zonana, H. V., and Norko, M. A. (1999). Sexual predators. *Psychiatric Clinics of North America, 22(1)*, 109–127.

# Part II

# Assessment

Chapter 6

# The clinical assessment of young people with sexually abusive behaviour

*Gary O' Reilly and Alan Carr*

## Introduction

This chapter outlines some basic ideas that can be used to plan and conduct a clinical assessment for a young person referred for problems with sexually abusive behaviour. It begins by considering key characteristics that reflect a good approach to clinical assessment with this population. It then considers aspects of motivation that are important in planning such assessments. It will outline the main areas usually covered during a clinical assessment and concludes with ideas on formulating information from the assessment, report-writing, and contracting for intervention. We use fictional case material to illustrate key points made regarding assessment throughout. The ideas contained in this chapter are drawn from a variety of sources including Beckett (1994), Graham *et al.* (1997), Becker (1998), APA Task Force (1999), Will (1999), and Sheerin and O' Reilly (2000), and O' Reilly (2001). Each of these authors provide useful information and ideas on conducting clinical assessments with young people who sexually abuse.

## Characteristics of a good assessment

Beckett (1994) starts his consideration of completing an assessment with adults who have committed sexual offences by outlining what he considers to be four characteristics of a good assessment. O' Reilly (2001) takes up this idea in relation to adolescents and suggests the following as key characteristics of a good clinical assessment:

1 It allows for the fact that the young person and his family can be at various points along a continuum from complete denial to acknowledgement of sexually abusive behaviour.
2 It is guided by clear theoretical models and research findings.
3 It aims to build a holistic understanding of the young person's life and therapeutic needs.
4 The assessment team strive to create a non-collusive collaborative relationship with the young person and his family.

5 The assessment team adopt therapist features that are linked with positive outcome. Marshall *et al.* (1999) have identified a number of these and they are listed in Table 6.1 below.
6 It incorporates strategies to motivate engagement in assessment and intervention.
7 It makes a distinction between the young person's unacceptable and harmful behaviours and the young person's underlying personality.
8 It conveys to the young person and his family that the crises and dilemmas they face are understood by the assessment team.
9 It offers hope when appropriate.
10 It assumes that most young people with sexually abusive behaviour will not be motivated to disclose full details of their offending behaviour during the assessment.
11 Strategies for the detection of the presentation of misleading information by the young person are appropriately incorporated into the assessment.
12 It has access to third party information such as victim statements to police, courts and social services.
13 Psychological testing is included as an integral part of the assessment.
14 It attempts a formulation of the strengths and weaknesses of the young person and his family that can be used to support them in rebuilding their lives in an abuse-free way.
15 It formulates a considered opinion of the degree of future risk of re-offending posed by the young person.
16 It concludes with feedback to the young person and his care-givers on the formulations reached as an outcome of the assessment and any recommendations for intervention that logically follow.
17 It concludes with the offer of a contract for intervention if this is the recommendation of the assessment team.
18 It shares information from the assessment with the child protection network and the judicial system.

*Table 6.1* Therapist features identified by Marshall, Anderson and Fernandez (1999) as reliably linked to a positive intervention outcome

| *Therapist features* | |
|---|---|
| • Empathic | • Encourages active participation |
| • Non-collusive | • Directive and reflective |
| • Respectful | • Encourages pro-social attitudes |
| • Appropriately self-disclosing | • Confident |
| • Warm and friendly | • Asks open-ended questions |
| • Appropriate use of humour | • Interested |
| • Sincere and genuine | • Deals with frustration and difficulties |
| • Communicates clearly | • Non-confrontational challenging |
| • Rewarding and encouraging | • Spends appropriate time on issues |

## Understanding the young person's current stage of motivation for participation in an assessment

O' Reilly *et al.* (2001) consider the usefulness of the Prochaska and Di Clemente Transtheoretical Model of Motivation (Prochaska and Di Clemente, 1983; 1986) for developing intervention techniques with young people who engage in sexually abusive behaviour. This model is also particularly helpful in understanding the level of motivation of young people as they attend for assessment. Prochaska and Di Clemente's model simply describes a person's motivation to tackle problematic behaviour as consisting of five potential stages. These are: *(1) A pre-contemplative stage of motivation*, where the person has not yet acknowledged that he has a problem that needs to be addressed. This lack of acknowledgement of a problem may reflect a variety of influences including denial of his offending behaviour, distorted thinking about the impact of the behaviour on those victimised, fear of the consequences of admitting to his behaviour, and shame. Di Clemente (1991) subdivides this stage into four subtypes of pre-contemplation based on individual characteristics of reluctance, rebelliousness, resignation and rationalisation. *(2) A contemplative stage of motivation*, where the young person acknowledges that he has a problem with sexually abusive behaviour and is in a position to think about the possibility of change. While such a person may be open to a consideration that change may be required this is not to say that they will necessarily view change as a positive thing. Instead their consideration of change may be such that they conclude that they do not wish to move in a direction where they will instigate change. *(3) A determination stage of motivation*, reflects a point where a young person has considered the need for change and has decided that change is indeed required. However, their determination to change does not mean that change will automatically follow, that the most appropriate form of change will be chosen, that positive changes will be maintained in the long-run, or that the young person will lose their ambivalence about change. Commitment to change in the determination stage may benefit from support. *(4) An action stage of motivation*, where a young person embarks on the implementation of his plans for changing his behaviour in a positive manner. In essence this may reflect a point in time where a young person seriously commits and begins to implement new behaviours, ways of thinking and ways of expressing his emotions that are opened up to him by a good intervention programme in conjunction with support from significant people in his life. *(5) A maintenance stage of motivation*, where the person is concerned with the continuation of changes that have successfully been made to address his problematic behaviour. In relation to addressing sexually abusive behaviour this can be equated to a relapse prevention stage of change.

It is our experience that young people present for assessment at intervention programmes at various points along this continuum of change. A key part of the assessment process is the formulation of ideas on where each individual lies along this model. If we can recognise where a young person is with regard to their readiness for change we can allow this to positively influence our thinking on how to approach him during the course of the assessment in a way that will facilitate him in moving from his presenting stage of motivation for change to the next. Di Clemente (1991) provides suggestions on how we might orientate our conversations with people at different stages of change in a way that will be more likely to be productive. These are included in Table 6.2.

*Table 6.2* Strategies to promote change at different points on the Prochaska and Di Clemente transtheoretical model of readiness for change

| *Strategies that may be helpful in promoting change in different stages of readiness for change* |
|---|
| *Pre-contemplation* |
| A person whose pre-contemplation is based on reluctance may be more likely to consider change when provided with individual feedback on their problem behaviour presented in a sensitive and empathic manner. |
| A person whose pre-contemplation is based on rebelliousness may be more likely to consider change when provided with choices that make sense to them regarding their problematic behaviour framed within a discussion on why change may be a good idea. |
| A person whose pre-contemplation is based on resignation may be more likely to consider change when provided with hope for the future and a discussion that explores barriers that are perceived to prevent change. |
| A person whose pre-contemplation is based on rationalisation may be more likely to consider change when their perspective is acknowledged and the limitations of their position are explored in a sensitive and non-confrontational style. |
| *Contemplation* |
| A person in a contemplative stage of change may be more likely to become determined to change when provided with a 'risk–reward analysis' of the potential costs and benefits of change. This should be developed from the perspective of the client. It can also be used to clarify the client's goals for change and explore how the barriers to change can be removed. The contemplation stage also allows an opportunity for the discussion of client ambivalence, the exploration of successes and failures in past attempts to change, and the promotion of an individual's sense of self-efficacy regarding his ability to cope with the challenges of change. |
| *Determination* |
| A person in the determination stage of change may benefit from assistance that shapes interventions that (a) support and strengthen commitment to change, (b) promote a realistic understanding of what change will be like, and (c) promote problem-solving skills that will assist change and help overcome barriers to change. |
| *Action* |
| A person in an action stage of change may be more successful if they are provided with (a) a public forum where they can make a commitment to change, (b) objective feedback on their plans and efforts in implementing change, (c) support during change, (d) the promotion of internal attributions regarding self-efficacy and change, (e) the provision of |

information on successful and flexible models of change, (f) external monitoring of change, and (g) skills training.

*Maintenance*
A person in a maintenance stage of change may be assisted by (a) clear relapse prevention plans and skills, (b) opportunities to reflect on changes made and unexpected barriers to change that have been encountered, (c) skills and opportunities to identify small slips that may lead to the re-emergence of problem behaviour, (d) emergency plans to deal with unexpected urges or opportunities to engage in problem behaviour, and (e) positive encouragement regarding constructive changes made to date.

## The structure and content of assessment

Graham *et al.* (1997) indicate that care needs to be given to structuring an assessment as this can play a vital role in ensuring that the young person can begin to view the process as positive and potentially helpful to him. In line with their ideas we have found that completing assessments across a number of sessions, including various combinations of involved individuals, the inclusion of psychometric testing, and contracting from the outset for feedback and potential intervention, provides a good structure around which a comprehensive assessment can be planned. The remainder of this chapter will outline the main features that can be used in such an assessment.

With regard to the content of an assessment with a young person who has sexually abused, the American Psychiatric Association Task Force (APA Task Force, 1999) outline the contents of what they regard as constituting a comprehensive assessment. Table 6.3 summarises the main areas they recommend for coverage by the assessment team. The questions outlined later in this chapter should be used to elicit information pertaining to each of these areas as appropriate for the individual concerned.

### *Assessment session 1: meeting with the young person and primary care-giver(s)*

The initial task in completing an assessment is to ensure that you contract with the young person and his parents or legal guardians for permission to complete the assessment. This allows an opportunity to outline and agree the content of the material to be covered during the course of the assessment and to ensure that all involved are clear and consent to the process. It also allows the clinical team completing the assessment to state clearly that their purpose in conducting the assessment is to reach a concluding point where there is a clear formulation of the young person's sexually abusive behaviour that suggests an appropriate plan for intervention.

As suggested by Graham *et al.* (1997), taking a developmental history can be useful to begin the information-gathering stage of an assessment for a number of reasons. Firstly, it is usually reassuring and less threatening for the

*Table 6.3* APA recommendations for the clinical assessment of a young person with sexually abusive behaviour

*APA Task Force recommendations for the main factors that should be included in an assessment of a young person with sexually abusive behaviour*

- Victim statements to police, social services, mental health professionals, etc.
- Background information including family history, educational history, medical history, psychosocial history and developmental history.
- Interpersonal relationship history.
- Sexual history including deviant sexual interests and the emergence of sexually aggressive behaviour over time.
- Reported use of deviant sexual fantasies and interests.
- The intensity of sexual arousal during the time surrounding each offence.
- The dynamics and process of victim selection.
- Use of coercion, force, violence and weapons.
- Behavioural warning signs.
- Identifiable triggers leading to inappropriate sexual behaviours.
- Thinking errors such as cognitive distortions or irrational beliefs.
- The spectrum of injury to the victim from the violation of trust, creation of fear to physical injury.
- Sadistic elements to the sexually abusive behaviour.
- Ritualistic and obsessive characteristics of the sexually abusive behaviour.
- Deviant non-sexual interests.
- History of assaultive behaviour.
- Issues related to separation and loss.
- Antisocial characteristics.
- Psychiatric diagnosis including disruptive behaviour disorders, affective disorders, developmental disorders, personality disorders, post-traumatic stress disorder, substance abuse disorder, and organic mental disorder.
- Ability to accept responsibility.
- Degree of denial or minimisation.
- Understanding wrongfulness.
- Concern for injury to victim.
- Quality of social, assertive and empathic skills.
- Family's response (from denial, minimisation, support, to ability to intervene appropriately).
- Exposure to pornography.
- History of sexual, physical and/or emotional victimisation.
- Ability to control deviant sexual interest.
- Knowledge and expression of appropriate sexual interests.
- School performance and educational level.
- Mental status examination.

young person and his family not to be directly asked about the sexually abusive behaviour during the first appointment. It can be very helpful to inform participants of this at the outset of the session. We usually begin by asking the young person directly how they felt about attending for the appointment. This usually elicits a variety of responses from "didn't mind coming" to "didn't want to come".

THERAPIST: Peter, do you mind if I ask you about how you felt about coming to the centre today for this assessment?
PETER: Eh . . . didn't want to come.

THERAPIST: What do you think today is going to be about?
PETER: About what happened with Eleanor. . . . It's over and won't happen again so I just want to get on with things.
THERAPIST: OK. Well, you are right, coming to the centre for this assessment is about what happened with Eleanor. Many of the young people who come to see us attend for similar reasons. We have learnt from them that most people feel like you seem to when they first come here. From what you have said already it sounds like you acknowledge what happened and have a clear idea that you do not want something similar to happen again. I think that is very good. Like you, most young people we have met who have had similar difficulties tell us when they first come here that they do not need any help. What we would like to do over the course of four or five meetings is to meet with you and important people in your life to try and understand from you what happened, and to try and understand how you are able to be so clear that it is not a problem that is going to recur for you. During the course of the assessment we hope to work chiefly on these two things understanding what happened and understanding the strengths you have or are beginning to develop that will help you and those people who support you to ensure that you have clear plans and strategies to avoid problems with sexually abusive behaviour in the future. Perhaps at the end of the assessment we will come to agree with you that you have a clear understanding of what happened and have clear plans about how to avoid repeating the behaviour again in the future. Perhaps we will find that there are areas of your understanding of what happened that it would be helpful for you to work some more on. If that's the case then we might be able to help you with this. Perhaps there will be things that other people in a similar situation to you have found helpful that you have not yet thought about. If this is the case then we would be happy to help you to learn about them. Does this sound OK to you?
PETER: I suppose.
THERAPIST: Good. Then today we would like to start by asking you and the other people here about your experiences growing up. This helps us to get to know you and them a little better. Some of the things we will ask about concern when you were a baby so you probably do not remember them. Other questions will be about what things have been like as you have grown up. These will be things like what going to school was like, what type of things you enjoy doing and who are the most

important people in your life. Do you think you will be able to help us with this type of stuff?
PETER: Suppose so.
THERAPIST: Good. It also means that we will not be asking you directly about what happened with Eleanor today. We will ask you about this later on when you have had the chance to get to know us a little better. Does this sound OK to you?
PETER: Yeah.

In introducing the assessment in this way a number of important things can be accomplished:

- An attempt is made to establish a co-operative and respectful working relationship with the young person that is characteristic of a cognitive behavioural model of practice.
- An attempt is made to establish a contract where the young person is an active participant in the assessment while receiving support from significant others. This establishes the format that will be aimed for in intervention when the young person will be an active participant in the programme while receiving support from significant others.
- The young person's perspective is acknowledged and used as a starting-point for contracting for the assessment: "From what you said already it sounds like you acknowledge what happened and have a clear idea that you do not want something similar to happen again. I think that is very good. Like you, most young people we have met."
- The young person is informed that others have faced similar difficulties and have received help from the assessment and intervention service.
- The young person is provided with positive reinforcement for his responses from the therapist: "*Good*", "*You are right*", "*I think that is very good*".
- An attempt is made to put the young person at ease by informing him that his abusive behaviour will not be addressed directly during the first appointment. This avoids eliciting the young person's strongest resistance to talking to the assessment team on their first meeting and allows the assessment to begin with topics which are usually less threatening for the young person and his family to discuss.
- The young person and his family are given a clear message that the assessment team wish to understand the young person in a broad way and are not solely interested in the abusive behaviour or in finding people to blame for what has happened.
- The content of the assessment is outlined.

- A number of potential outcomes to the assessment are signalled starting from the feedback meeting. These range from no further contact with the service to working on developing a better understanding of the build-up to the abusive behaviour to developing relapse prevention plans and skills.

A number of authors (Carr, 1999; Gillberg, 1995; Sheerin and O' Reilly, 2000) describe the main areas that are usually covered while completing a developmental history. Broadly speaking the aim of collecting developmental information is to gain an understanding of the developmental pathway that has been followed by an individual so we can begin to construct a formulation of potential predisposing, precipitating and maintaining factors that provide a context to the young person's sexually abusive behaviour. It should also identify individual strengths that may be important in planning for the prevention of further sexually abusive behaviour. The main areas that are usually enquired about during a developmental interview are outlined in Table 6.4.

*Table 6.4* Assessment session 1

*Main areas covered in a developmental interview during assessment session 1*

*Development during infancy and early childhood*

- Mother and child's health status during pregnancy.
- Any complications during delivery.
- Mother and child's health after delivery.
- Any disruptions to parental bonding after delivery due to health difficulties or other factors.
- Child's temperament as an infant.
- Child's pattern of sleeping as an infant.
- Child's pattern of feeding as an infant.
- Child's accomplishment of main motor milestones including ages for sitting-up, crawling, standing, walking with assistance and walking independently.
- Any unusual features of motor development such as delay in motor development or not crawling, unusual gait or attendance with an occupational therapist for assessment and intervention.
- The child's level of activity as reflected in their accomplishment of different stages of motor development (inactive, normal, overactive).
- Child's accomplishment of main speech and language milestones including ages for babbling, first words, two-word combinations, and use of sentences.
- Any unusual features of speech and language such as delayed speech, articulation difficulties or attendance with a speech and language therapist for assessment and intervention.
- Accomplishment of toilet training and any difficulties with toileting such as encopresis or enuresis.
- Any significant separations from primary care-givers during infancy and early childhood.
- Opportunities for the development of social skills in early childhood through contact with siblings, members of the extended family, peers and family friends.
- Any unusual features of social skills development.
- Any general behaviour difficulties.
- Any sexualised behaviour difficulties.

*Main areas covered in a developmental interview during assessment session 1*

- Any difficulties in learning rules of social behaviour.
- Any difficulties in the regulation of affect such as temper tantrums.
- Any significant emotional difficulties.
- Any significant family events or difficulties during early childhood.
- Attendance at pre-school including the child's reaction to separation from primary care-givers, relationships formed with teachers, relationships formed with peers, and response to pre-school rules and tasks.
- Any additional strengths from infancy and early childhood not previously identified.
- Any other important information from infancy and early childhood.

*Development during middle and late childhood*

- Attendance at primary school including the child's reaction to separation from primary care-givers, relationships formed with teachers, relationships formed with peers, and response to primary school rules and tasks.
- Any significant behavioural problems in primary school.
- General academic performance in comparison to peers in primary school.
- Any significant general or specific learning difficulties in primary school.
- Any additional educational resources made available during primary school.
- Any change in class or school.
- Relationships developed with peers outside of primary school.
- Relationships with siblings and adult family members.
- The general development and expression of social skills in middle and late childhood.
- Any significant family events or difficulties during middle or late childhood.
- Any significant life events influencing development during middle or late childhood.
- Any significant general behavioural problems.
- Any sexualised behavioural difficulties.
- Any significant emotional problems.
- Any additional strengths from middle and late childhood not previously identified.
- Any other important information from middle and late childhood.

*Development during adolescence*

- Attendance at secondary school including the child's reaction to separation from primary care-givers, relationships formed with teachers, relationships formed with peers, and response to secondary school rules and tasks.
- Any significant behavioural problems in secondary school.
- General academic performance in comparison to peers in secondary school.
- Any significant general or specific learning difficulties in secondary school.
- Any additional educational resources made available during secondary school.
- Any change in class or school.
- Relationships developed with peers outside of secondary school.
- Relationships with siblings and adult family members.
- The general development and expression of social skills in adolescence.
- Development of interest in age appropriate relationships that have a sexual dimension.
- Any significant family events or difficulties during adolescence.
- Any significant life events influencing development during adolescence.
- Any significant general behaviour problems.

- Any sexualised behaviour problems.
- Any significant emotional problems.
- Use of alcohol or drugs.
- Use of pornography.
- Any additional strengths from adolescence not previously identified.
- Any other important information from adolescence.

*Medical history*

- Any current medical conditions.
- Any current medication.
- Any significant past medical conditions.
- Any past hospitalisations.
- Any significant past head injuries.
- Any past genital injuries.
- Any allergies.
- Any significant family medical history.

### *Assessment session 2: meeting with primary care-giver(s)*

The second session can usefully be used to meet with the young person's primary care-giver(s). There are a number of potential advantages to having such an appointment. These include the following:

- It allows the primary care-giver(s) an opportunity to talk about any important issues that they may feel uncomfortable discussing in the presence of the young person.
- It introduces or confirms the idea that a key part of successful assessment and intervention that aims to support a young person in refraining from further sexually abusive behaviour is contributed by the care-giver(s), and that the assessment and intervention team would like to support them in this.
- It provides an opportunity for the identification of care-giver resources that may be supportive of the young person in his efforts to effectively deal with his sexually abusive behaviour.
- It provides an opportunity to assess the primary care-giver(s)' readiness to support the young person in addressing and preventing their sexually abusive behaviour.
- It allows an opportunity for the assessment team to further cement their working alliance with the primary care-giver(s).
- It allows an opportunity to explore in more detail whether family dynamics such as a coercive style of interaction as identified by the Barbaree *et al.* (1998) model have been a part of the young person's experience and need to be integrated into the intervention plan.

The main content areas that can be covered in this part of the assessment are outlined in Table 6.5.

*Table 6.5* Assessment session 2

| *Main areas covered in assessment session 2 with the young person's primary care-givers* |
| --- |
| • Obtaining a detailed genogram of members of the young person's immediate and extended family and other important people who are not family members. A detailed guide for constructing genograms can be found in Carr (2000).<br>• Areas of strength and family coping skills.<br>• Personal strengths of the young person referred with sexually abusive behaviour problems.<br>• Difficult problems that have been faced by the family and effective and non-effective coping skills that have been utilised to manage these.<br>• Any additional current difficulties that are being faced by the family.<br>• Close, positive relationships within the family system.<br>• Negative and conflictual relationships within the family system.<br>• The care-giver's understanding of the young person's account of his sexually abusive behaviour.<br>• The level of acceptance by the primary care-givers of the young person's responsibility for his sexually abusive behaviour.<br>• The care-giver's availability and capacity for supervision of the young person.<br>• The care-giver's attitude towards the provision of assessment and intervention for the young person.<br>• The care-giver's opinion on the level of readiness of the young person for assessment and intervention.<br>• The level of awareness of the young person's sexually abusive behaviour within the extended family system and within the broader community.<br>• The primary care-giver's attitude towards participation in parents' work as part of the young person's intervention programme.<br>• Any immediate or extended family history of substance abuse, mental health difficulties, sexual victimisation, physical violence, sexually abusive behaviour difficulties, and criminality.<br>• Positive goals for the future. |

In conducting this type of interview the assessment team need to exercise sensitivity and good judgement in discussing difficult life experiences for the family at a level and a pace that is set by the young person's primary care-givers. An important balance needs to be struck between respectfully identifying difficult areas in a family's experience while also identifying strengths and coping mechanisms that have been utilised by the family. At the end of this part of the assessment it is helpful to draw the discussion to a conclusion by considering what the primary care-givers regard as a positive future developmental pathway for the young person. This can help to conclude the meeting on a positive note and also to begin to co-construct a concrete expression of clear and healthy goals for the young person. Questions such as "Given all we have discussed so far in the assessment if you had three positive goals or wishes for Peter for his future what would they be?" can facilitate a useful concluding discussion for the meeting.

### *Assessment session 3: individual meeting with the young person*

The third session of the assessment allows an opportunity for the young person to be seen individually. There are a number of tasks that can be completed during this meeting. Further efforts can be made to build on whatever level of working relationship was established during the first appointment. It also allows for the assessment of individual strengths and difficulties (acknowledgement of abusive behaviour, readiness for change, low mood, conduct problems, or attention and concentration problems). It also allows for the introduction of a discussion of sexual behaviour, experiences and attitudes separate from the young person's abusive behaviour. This allows the assessment team to begin to understand the developmental pathway that the young person's sexuality has been following. It further provides an opportunity for the young person to disclose any negative or abusive sexual experiences that they have had in the past in the context of a discussion other than one concerning their own abusive behaviour. Finally, a discussion on sexuality at this point prepares the ground for the assessment of the young person's sexually abusive behaviour during the fourth and final appointment.

Table 6.6 outlines the main content areas that can be covered during the course of assessment session 3. It begins with a gradual discussion of interests and activities. The questions on sexuality and sexual development are those suggested by Becker (1998) as constituting a comprehensive sexual development history. In approaching this part of the interview Becker makes a number of sensible and helpful recommendations to make the discussion less embarrassing for the young person, which include: (1) Inform the young person that as part of your work you have completed many similar assessments in the past (if this is the case) and that there is nothing to be embarrassed about. (2) Remind the young person that the purpose of the assessment is to gain a good understanding of him and the type of assistance that it will be most helpful for him to receive. (3) Be aware of your body language and responses given to the content of what the young person may say to ensure that this does not provide negative feedback to the young person. In asking about past sexual experiences Becker suggests that presenting questions to the young person in a neutral fashion such as "When was the first time you touched someone in a sexual way?" or "When was the first time someone touched you in a sexual way?" allows the interviewee to disclose normative experiences but also to disclose information on non-normative or abusive experiences without being directly prompted to do so.

Table 6.6 Assessment session 3

| *Main areas covered in assessment session 3* |
| --- |
| *General areas covered in interview 3*<br>• The young person's interests, hobbies, likes and dislikes.<br>• Important friendships in the young person's life.<br>• Activities engaged in by the young person with friends and peers.<br>• Any socialisation difficulties reported by the young person.<br>• Any conduct disorder type behaviour engaged in by the young person individually or with peers.<br>• Any difficulties with low mood experienced by the young person and approaches used to manage them.<br>• Any difficulties with strong angry feelings experienced by the young person and approaches used to manage them.<br>• Any difficulties with conflict and aggression experienced by the young person and approaches used to manage them.<br>• Any difficulties with attention and concentration experienced by the young person and approaches used to manage them.<br>• Use of alcohol and drugs.<br>• Use of pornography. |
| *Comprehensive sexual history*<br>• What age was the young person the first time they had a "crush" on someone? Who was that person and what were the circumstances?<br>• What age was the young person the first time they kissed someone? Who was that person and what were the circumstances?<br>• What age was the young person the first time they saw a male naked? Who was that person and what were the circumstances?<br>• What age was the young person the first time they saw a female naked? Who was that person and what were the circumstances?<br>• What age was the young person the first time they touched someone in a sexual way? Who was that person and what were the circumstances?<br>• What age was the young person the first time someone touched them in a sexual way? Who was that person and what were the circumstances?<br>• The young person is invited to provide information on each person with whom they have had any form of sexual contact. Information sought should clarify who each person was, what age they were, the level of activity engaged in and whether the activity was wanted or unwanted by either party. If it becomes apparent that the young person has been the victim of sexually abusive behaviour then the appropriate child protection guidelines should be fully followed in relation to this. |

## Assessment session 4: individual meeting with the young person

In the final assessment interview meeting the primary objective is to gain an understanding of the specifics of the young person's sexually abusive behaviour that will allow us to construct a formulation of his difficulties and so suggest an appropriate plan for intervention. This is potentially the most difficult of the assessment meetings for the young person and every effort should be made to facilitate him in as full a participation as is possible for him. Each of the characteristics of a good assessment outlined at the start of this chapter have a particular relevance at this point. In beginning this appointment it can be helpful to remind the young person of some important facts that established the basis for the contract for the assessment including that the purpose of the assessment is not to make judgements about him and his abusive behaviour, to chastise him for his behaviour, or to cause him embarrassment. Instead the purpose is to work with the young person to build up an understanding of what has happened and to develop a strategy to support him in developing clear plans and skills that will make his behaviour safe in the future.

In asking the young person about his sexually abusive behaviour the assessment team need to exercise good judgement with regard to how many offences they discuss in detail if the young person has more than one known offence. In general it can be useful to establish how many offences the young person has perpetrated and to discuss in detail the most recent offence. It should be established if this represents a typical incidence, if not detail about a typical incident should be included in the assessment. It is usually also instructive to ask for detail about the first offence.

Table 6.7 outlines the main areas that can be covered during assessment interview 4. It is designed to facilitate the construction of a formulation of the young person's abusive behaviour that informs the planning of appropriate interventions using cognitive behavioural and relapse prevention models. It is also informed by Lane's cycle of offending model (Lane, 1997). Consequently it attempts to elaborate a comprehensive picture of the offence by detailing antecedent factors, abusive behaviour related factors, and consequential factors following on from the abusive behaviour. Questioning concentrates on inviting the young person to discuss situations, thoughts, feelings and behaviours.

On concluding assessment session 4 it can be helpful to provide the young person with positive feedback that reinforces his participation to date that may help to encourage his continued involvement with the team as they work towards establishing a contract for intervention if this is to be the outcome of the assessment. This positive feedback should be encouraging but realistically reflect the level of participation that the young person has been able to provide. A client who has struggled to cooperate with the assessment might appropriately receive feedback that provides encouragement by acknowledging his level of involvement with the process to date, his struggle with achieving a fuller level of participation but also signposts the potential benefits of participation in intervention from his current position:

*Table 6.7* Assessment session 4

| *Main areas covered in assessment session 4* |
|---|

*Antecedents to the sexually abusive behaviour*

- Where was the young person before the offence took place? Who else was around or nearby?
- What was the young person doing before the offence?
- What was the young person thinking before the offence?
- How was the young person feeling before the offence?
- When did the young person start to think about offending (including pre-offence fantasy)?
- How did the young person set up the offence situation?
- How did the young person select the person whom they assaulted?
- What steps did the young person take to avoid detection?

*Abusive behaviour*

- Where did the offence take place? Who else was around or nearby?
- What behaviours did the young person engage in during the offence?
- How did the young person feel during the offence?
- What thoughts were going through the young person's mind during the offence?
- What did the young person notice about the reaction of the person who was assaulted during the offence?
- What methods of coercion were used by the young person during the assault?

*Consequences*

- What did the young person do after the offence?
- How did the young person feel immediately after the offence?
- What thoughts were going through the young person's mind immediately after the offence?
- What did the young person notice about the reaction of the person who was assaulted after the offence?
- What did the young person say or do to the person who was assaulted in an effort to prevent detection of their abusive behaviour?
- What other steps did the young person take to avoid detection?
- What thoughts went through the young person's mind as he took steps to avoid detection or after a period of time had passed?
- How did the young person feel as he took steps to avoid detection or after a period of time had passed?
- How was the young person's offence discovered?
- How did the young person feel about and respond to the discovery of his abusive behaviour?
- The young person's understanding of the harmfulness and illegality of his abusive behaviour.
- How did others respond to the discovery of the young person's abusive behaviour?
- How does the young person feel about his abusive behaviour now?
- What does the young person recognise as risky thoughts, feelings, behaviours and situations now? How does he manage these?
- What does the young person think and feel about his participation in assessment? Has there been any change in his attitude since his first attendance?
- What does the young person think and feel about participating in intervention?
- What does the young person think and feel about his care-givers' participation in intervention in support of him?

*Concluding questions*

- How does the young person feel about the future with and without intervention?
- What positive wishes does the young person have for his future?

THERAPIST: Thank you Peter for coming to meet us today and for the other times when you came to see us recently. We are glad that you did this. We understand that this is a difficult assessment to take part in, so well done on seeing it through to completion. It's been clear to us that today was more difficult for you than our other meetings. It seems you have found it a struggle to understand and tell us about your understanding of your sexually abusive behaviour difficulties. A thought that occurs to me at this point is that if you were offered a place on an intervention programme an important area the team could try to help you with is developing your understanding of what happened. You could then use this understanding to help you further with the goal that you have set yourself of avoiding problems with sexually abusive behaviour in the future. I know they have been able to help people in this way before. Do you think this approach might be helpful to you if it is available?

In contrast a young person who has been better able to cooperate with the assessment and has expressed clearly a reasonable first account of his abusive behaviour and states a wish to participate in intervention might be given feedback that not only provides him with encouragement but introduces him to some of the tasks he will complete during intervention:

THERAPIST: Thanks Peter for the way you have taken part in the assessment. Understanding and admitting what happened is an important part in reaching your goal of not repeating your abusive behaviour. The treatment team have a lot of experience in helping people further develop their understanding of their abusive behaviour. I am confident that they will also be able to help you with this. There are also other positive skills that they can teach you that will help you to keep clear of problems with sexually abusive behaviour in the future. These include helping you with your understanding of the harmful impact of your abusive behaviour on the person you assaulted, on her family, your family and on you. They can also help you to build up what's called a Relapse Prevention Plan. This is a personal plan and a collection of useful practical skills, like anger management skills, that the team help you develop that you can use to avoid further problems with sexually abusive behaviour. If there is a place available on the intervention programme for you I think you can do very well there.

### *Case example*

Below is a written report following the style of assessment outlined in this chapter. The case example for Peter Hill is fictional but we hope realistic. Figure 6.1 provides a genogram for the Hill family while Figure 6.2 provides a diagram summarising the case formulation. The approach to case formulation utilised emphasises predisposing, precipitating, maintaining and protective factors and follows the model for formulating clinical problems developed by Carr (1999).

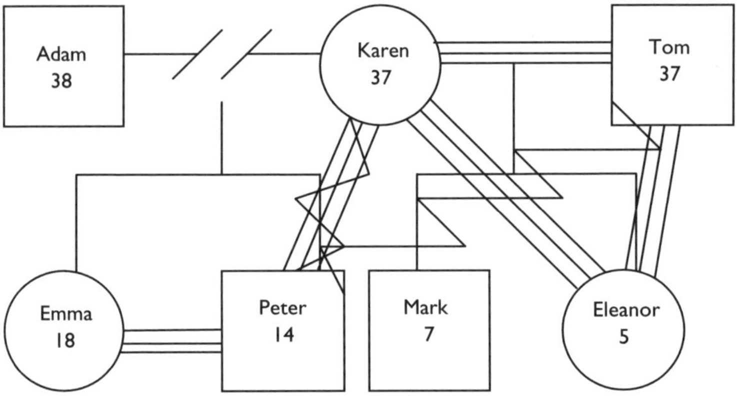


*Figure 6.1* Genogram for Peter Hill and family.

*Name:* Peter Hill.

*DOB:* 15/11/1988. *CA:* 14 years.

*Date of Report:* 16/11/2002.

*Family Composition*

Karen McKenzie – mother, 37 years.

Tom McKenzie – step-father, 37 years.

Adam Hill – father, 38 years.
Emma Hill – sister, 18 years.
Peter Hill – referred client, 14 years.
Mark McKenzie, half-brother, 7 years.
Eleanor McKenzie, half-sister, 5 years.

*The nature of this report*
This report outlines the findings from a comprehensive assessment with Peter Hill (14 years), his mother Karen McKenzie, and his step-father Tom McKenzie following confirmed allegations that he had sexually abused his half-sister Eleanor (5 years). The information in this report is drawn from the following sources: the letter of referral from Jim Burns (Social Worker); the CSA assessment reports from the Community Care Social Work Team; individual and joint assessment sessions with Peter, Karen and Tom; and psychological testing with Peter.

*Reason for referral*
Peter Hill was referred for assessment by Jim Burns, Community Care Social Worker. In his letter of referral Jim stated the reason for referral as follows:

> *Peter Hill, 14 years, has admitted to sexually abusing his 5-year-old half-sister Eleanor on three separate occasions. His abusive behaviour came to light when Eleanor told her mum that that Peter had been "doing bold things" to her when babysitting. Karen took Eleanor to her local General Practitioner who made a referral to Community Care Social Services. At an assessment meeting with two social workers Eleanor repeated that Peter had been "doing bold things" to her while he was babysitting. She disclosed that this included touching her vagina with his hand and getting her to touch his penis. Eleanor reports that Peter behaved in this way "a few times" but was unable to specify how many. When confronted by his mum and step-father Peter initially denied Eleanor's allegation. However, after the family went to their General Practitioner Peter admitted to his mum that "something happened". During an interview with the social work team Peter admitted that Eleanor's allegations that he had sexually abused her were correct. According to Peter he touched Eleanor on the vagina on three separate occasions. These incidents occurred while he was babysitting Eleanor and their brother*

*Mark while both parents were at work. Peter denies getting Eleanor to touch him. He reports that he engaged in the abusive behaviour because he was curious to see what it would be like.*

*The family are willing to accept a referral for Peter for an assessment of his sexually abusive behaviour. However, they have decided against making a formal complaint to the police. Consequently, although the police have been made aware of the incidents through community care notification, no charges are pending at present. Peter is currently residing in a Health Service Residential Home on a voluntary care basis. I would be grateful if your team could see Peter and his family for assessment with a view to his participation in the adolescent intervention programme.*

*Developmental history*

During the course of the assessment the following developmental information regarding Peter was reported.

Peter was born 5 weeks before full-term. He had a low birth-weight of 3 lbs. Following delivery Peter was placed in an incubator for three weeks. On discharge from hospital Peter is reported to have been a healthy baby. He attained motor and speech and language milestones within normal limits. He is reported to have been a "hyper" child who "was always on the go and into everything, and constantly demanded attention".

Karen reports that Peter's first two years of childhood were the final two years of her marriage to his father Adam. She reports that this time was marked by a significant amount of marital conflict. She indicated that Adam had alcohol abuse problems and that when he was drunk he would frequently become violent towards her and at times towards their two children. Karen explained that during her initial separation and subsequent divorce from Adam she became depressed and was prescribed anti-depressant medication by her General Practitioner for roughly one year. Since this time she has not had any recurrence of depressive symptoms. However, she acknowledges that this was a particularly difficult time for Peter and his older sister Emma and that both children spent long periods of time staying with Karen's sister Frances.

Peter began to attend his local National School at four years of age. His teachers reported that he had significant behavioural problems throughout his time in primary school. In particular his behaviour is reported to have been characterised by poor concentration, overactivity, excessive talking, frequently leaving his seat during class, and significant levels of fighting with classmates. Peter reports that he did not like primary school and that he was bullied by other pupils. Academically his performance during this time is described as "low-average". From second class onwards he attended a remedial teacher three times per week for additional tuition for reading and mathematics. At eight years of age Peter was referred by his school to the local child guidance service where he was assessed and diagnosed with Attention Deficit Hyperactivity Disorder. Peter was prescribed Ritalin and consequently enjoyed significant improvements in his concentration and general behaviour in school.

Peter enrolled at his local secondary school at twelve years of age. Although he has not experienced the same behavioural problems that he encountered during primary school he continues to have difficulty in establishing and maintaining friendships with peers.

*Psychosexual development*

Peter reports that he had his "first crush" when he was eleven years of age. He reports that this was on a girl in his class who was the same age. He indicated that he has had two girlfriends but was unable to recall their names. He reported that he went out with each of these girls for just a few days and his level of intimacy with them involved kissing. Peter reports that he is only sexually attracted to females and that there is usually no age difference between him and the girls he likes. Peter indicated that he has not had a sexual experience that made him feel uncomfortable or which he regards as abusive. He reports that he has never seen "adult" films or magazines. His parents report that Peter did not engage in any sexualised behaviour as a child that was a source of concern to them.

*Family history*

As noted previously Karen reported significant difficulties, including intra-familial violence, in her relationship with her first husband Adam. She also described her family of origin as follows. Her mother Laura died when Karen was four years of age. Karen left home at seventeen years of age when she met Adam. She reports that initially things went well in her relationship with Adam but their relationship deteriorated with his increasing alcohol abuse. Karen explained that it is her understanding that Adam's father Steve also had an alcohol abuse problem and that Adam's brother Ken has served a prison sentence for car theft.

Karen reports that when Peter was six years of age she met her current partner Tom. The couple have been married seven years and have two children, Mark (6 years) and Eleanor (5 years). Karen indicated that since she met Tom the couple have enjoyed a stable and satisfying relationship. Prior to Eleanor's disclosure of Peter's abusive behaviour they have not encountered any significant problems within their family.

Karen, Tom and Peter report the following features of relationships within the family. Karen and Tom report that their relationship is close, mutually supportive with little conflict. Eleanor enjoys a close relationship with both her parents. Karen describes herself as particularly close to her sister Frances who has been very supportive of her in the past. Karen indicated that she deliberately has no contact with her first husband Adam and that he has chosen not to have any contact with Peter or Emma. Peter is reported to have a close relationship with his older sister Emma. Prior to the disclosure of Peter's sexually abusive behaviour he was seen as having a reasonable relationship with his stepfather Tom and his two half-siblings. However, since then there has been a considerable amount of strain in the relationships between all family members.

*Peter's account of his sexually abusive behaviour*

During the course of this assessment Peter acknowledged that he sexually abused Eleanor on three separate occasions over a one-month period. He reports that the incidents took place while he was babysitting in the evening time while both Karen and Tom were at work. In describing the incidents Peter reported that they "just happened" and was unable to acknowledge any thoughts, feelings or actions that were part of the build-up to his abusive behaviour. He acknowledges touching his sister but denies getting her to touch him. After the abusive incidents he felt guilty and was afraid of getting caught. He told Eleanor not to tell anyone what he had done or they would both get into trouble. Peter reported that at the time he knew his behaviour was wrong because it was "bad" for his sister. However, he was unable to be specific about the way in which it is bad for her. With regard to his future risk Peter reported that he views himself as low risk of reoffending because he has "learnt a lesson from what has happened". However, he was unable to describe any changes he has made to his relationships or behaviour that reflect the lessons he feels he has learnt. Peter reports that he is unsure if he needs to attend an intervention programme but is prepared to do so if this is a recommendation from the assessment.

*Psychometric assessment*
As part of this assessment Peter completed the Adolescent Sexual Offender Assessment Pack (ASOAP). The ASOAP is a battery of psychological tests currently being developed for use with adolescents who have engaged in sexually abusive behaviour. It is designed to measure personality, offence-specific, and socially desirable responding factors thought to be related to sexually abusive behaviour. In some instances a young person's current level of functioning on the questionnaires is compared to a preliminary pool of normative data collected from non-offending adolescents. In most instances the current normative data is based on adult non-offenders. Consequently, considerable caution is required in interpreting the results. However, the findings reported below regarding Peter have been discussed with him and he indicates that he feels they are accurate. They are also consistent with our clinical opinion of Peter based on his assessment.

The results from Peter's completion of the ASOAP questionnaires indicate the following.

- An average level of honesty in responding to general behaviour and personality questionnaires.
- An average level of honesty in responding to questionnaires relating to sexual behaviour and sexual behaviour problems.
- Low self-esteem.
- An external locus of control (i.e. tends to place responsibility for own behaviour externally).
- Difficulties in cognitively taking the perspectives of others.
- Impulse control problems.
- Anger management difficulties, particularly through high levels of verbal and physical expression of anger.
- Victim empathy distortions specific to his sister Eleanor.
- An absence of global cognitive distortions regarding children and sexuality.
- The acknowledgement of previously undisclosed sexual behaviour problems of peeping and masturbating while secretly watching somebody.

*Summary and recommendations*

In summary, Peter Hill is a 14-year-old who has acknowledged sexually abusing his five-year-old half-sister Eleanor on three separate occasions over a one-month period. He admits to touching her in an inappropriate manner but denies that his abusive behaviour included getting his sister to touch him despite the fact that this was clearly reported by his sister during her disclosure. During the course of this assessment Peter and his family have identified a number of important predisposing, precipitating and maintaining factors that may have had a role in the development of his sexually abusive behaviour. These are outlined above and summarised in Figure 1 which accompanies this report along with a number of strengths that the family hope will help Peter work towards developing an abuse-free lifestyle in the future. Peter has shown a moderate degree of motivation to change his abusive behaviour during this assessment and has agreed to participate in a group-based intervention programme for young people who have engaged in sexually abusive behaviour. We strongly recommend that during his participation in this programme, Peter's work should have a particular emphasis on the following.

- Improving Peter's moderate degree of motivation to acknowledge and change his abusive behaviour.
- An acknowledgement by Peter of the full extent of his sexually abusive behaviour.
- The development of an understanding and acknowledgement of the emotional, cognitive and behavioural build-up to his abusive behaviour.
- Appropriate psycho-education on the effects of sexually abusive behaviour on people.
- The development of an appropriate awareness of the damaging effects of his abusive behaviour on Eleanor and other members of the family.
- The development of clear relapse prevention plans and skills.
- Building self-esteem.
- Building appropriate social skills.
- Encouraging perspective-taking skills.
- Developing impulse-control skills.
- Life story awareness work.
- Anger awareness and the development of anger management skills.

- Healthy relationship and sexuality education.

Joseph Lane,
Clinical Psychologist.

Mary Street,
Social Worker.

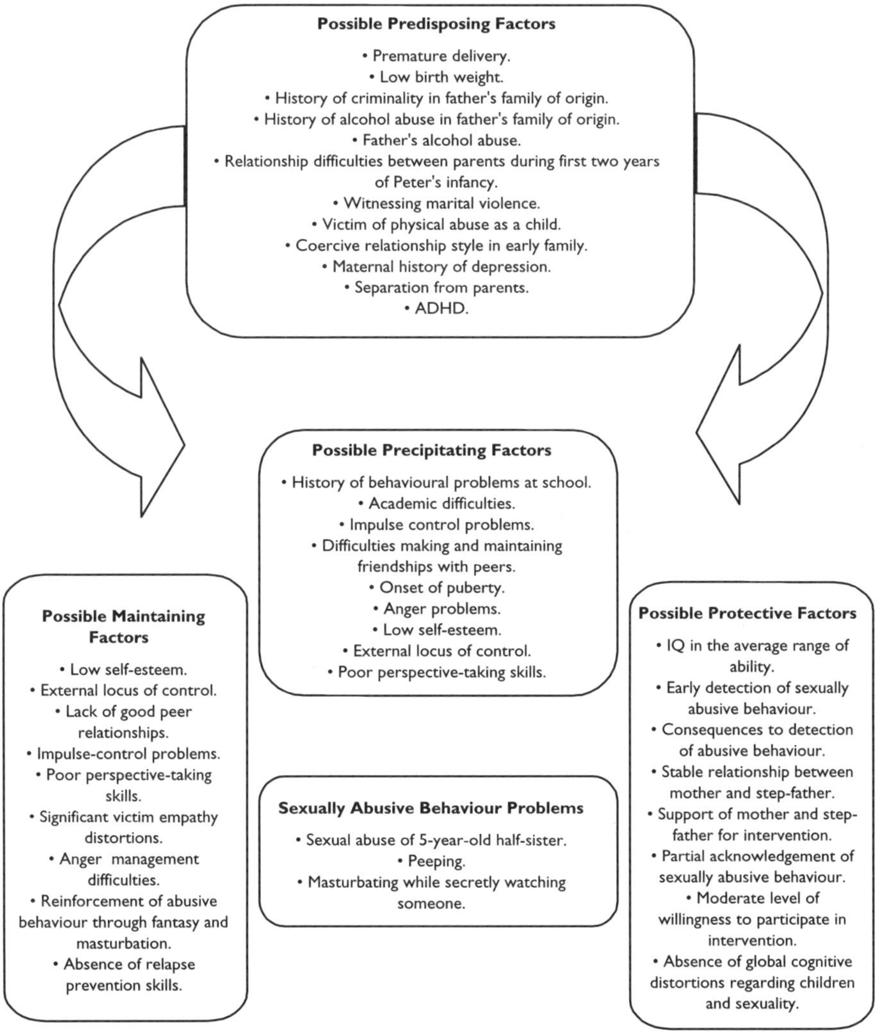


*Figure 6.2* Formulation diagram for Peter Hill.

| Contract for Intervention for Peter Hill | |
|---|---|
| I, Peter Hill, agree to take part fully in the weekly intervention programme.<br><br>I agree to work on the following as my main goals:<br>• Improving my motivation to acknowledge and change my abusive behaviour.<br>• Acknowledging the full extent of my sexually abusive behaviour.<br>• The development of an understanding and acknowledgement of the emotional, thinking and behavioural build-up to my abusive behaviour.<br>• Learning about the harmful effects of abusive behaviour on people.<br>• Learning about the harmful effects of my abusive behaviour on Eleanor and other members of my family.<br>• The development of clear relapse prevention plans and skills.<br>• Building self-esteem.<br>• Building social skills.<br>• Learning perspective-taking skills.<br>• Learning impulse-control skills.<br>• Life story awareness work.<br>• Anger awareness and the development of anger management skills.<br>• Learning about healthy relationship and sexuality.<br><br>I understand and agree to keep the all of the rules of the programme, including:<br>Strict confidentiality<br>No aggressive behaviour towards people or property<br>No disrespectful behaviour towards staff or other people on the programme<br>No meeting other people on the programme outside of group<br><br>Signed:<br><br>________________<br>Peter Hill | <br><br><br><br><br><br><br><br><br><br><br><br><br><br><br><br><br><br><br><br><br><br><br>________________<br>Date |
| I, Karen McKenzie, mother of Peter Hill, agree to support Peter in his work on the intervention programme and will be attending the Parents Programme as part of my support. I fully agree with the goals he has indicated that he is going to work towards.<br><br>________________<br>Karen McKenzie | <br><br>________________<br>Date |
| On behalf of the intervention team we agree to fully help Peter achieve the goals he has outlined above.<br><br>________________<br>Joseph Lane<br>Clinical Psychologist<br><br>Date: | <br><br>________________<br>Mary Street<br>Social Worker |

*Figure 6.3* Contract for Intervention for Peter Hill.

## *Feedback and contracting for intervention*

The final stage in a formal assessment of sexually abusive behaviour problems is the provision of feedback on problem formulation to the young person and his care-givers. This should form the basis for the negotiation and agreement of a plan for the young person and his family that logically follows from the formulation. The formulation model outlined in Figure 6.2 gives a structure around which feedback can be given. At the conclusion of this meeting all concerned should be clear on the formulation, and where possible working toward the intervention goals outlined in the report should be agreed. These goals should be outlined in a contract for intervention signed by the young person, key family members and the intervention team. An example of a contract, including some key rules of the intervention programme such as confidentiality, respectful behaviour and no aggression, is given in Figure 6.3.

## Summary

In this chapter we have tried to outline an approach to the assessment of young people with sexually abusive behaviour problems which is informed by theory and research. We have also attempted to incorporate simple strategies to maximise the young person's motivation to participate in the assessment process. Clear guidelines on content and structure for assessment interviews were outlined. A case example was provided to illustrate how information from the assessment can be formulated to integrate and summarise findings and set intervention goals.

## References

APA Task Force (1999). *Dangerous Sex Offenders: A Task Force Report of the American Psychiatric Association*. Washington: American Psychiatric Association.

Barbaree, H., Marshall, W., and McCormack, J. (1998). The development of deviant sexual behaviour among adolescents and its implications for prevention and treatment. In *Understanding, Assessing and Treating Juvenile and Adult Sex Offenders: A Special Issue of the Irish Journal of Psychology, 19(1)*, 1–31. Dublin: Psychological Society of Ireland.

Becker, J. (1998). The assessment of adolescent perpetrators of childhood sexual abuse. In *Understanding, Assessing and Treating Juvenile and Adult Sex Offenders: A Special Issue of the Irish Journal of Psychology, 19(1)*, 68–81.

Beckett, R. (1994). Assessment of sex offenders. In T. Morrison, M. Erooga and R. Beckett (eds), *Sexual Offending Against Children: Assessment and Treatment of Male Abusers*. London: Routledge.

Carr, A. (1999). *The Handbook of Child and Adolescent Clinical Psychology: A Contextual Approach*. London: Routledge.

Carr, A. (2000). *Family Therapy: Concepts, Process and Practice*. Chichester: Wiley.

Di Clemente, C. (1991). Motivational interviewing and the stages of change. In W. Miller and S. Rollnick (eds), *Motivational Interviewing: Preparing People to Change Addictive Behaviour*. New York: Guilford Press.

Gillberg, C. (1995). *Clinical Child Neuropsychiatry*. Cambridge: Cambridge University Press.

Graham, F., Richardson, G., and Bhate, S. (1997). Assessment. In M. S. Hoghughi,

S. R. Bhate and F. Graham (eds), *Working with Sexually Abusive Adolescents*. California: Thousand Oaks Press.

Lane, S. (1997). In Ryan, G. and Lane, S. (eds), *Juvenile Sexual Offending: Causes, Consequences, and Correction*, 2nd edn. Lexington: Lexington Books.

Marshall, W., Anderson, D., and Fernandez, Y. (1999). *Cognitive Behavioural Treatment of Sexual Offenders*. Chichester: Wiley.

O' Reilly, G. (2001). Adolescents who sexually abuse others. In Kevin, Lawlor (ed.), *The End of Innocence: Child Sexual Abuse in Ireland*. Dublin: Oak Tree Press.

O' Reilly, G., Morrison, T., Sheerin, D., and Carr, A. (2001). A group based module for adolescents to improve motivation to change sexually abusive behaviour. *Child Abuse Review, 10*, 150–169.

Prochaska, J., and DiClemente, C. (1983). Stages and processes of self-change of smoking: towards an integrative model of change. *Journal of Consulting and Clinical Psychology, 51*, 390–395.

Prochaska, J., and DiClemente, C. (1986). Towards a comprehensive model of change. In W. Miller and N., Heather (eds), *Treating Addictive Behaviours*. New York: Plenum.

Sheerin, D., and O' Reilly, G. (2000). Treatment of adolescent sexual offenders part 1: Assessment and treatment approaches. *Modern Medicine, 30(3)*, 49–54.

Will, D. (1999). Assessment issues. In M. Erooga and H. Masson (eds), *Children and Young People Who Sexually Abuse Others*. London: Routledge.

Chapter 7

# The psychophysiological assessment of juvenile offenders

*Judith V. Becker and Cathi Harris*

## Introduction

The purpose of this chapter is to review the empirical literature on the use of various physiological assessment techniques with adolescent sexual offenders, including the penile plethysmograph, the Abel Screen, and the polygraph. Physiological measures have been utilised in the assessment of youthful and adult sexual offenders. These measures are useful in guiding treatment planning and informing risk management. Specific to treatment planning, these measures are often helpful in addressing the issue of denial and minimisation of sexual offending behaviour. It is important for clinicians and the general public alike to understand the motivation for youth denying and/or minimising such behaviour. Our society at large has an extremely negative and punitive response when a disclosure occurs regarding sexual offending behaviour for both juveniles and adults. The response of society and the possible consequences to the juvenile of disclosing can greatly impact the amount of information that a juvenile is willing to disclose. With the use of physiological assessment instruments clinicians can become more informed in their formulations than when they rely solely on the self-report and disclosure offered by a person who has engaged in sexually abusive behaviour. Three methods of psychophysiological assessment are described below: the plethysmograph, the Abel Screen, and the polygraph. For each method research data, advantages and limitations will be outlined.

## Plethysmograph

Phallometric assessment is frequently used as part of an overall battery for sexual offenders, to measure deviant arousal. The procedure involves measuring changes in penile tumescence utilising a penile plethysmograph, while the individual is presented a variety (deviant and non-deviant) of sexual stimuli either visually or auditorily. The relative magnitude of the individual's responses reflects the amount of sexual interest associated with the specific stimuli (Becker and Murphy, 1998). Murphy and Barbaree (1988) provide a comprehensive review of the literature on phallometric assessment and address the psychometric properties of plethysmography.

While phallometry is the best objective measure of male sexual arousal, there are limitations to its use. These include a lack of standardised administration and interpretation procedures, a lack of standardised normative data to guide the interpretation of results, and a susceptibility to individuals faking their results (Barker and Howell, 1992). The majority of public literature on phallometry involves male adult sexual offenders. There are a limited number of published studies on the use of this form of assessment with adolescent sexual offenders which will be described below.

The Association for the Treatment of Sexual Abusers (ATSA), in its publication, *Practice Standards and Guidelines for Members of the Association for the Treatment of Sexual Abusers* (ATSA, 2001), provides guidelines for the use of phallometry. These guidelines state, "phallometric testing should not be used as the sole criterion for estimating risk for engaging in sexually abusive behaviour, recommendations to release clients to the community, or decisions that clients have completed a treatment programme. Phallometric test results should be interpreted in conjunction with other relevant information. Phallometric test results should not be used to make inferences about whether an individual has or has not committed a specific sexual crime" (p. 40). Phallometric assessment should also never be utilised without the consent of the person being evaluated. The authors recommend that when utilising this form of assessment with adolescents, the consent both of the adolescent and of the parents or guardian should be obtained.

Becker, Hunter *et al.* (1992) demonstrated the reliability of audiotaped phallometric stimuli with adolescent sexual offenders. Adolescents from two distinct clinical settings (residential and outpatient) were presented nineteen audiotaped stimuli cues on two separate occasions. The audiotapes were developed specifically for an adolescent population. The stimuli consisted of two-minute verbal portrayals of sexual interactions between an adolescent and other individuals. The cues covered the following themes: voyeurism, coercion of male victims of varied ages, coercion of female victims of varied ages, age-appropriate consensual female, age-appropriate consensual male, incest, frottage, exhibitionism, rape, a neutral cue, and two cues describing non-sexual assault of a female and non-sexual assault of a male. Penile responses were recorded while the adolescent listened to the tapes (for a more detailed description of the procedure utilised and specific audiotape cues, see Becker and Kaplan (1988)). All scores were recorded as millimetres of change from baseline and then transformed to z-scores. Data were analysed using Pearson correlation measures. Significant correlations were found for all cues except incest with a female child, exhibitionism, rape of an adult and frottage.

Becker *et al.* (1989) assessed a number of variables to ascertain whether they were associated with greater degrees of erectile responding. Adolescents from two clinical sites listened to audiotaped descriptions of sexual interactions with either a male or a female while erection responses were monitored. Those adolescents who had a history of being sexually abused and whose victims were males had higher deviance scores on a paedophile index than those who had no history of being sexually abused. At one of the clinical sites, the paedophile indexes were lower for those adolescents who had been sexually abused and who had female victims. This was not true for the other site.

Becker, Kaplan and Tenke (1992) evaluated the erection responses of adolescents who had committed sexual offences and were referred for evaluation or treatment. All had either sexually abused or assaulted female victims. Their erectile responses to audiotaped cues were monitored. Results indicated that those adolescents who had a history of abuse, either physical or sexual, showed more arousal to both deviant and non-deviant cues than those without an abuse history. As part of this study, an attempt was made to classify respondents based on their response profiles to all cues in which female targets were portrayed, except for the assault and incest cues. The respondents were classified as non-responders if they failed to respond (less than 20% full erection) to cues depicting any category. Respondents were classified as non-discriminators if responses to female stimuli were above 20 per cent full erection and the difference between responses to all age groups was 25 per cent or less. Adolescents were classified into one of five categories based on erection response: child, peer, adult, adult–child, or non-discriminator. Results indicated that the age-response profiles for participants were clearly distinguishable and supported the validity of the classification procedure. Of the sample 30 per cent were non-responders; 36 per cent were responsive to child cues; 33 per cent to peer or adult cues. The study also examined erectile responses relative to whether an adolescent admitted or denied the offence for which he had been arrested. Fifty-eight per cent of those who denied having committed the offences were non-responders. In conclusion, the authors noted that based on erectile response profiles adolescent sexual offenders are a heterogeneous population, and that plethysmography may be of limited utility with those offenders who deny their offences. Furthermore, one needs to use caution when interpreting phallometric data of those adolescents who present with a history of abuse.

Phallometry was utilised by Hunter and Goodwin (1992) to assess the clinical utility of satiation therapy with juvenile sexual offenders. Thirty-nine adolescent sexual offenders receiving treatment in a residential treatment programme served as participants. Results indicated that twenty-seven youths showed a significant decline in their percentage deviance scores from baseline to nine-month treatment interval using verbal satiation and other therapies. These authors report that twelve youths remained relatively refractory. The age of the adolescent was the only variable reported to predict response to treatment. Specifically, the older youths demonstrated more of an ability to lower their deviant arousal while maintaining high arousal to stimuli depicting consensual, age-appropriate sexual activity. The authors concluded that age as a variable warrants further investigation and hypothesised that the older the adolescent is, the greater the capacity for suppression of response. Similarly, in looking at arousal, Kaemingk *et al.* (1995) found a correlation between age and sexual arousal. Younger participants experienced greater arousal.

In another study, the Adolescent Sexual Interest Cardsort (ASIC), a self-report measure of sexual interest, based on a revision of the one developed by Gene Abel, was administered to two samples of thirty-eight juvenile sexual offenders to assess its test–retest reliability and concurrent validity (Hunter *et al.*, 1995). This instrument was correlated with phallometrically-measured arousal by correlating the average client response on the ASIC with his average maximum tumescence response to phallometric assessment of fourteen common stimulus categories. Statistically significant test–retest correlations using the Pearson R method were demonstrated for sixty of the sixty-four items on the ASIC (the correlations ranged from $r = 0.44$ to 0.98). When the adolescents' ratings of sexual interest via the ASIC were correlated with phallometric responses to similar categories of stimuli, significant correlations were found for only four of the fourteen categories which were examined, suggesting little correspondence between client report of sexual interest on the ASIC and phallometric assessment of the same. These authors concluded that there appears to be little correspondence between phallometric and self-report measures of sexual arousal in the adolescent sexual offender population. A recommendation was made that clinicians should use caution and not view self-report measures of sexual arousal interchangeably with phallometry in the evaluation of deviant sexual arousal and interest.

More recently, Murphy *et al.* (2001) investigated the relationship between offender and offence characteristics, including gender of victim, history of sexual abuse, history of physical abuse, race, and interaction between these factors, in the prediction of physiologically measured sexual arousal to deviant and non-deviant stimulus categories in a sample of seventy-one adolescent sexual offenders. Those authors utilised the stimuli developed by Becker, Hunter *et al.* (1992), and found that the strongest relationships with sexual arousal measures occurred in reference to the gender of the victim, and race. Subjects who had male victims tended to respond more than subjects with female victims. Race was negatively correlated with the arousal measures. African-American adolescents showed less responding to all stimuli compared to Caucasian subjects. There was an interaction effect for history of sexual abuse and gender of victim. Subjects who had been abused and who had at least one male victim had higher levels of arousal. These results relative to sexual abuse and high levels of arousal are similar to Becker *et al.* (1989). The authors concluded that their data suggests that adolescent offenders who had been victims of sexual abuse and who target male victims need to be prioritised in terms of receiving intensive treatment.

In conclusion the use of plethysmography with adolescent sexual offenders remains somewhat controversial. The limited research conducted to date would indicate the following. This procedure might have its greatest utility with older adolescents who target male victims and who have acknowledged engaging in norm-violating sexual behaviours. The studies conducted by Kaemingk *et al.* (1995) and Hunter *et al.* (1995) indicate that the younger the adolescent, the higher the observed level of arousal (however, this finding was not supported by the Murphy *et al.* study (2005)). It is not recommended that this form of assessment be used with very young adolescents. If a clinician is to use this form of assessment it should be used following the ATSA (2001) guidelines. Clearly, more research is needed to fully evaluate the utility and validity of phallometric assessment with an adolescent population. Valid data on adolescent sexual arousal patterns are useful to the clinician in structuring treatment programmes. If arousal management techniques are utilised as part of a treatment programme, it is important for the clinician to know the extent of deviant as well as non-deviant sexual arousal of the young people concerned.

## Abel screen

Given the intrusiveness of phallometric testing, alternative measures for assessing sexual interest have been proposed. Such measures have been called Viewing Time or Visual Reaction Time. Quinsey *et al.* (1993) provided a review of the literature supporting viewing time as a measure of sexual interest. Significant correlations were found between viewing times and ratings of sexual attractiveness among "normal" subjects. Quinsey *et al.* (1996) found that viewing time correlated with ratings of sexual attractiveness and phallometrically measured age and gender preferences. Quinsey and Lalumiere (2001) have noted that in utilising a viewing time measure it is essential that the client remain unaware that viewing time is being recorded. These authors note however that by not taking this issue into account, ethical concerns and serious practical issues arise that compromise the validity of this technique.

Abel *et al.* (1998) assessed the reliability and validity of visual reaction times and plethysmography in groups of individuals with sexual interest in children of various ages and genders. Fifty-six participants completed both phallometric and visual reaction time measurement. Participants in the study were between the ages of eighteen and forty-nine. Phallometric measurement included the presentation of four slides in each of eleven categories, including males and females aged four, eight, twelve, sixteen and twenty-two years and slides of landscapes. Visual reaction time included seven slides in each of six categories, including males and females aged eight-to-ten, fourteen-to-seventeen, and over twenty-two years. The authors report that both visual reaction time and phallometry demonstrated good reliability. Visual reaction time and plethysmography evidenced consistent results within the six slide categories used. Furthermore, the authors reported that the findings of their study lend strength to the validity of both measures. It was concluded by these authors that both methodologies were helpful in determining sexual interest. Visual reaction time was reported to be an effective, non-invasive and cost-efficient means of determining sexual interest.

Fischer and Smith (1999) described as weak the evidence regarding the reliability and validity of the use of visual reaction time for adults. They also questioned the reliability and validity of the measure for use with adolescents. However, Letourneau (2002) also assessed the validity and reliability of visual reaction time as a measure of sexual interest. Participants in that study consisted of fifty-seven sexual offenders who were incarcerated in a military prison. Participants completed self-report measures of sexual interest and underwent Visual Reaction Time (VRT) and penile plethysmography (PPG) assessment. Letourneau reported that with respect to internal consistency, results were acceptable for both VRT and PPG. Convergent validity was assessed in this study. Results indicated that VRT and PPG results were significantly correlated for all stimulus categories except for the female adolescent stimulus category. The possible reason for the lack of correlation is that audio stimulus cues were utilised as part of the plethysmographic assessment, and there was a lack of identification of age ranges for the child stimuli. Consequently there was no "female adolescent" category, and Letourneau noted that the female child stimuli were used in that analysis. Results indicated that both VRT and PPG identified those offenders who had targeted young boys. VRT identified offenders against adolescent girls. Neither VRT nor PPG identified offenders against adult women at a statistically significant level. Surprisingly, men who had female child victims evidenced lower arousal to female child stimuli as assessed by the PPG; VRT did not attain statistical significance in identifying offenders against young girls. Results indicated that every offender, regardless of his index offence, evidenced high interest to the adolescent female slides presented as part of VRT.

In a study by Smith and Fischer (1999) eighty-one adolescent males, forty-one of whom were identified as sexual perpetrators, were assessed. Participants were administered the Abel Assessment for Interest in Paraphilias (AAIP) on two occasions. The authors reported that the test–retest data did not support the reliability of the AAIP for use with adolescents. Furthermore, they report that the diagnostic validity data showed that the ability of the AAIP in determining specific deviant attractions within the adolescent perpetrator group was "poor". Specifically, the authors report that this form of assessment is not useful in diagnosing the specific paraphilic tendencies of the juvenile sexual offenders in the sample. Further research with other populations and other samples was recommended by the authors.

In a recent unpublished manuscript Abel, Jordan, Rouleau, Emerick, and Barboza-Whitehead assessed the validity of the Abel Assessment for Sexual Interest (AASI), attempting to classify male adolescent child molesters. The

AASI provides data on the subjective ratings of sexual interest, visual reaction time to twenty-two categories of sexual stimuli and a sexual offender-specific questionnaire, which the respondent completes. A large sample size was utilised, selected from over 400 adolescent males who had victimised either male or female children between 1994 and 2001. Using both VRT and a self-report questionnaire about sexual interests, the authors found a sensitivity of 68 per cent and a specificity of 66 per cent in classifying molesters of girls; and a sensitivity of 66 per cent and a specificity of 69 per cent in classifying molesters of boys. This represents an increased utility of the AASI over using VRT alone. It is of note that the results of this study appear to contradict the previously reviewed studies assessing the utility of the VRT procedure – the large sample size and addition of a self-report questionnaire may have contributed to the improvement in results.

In conclusion, the Abel Screen, a tool assessing sexual interest based on visual reaction time, can be utilised with adolescent offenders to inform clinicians of sexual interests and in classification.

## Polygraph

Frequently, sexual offenders will deny or minimise the extent of fantasies or behaviours that involve themes including minors or force. In an attempt to ascertain whether the material provided in a clinical interview is accurate, some clinicians utilise polygraphy. The polygraph has also been used to monitor whether the offender is adhering to conditions of his probation.

The term "polygraph" comes from Greek words, poly meaning "many" and graph meaning "to write". It is a device that displays, either via ink pens on a chart or computer visual display, representations of various physiologic activities. The physiological activities most commonly measured are respiration, blood pressure and palmar sweating (Ben-Shakhur and Furedy, 1990). Sensors are placed on different parts of the body. A blood pressure cuff is placed around the biceps; electrodes are placed around the fingers, and pneumatic tubes to the chest and stomach. The polygraph amplifies signals that are picked up from the sensors, thus measuring physiologic activity and changes in activities (Vrij, 2000). It has been assumed that changes in physiological activity are associated with arousal and that individuals who are lying will evidence more arousal than those individuals who are telling the truth (Vrij, 2000). Although the polygraph has been referred to as a "lie detector", it does not however detect lies. It assesses physiological arousal that may be the result of a lie (Saxe, 1991). In the United States, outcomes of polygraph tests may be used in criminal court cases; however, they are inadmissible in some states. It is not used in many other jurisdictions outside the United States (Vrij, 2000).

Vrij (2000) reports, "field studies examining the accuracy of polygraph tests have shown that these tests make substantial numbers of mistakes" (p. 205).

He continues, "Given the number of mistakes made in polygraph tests, I think that polygraph outcomes should not be allowed as a substantial piece of evidence in court." ATSA, in its publication, *Practice Standards and Guidelines for Members of the Association for the Treatment of Sexual Abusers* (ATSA, 2001), notes, "polygraph examinations have become a common part of the treatment and risk management of convicted sexual offenders who are under the supervision of probation/parole officers. Polygraph examinations can provide information, about the client's instant offense(s), sexual history, violations of treatment or supervision conditions, and unreported offenses" (p. 44). ATSA recommends that standards and guidelines of recognised polygraph organisations should be followed by examiners.

There are relatively few empirical articles published on the use of polygraphy with sexual offenders. Blasingame (1998) conducted a literature review for the purpose of evaluating research findings regarding the use of the polygraph with sexual offenders. In that review, Blasingame reports, "inconsistent empirical data from various studies provide a challenge to the validity and reliability of the polygraph procedure" (p. 37). A number of treatment providers have reported, however, that the use of polygraphy has enhanced the disclosures made during the pre-test interview before the polygraph was actually administered. It was also noted that the use of periodic polygraphs may have a strong deterrent effect, that is, an offender knowing that he may be polygraphed may be more likely to adhere to the conditions of probation or parole. It was noted by that author that empirically based standards for use and interpretation of polygraphy results were found to be lacking. Blasingame presents guidelines for the use of polygraphy with sexual offenders.

Ahlmeyer *et al.* (2000) reported on the results of polygraph examinations of thirty-five inmates and twenty-five parolees under the jurisdiction of the Colorado Department of Corrections. All participants in the study had committed sexual offences. Information was obtained on the number of victims and offences from their pre-sentence investigative report and sexual history disclosure form. The men had undergone two consecutive polygraph examinations. Those authors reported that 80 per cent of the polygraphs administered were found to be deceptive, 15 per cent were non-deceptive, and 5 per cent were inconclusive. The research indicated that inmates admitted to a greater number of victims and offences on average than did those men who were on parole. Those offenders who were non-deceptive as to their results on the first polygraph had more admitted offences than those offenders who were in the deceptive group. Overall, the authors report "dramatic increases in the number of admitted victims and offences were found for inmates, but not for parolees, across each source" (p. 123). Of interest, however, is that the number of victim and offence admissions declined substantially on the second polygraph examination for both the offenders and the parolees. These authors concluded that their results support the polygraph as an effective intervention for eliciting admissions of past sexual offending behaviours.

One article on the use of polygraphy with adolescent sexual offenders was found in the empirical literature (Emerick and Dutton, 1993). Seventy-six adolescent males between the ages of ten and eighteen participated in the study. All of the youths had been reported for or adjudicated for a sexual crime. The procedure in this study involved a review of each participant's assault history, as documented in official legal and clinical records. Each youth underwent a clinical interview, and finally, the above-mentioned information was provided to the polygrapher prior to the pre-test polygraph interview and confirmation testing. Eight of these youths denied having committed an offence and sixty-eight acknowledged a history of "hands-on" sexual assaults. When the data were analysed, the authors found significant differences across the three data sources for a number of the assault history factors. The participants' self-report changed significantly during the confirmation polygraph. It was reported that the participants tended to acknowledge assault behaviours alleged by collateral source; however, the data contained in collateral information understated the range of assault behaviours that these youths had engaged in. The authors caution against the generalisation of their data to all adolescent offenders, given that the youth in their sample were considered "high risk" and consequently may not be representative of the adolescent sexual offender population in general.

## Summary and conclusions

It is important for a clinician to obtain an accurate sexual history from juvenile offenders prior to formulating an individualised treatment approach for these youths. To date, evaluations have consisted of review of collateral information, a clinical interview and, in some cases, the administration of various paper and pencil instruments. In an attempt to obtain objective information regarding the youth's sexual interests and/or arousal patterns, clinicians have utilised the Abel Screen and, in some cases, phallometry. There is relatively little published data available on the use of the Abel Screen. As noted above, Fischer had utilised this procedure and raised questions regarding the validity and reliability. More recently, unpublished studies by Gene Abel and colleagues, utilising a large sample, provides data that support the use of this assessment tool as part of an overall assessment. Hopefully, more studies will be conducted in the future evaluating the effectiveness of the Abel Screen in assessing the sexual interests of a juvenile population. Nonetheless, the present data presented by Abel appears promising.

The data to date on using phallometric measures with an adolescent sexual offender population appears to indicate that there is considerable fluidity in an adolescent responding to these procedures. The use of phallometric assessment appears to have greater utility when assessing adolescent males who have targeted male minors as their victims. The data is somewhat mixed regarding history of sexual abuse and phallometric test results. More research is called for assessing the utility of phallometric assessment with juveniles. It would appear that it might not be appropriate to use this form of assessment with all juvenile offenders, but that decisions should be made as to whether it should be used based on the age and type of behaviours that have been alleged.

Finally, only one published study was found assessing the utility of the polygraph with a juvenile sexual offender population. Controversy has existed in the field regarding the use of the polygraph in general, and particularly in forensic cases. More research needs to be conducted regarding the validity and reliability of the use of this instrument as part of assessment with a juvenile population.

This chapter has reviewed the use of three physiological assessment instruments with juvenile sexual offenders. Each offers some potential utility and informs the clinician on treatment planning and risk management. In addition, they assist the clinician in obtaining information which the adolescent may find difficult to disclose due to societal judgement. Although these instruments are extremely useful, what appears to be important to facilitate disclosure is creating a safe environment in which a youth is willing to disclose his sexual history and to be able to obtain from the juvenile a commitment to changing behaviours. Establishing a trusting relationship and good rapport with a juvenile and informing him of the benefits to their being open, honest, disclosing and receiving treatment is also helpful to facilitate disclosure. It is also important to let the juvenile know the benefits to him of working to change inappropriate fantasies and behaviours. Finally, any assessment that is conducted with a juvenile should be comprehensive in nature. It should begin with a review of victim statements, and any other collateral information. It should obtain the consent of the juvenile to conduct a comprehensive clinical evaluation, including a comprehensive sexual history, and involve the administration of standardised instruments that have known reliability and validity. An ultimate goal is to provide the best possible assessment and treatment to a youth who has engaged in sexual offending behaviour, thereby restoring the youth to society as a productive individual while maintaining the safety of our society.

## References

Abel, G., Huffman, J., Warberg, B., and Holland, C. L. (1998). Visual reaction time and plethysmography as measures of sexual interest in child molesters. *Sexual Abuse: A Journal of Research and Treatment, 1(2)*, 81–95.

Ahlmeyer, S., Heil, P., McKee, B., and English, K. (2000). The impact of polygraphy on admissions of victims and offenses in adult sexual offenders. *Sexual Abuse: A Journal of Research and Treatment, 12(2)*, 123–138.

ATSA (2001). *Practice Standards and Guidelines for Members of the Association for the Treatment of Sexual Abusers*. Oregon: Association for the Treatment of Sexual Abusers.

Barker, J. G., and Howell, R. J. (1992). The plethysmograph: A review of recent literature. *Bulletin of the American Academy of Psychiatry and the Law, 20(1)*, 13–25.

Becker, J. V., and Kaplan, M. S. (1988). The assessment of adolescent sexual offenders. In R. J. Prinz (ed.), *Advances in Behavioral Assessment in Children and Families*, vol. 4. Greenwich, CT: JAI, pp. 97–118.

Becker, J. V., and Murphy, W. D. (1998). What we know and do not know about assessing and treating sex offenders. *Psychology, Public Policy and Law, 4(1/2)*, 116–137.

Becker, J. V., Hunter, J. A., Stein, R. N., and Kaplan, M. S. (1989). Factors associated with erection in adolescent sex offenders. *Journal of Psychopathology and Behavioral Assessment, 1(4)*, 353–361.

Becker, J. V., Hunter, J. A., Goodwin, D. W., Kaplan, M. S., and Martinez, D. (1992). Test–retest reliability of audiotaped phallometric stimuli with adolescent sexual offenders. *Annals of Sex Research, 5*, 45–51.

Becker, J. V., Kaplan, M. S., and Tenke, C. E. (1992). The relationship of abuse history, denial and erectile response: Profile of adolescent sexual perpetrators. *Behavior Therapy, 23*, 87–97.

Ben-Shakhur, G., and Furedy, J. J. (1990). *Theories and Applications in the Determination of Deception*. New York: Springer Verlag.

Blasingame, G. D. (1998). Suggested clinical uses of the polygraph in community-based sexual offender treatment programs. *Sexual Abuse: A Journal of Research and Treatment, 10(1)*, 37–45.

Emerick, R. L., and Dutton, W. A. (1993). The effect of polygraphy on the self-report of adolescent sex offenders: Implications for risk assessment. *Annals of Sex Research, 6*, 83–103.

Fischer, L., and Smith, G. (1999). Statistical adequacy of the Abel Assessment for Interest in Paraphilias. *Sexual Abuse: A Journal of Research and Treatment, 11(3)*, 195–205.

Hunter, J. A., and Becker, J. V. (1994). The role of deviant sexual arousal in juvenile sexual offending: Etiology, evaluation and treatment. *Criminal Justice and Behavior, 21(1)*, 132–149.

Hunter, J. A., Becker, J. V., and Kaplan, M. S. (1995). The Adolescent Sexual Interest Cardsort: Test–retest reliability and concurrent validity in relation to phallometric assessment. *Archives of Sexual Behavior, 24(5)*, 555–561.

Hunter, J. A., and Goodwin, D. W. (1992). The clinical utility of satiation therapy with juvenile sexual offenders: Variations and efficacy. *Annals of Sex Research, 5*, 71–80.

Kaemingk, K. L., Koselka, M., Becker, J. V., and Kaplan, M. S. (1995). Age and adolescent sexual offender arousal. *Sexual Abuse: A Journal of Research and Treatment, 7(4)*, 249–257.

Letourneau, E. J. (2002). A comparison of objective measures of sexual arousal and interest: Visual reaction time and penile plethysmography. *Sexual Abuse: A Journal of Research and Treatment, 14(3)*, 307–323.

Lykken, D. T. (1998). *A Tremor in the Blood: Uses and Abuses of the Lie Detector*. New York: Plenum Press.

Murphy, W. D., and Barbaree, H. E. (1988). *Assessment of Sexual Offenders by Measures of Erectile Response: Psychometric Properties and Decision-Making*, Monograph Order No. 86MO506500501D. Rockville, MD: National Institutes of Health.

Murphy, W. D., Dilillo, D., Haynes, M. R., and Steere, E. (2002). An exploration of factors related to deviant sexual arousal among juvenile sex offenders. *Sexual Abuse: A Journal of Research and Treatment, 13(2)*, 91–102.

Quinsey, V. L., and Lalumiere, R. E. (2001). *Assessment of Sexual Offenders Against Children*, 2nd edn. American Professional Society on the Abuse of Children Study Guides, 1. Thousand Oaks, CA: Sage.

Quinsey, V. L., Rice, M. E., Harris, G. T., and Reid, K. (1993). The phylogenetic and ontogenetic development of sexual age preferences in males: Conceptual and measurement issues. In H. E. Barbaree, W. L. Marshall and S. M. Hudson (eds), *The Juvenile Sex Offender*. New York: Guilford Press, pp. 143–163.

Quinsey, V. L., Earls, C. N., Ketsetzis, M., and Karamanoukian, A. (1996). Viewing time as a measure of sexual interest. *Ethology and Sociobiology, 17*, 341–354.

Saxe, L. (1991). Science and the GKT Polygraph: A theoretical critique. *Integrative Physiological and Behavioral Science, 26*, 223–231.

Smith, G., and Fischer, L. (1999). Assessment of juvenile sex offenders: Reliability and validity of the Abel Assessment for Interest in Paraphilias. *Sexual Abuse: A Journal of Research and Treatment, 11(3)*, 207–216.

Vrij, A. (2000). *Detecting Lies and Deceit: The Psychology of Lying and the Implications for Professional Practice*. New York: John Wiley.

Chapter 8

# Comparisons between juvenile and adult sexual offenders on the multidimensional assessment of sex and aggression

*Raymond A. Knight*

## Introduction

The serious societal problem of juvenile sexual offending has elicited concern from community, clinical, legal and research quarters (Barbaree *et al.*, 1993). Juveniles account for 30 to 60 per cent of cases of child molestation and 20 to 30 per cent of the rapes reported each year in the United States (Brown *et al.*, 1984; Fehrenback *et al.*, 1986). The widespread concern about juvenile sexual offending has unfortunately not been adequately matched with a sufficient empirical scrutiny of juvenile sexual coercion, and much of the existing research is riddled with methodological flaws (Becker and Hunter, 1997; Knight and Prentky, 1993).

There is a growing body of research on adult sexual offenders, but the generalization of adult findings to juveniles is problematic and requires empirical support. Some data indicate that most sexually aggressive juveniles will not continue their coercive offending into adulthood (Weinrott, 1996), especially if they are provided adequate treatment and supervision. Other data indicate, however, that certain patterns of juvenile offending may portend chronic sexual aggression that persists into adulthood (Knight and Prentky, 1993). Several recent studies provide evidence that incarcerated juvenile and adult sexual offenders show marked similarities and suggest that adult offenders might provide a reasonable model for these institutionalized juvenile offenders. Knight and Cerce (1999) found similar patterns in the covariations among critical factors related to sexual aggression in incarcerated adolescent and adult sexual offenders and also in generic criminal and community samples. In addition, Johnson and Knight (2000) found that with some modifications Malamuth's (Malamuth *et al.*, 1993, 1991) two-path confluence model of sexual coercion against females in college populations showed substantial predictive validity in an incarcerated juvenile sexual offender sample. Knight (1997) improved on Malamuth's two-path model and validated a three-path aetiological model of sexual coercion against women on a sample of 275 adult sexual offenders. Knight and Sims-Knight (in press b) demonstrated that this three-path model generalized well to a sample of adult community controls, and in a subsequent study they found that the model predicted sexual coercion against women or age-appropriate females in a sample of institutionalized juvenile offenders (Knight and Sims-Knight, in press a).

All of these studies dealt with the covariation among critical variables rather than absolute differences in the levels. The purpose of the present chapter is to explore the differences between incarcerated juvenile offenders and incarcerated adult offenders on a number of domains that have been found important in assessing sexually coercive behaviour. We compared adult offenders (n = 452) to the juvenile offenders (n = 227) both on selected rationally constructed scales and on thirty-two scales derived factor analytically from eight of the domains assessed by the Multidimensional Assessment of Sex and Aggression (the MASA). The MASA is a computerized inventory designed to gather self-report data on multiple domains related to sexual coercion (Knight and Cerce, 1999; Knight *et al.*, 1994).

Knight and Prentky's (1993) retrospective study of adult sexual offenders provided us with several a priori hypotheses to test in the present study. This study attempted both to explore the usefulness of adult taxonomic models for juvenile offenders and to search for identifying characteristics of juvenile onset sexual offenders that might ultimately serve as risk factors for the continuance of sexually aggressive behaviour into adulthood. They used both archival codings and responses to a computerized developmental inventory to divide their adult sexual offenders into those who had begun their sexually coercive behaviour in adolescence (juvenile onset group) and those who began their offending as adults (adult onset group). The juvenile onset group was distinguished from the adult onset group by a lower general level of social competence, by their higher frequency of antisocial behaviour, especially juvenile antisocial behaviour, and by the higher frequency of childhood sexual abuse that they had experienced.

Knight and Prentky's (1993) data suggested the possibility that these three variables might be important in identifying juvenile offenders who are more likely to continue their sexual coercive behaviour into adulthood. Some data (Righthand *et al.*, 2001; Zakireh, 1999) have suggested that juveniles with a high probability of continuing their offending into adulthood may be overrepresented in incarcerated samples. Because our juvenile sample comprised incarcerated offenders, we would expect in the present study that these juveniles would be higher than generic adult sexual offenders on variables measuring these three domains.

## Method

### *Participants*

The 227 juvenile sexual offenders in this study were sampled from residential treatment facilities in four states (Maine, Massachusetts, Minnesota and Virginia). The 452 adult sexual offenders were incarcerated in prisons in three states (Massachusetts, Minnesota and New Jersey). The penal facilities for the adults ranged from generic prisons to treatment programmes for committed sexual offenders.

Descriptive data for the samples are presented in Table 8.1. The juvenile sample ranged in age from eleven to eighteen years ($M$ = 16.09, $SD$ = 1.59). The adults ranged in age from nineteen to sixty-eight years ($M$ = 39.02, $SD$ = 10.68). Table 8.1 indicates that the distribution of races for the two samples differed slightly (c, $\Rightarrow c^2$ (5) = 15.35, $p < .01$). As can be seen in the table, African-Americans and "Other" races were slightly overrepresented in the juvenile sample relative to the adults, and Asians and Caucasians was slightly underrepresented. The largest difference between the samples in any single race category, however, was less than 6 per cent (5.6% "Other" category). Both adults and juveniles had histories of arrests and incarcerations. Residencies in treatment programmes with enforced limitations on freedom were counted as incarcerations for the juveniles. For both samples the present arrest and incarceration were included in the totals. Not surprisingly, the adults had been both arrested and incarcerated significantly more times than the juveniles ($F(1,618)$[1] = 7.79, $p < .01$ and $F(1,613)$ = 8.14, $p < .01$, respectively). The adult offenders comprised four subgroups 157 rapists (all victims seventeen years of age or older); 148 child molesters (some extrafamilial

*Table 8.1* Descriptive characteristics of the juvenile and adult samples

| | | *Juveniles (n = 227)* | *Adults (n = 452)* |
|---|---|---|---|
| *Age* | Mean | 16.09 | 39.02 |
| | Standard deviation | 1.59 | 10.68 |
| *Race* | African-American | 8.8% | 4.5% |
| | Asian | 9.2% | 13.3% |
| | Caucasian | 30.4% | 35.3% |
| | Hispanic | 37.0% | 36.0% |
| | Native American | 3.5% | 5.4% |
| | Other | 11.0% | 5.4% |
| *Number of times arrested* | Mean | 4.47 | 6.67 |
| | Standard deviation | 10.00 | 9.10 |
| *Number of times incarcerated* | Mean | 2.99 | 4.44 |
| | Standard deviation | 5.15 | 6.30 |

victims, with all victims sixteen years old or younger); 117 incest offenders (all intrafamilial victims, with all victims sixteen years old or younger); and thirty mixed-age offenders (victims both above and below seventeen years of age).

### Procedure

*Multidimensional Assessment of Sex and Aggression* All offenders were administered either Version 3, 4 or 5 of the MASA. All of the juveniles and 307 of the adults were administered the computerized form of the inventory, and 145 of the adults were administered a paper-and-pencil form of Version 3. The MASA is a self-report inventory that comprises items assessing social competence, juvenile and adult antisocial behaviour and aggression, expressive aggression, sadism, proneness to anger, offence planning, sexual fantasies and behaviour, paraphiliac fantasies and behaviour, pornography exposure, and early life experiences such as physical/sexual abuse, caregiver interaction, and alcohol/drug abuse (Knight and Cerce, 1999; Knight *et al.*, 1994).

We have previously described the methodological details for constructing the original MASA (Knight *et al.*, 1994). In brief, it involved: (a) specifying multiple domains that were critical for the assessment of rape, (b) generating an extensive item pool covering all these domains, (c) rating by experienced clinicians the appropriateness of items for each domain, (d) selecting the most suitable items for each domain, (e) rewriting chosen items to maximize their relevance to particular domains, (f) assessing domain coverage, (g) creating supplemental items for areas that were not adequately represented, and (h) testing the reliability and validity of the original version of the MASA on 127 Massachusetts Treatment Center (MTC) sexual offenders. In general, these scales showed adequate to high test–retest reliabilities (86% of the a priori scales equalled or exceeded .70, and 57% of the scales equalled or exceeded .80) and internal consistencies (94% of the scales had alphas greater than .70, and 80% had alphas greater than or equal to .80). With the exception of the scales assessing sexual deviance, drive, fantasy, sadism and offence planning, which were not adequately described in the archival files, MASA scales have had moderate to high correlations with companion scales derived independently from archival records (Knight *et al.*, 1994).

The MASA was originally developed to supplement our coding of archival records, which we had found significantly lacking in the area of sexual behaviour, cognitions and fantasies. As we expanded our subject pool to include institutions other than MTC, we had to expand the coverage of the MASA, because the records at these institutions lacked the information that we needed for our investigations. Consequently, the first version of the MASA assessed all of the domains cited except for developmental questions. In subsequent versions we have added a detailed developmental interview and assessments of other components of thought and behaviour that were hypothesized to be critical in the development and assessment of sexual coercion. The additions relevant to the study reported here include assessments of components of Factor 1 (Emotional Detachment/Arrogant and Deceitful Personality) of the Psychopathy Checklist (Hare *et al.*, 1990; Harpur *et al.*, 1988, 1989).

Selection of all offenders for testing involved a two-step process. Potential volunteers were identified and approached by on-site institutional personnel. In some prisons, this involved advertising, and in other prisons participants were contacted directly by programme personnel. When the research team arrived at the prison to administer the MASA, interested participants gathered in groups of six to fifteen participants. They were informed in detail about the nature of the study, about the kinds of questions they would be asked, about the protection of confidentiality that they were guaranteed, about the Certificate of Confidentiality that we had been awarded by the National Institute of Mental Health, and about the fee they would be paid for their participation ($18). Participants were not asked to put their name or their prison identification number on any part of MASA. Only a randomly assigned research identification number was used. A master list linked the research numbers to names to provide a link to supplemental information that was abstracted from their criminal records and for purposes of payment. After the information abstraction and payment, the master list was destroyed. A strong plea was made for honesty, and the potential future benefits of improved assessment for sexual offenders was emphasized.

After informed consent statements had been explained and signed both by the offender and by a member of the research team, either the paper-and-pencil version of MASA was distributed and a standard set of instructions was given or the participant was seated at a computer, which provided a tutorial on how to answer the MASA, a check that the participant understood the directions, and a brief fourth grade level reading test. The MASA Versions 3, 4 and 5 have been written for a fourth grade reading level. For those offenders who had difficulty reading and/or comprehending the questions, a member of the research team read the inventory to them in a private room. The MASA measures response latency, and extensive testing with college students has yielded estimates of the minimum amount of time required to read items. Participants whose response latencies indicated they were not spending adequate time to read the questions, or who gave improbable answers to specially created items, were eliminated from the data analyses.

*MASA Factor and Rational Scales* As can be seen in the left column in Table 8.2, the present study involved comparisons of level differences between groups on summative scales that were either factor analytically derived (8 domains; see Knight and Cerce, 1999) or rationally constructed (5 domains). Table 8.2 presents for juvenile and adult offenders separately the average internal consistencies for the scales in each of twelve of the thirteen domains assessed. Six early developmental scales (all four scales in the sexual abuse

*Table 8.2* Average internal consistencies for juveniles and adults for the domains assessed

| *Scale type* | *Domain* | *Juveniles* | *Adults* |
|---|---|---|---|
| *Factor scales* | Juvenile antisocial (n = 6)[a] | .862[b] | .867 |
| | Expressive aggression (n = 2) | .797 | .886 |
| | Pervasive anger (n = 4) | .808 | .842 |
| | Sadism (n = 3) | .772 | .821 |
| | Sexualization (n = 3) | .683 | .784 |
| | Paraphilias (n = 4) | .784 | .863 |
| | Pornography exposure (n = 4) | .854 | .897 |
| | Offence planning (n = 6) | .860 | .874 |
| *Rational scales* | Social competence (n = 3) | .773 | .786 |
| | Emotional detachment (n = 3) | .722 | .762 |
| | Arrogant/deceitful (n = 4) | .673 | .603 |
| | Sexual abuse (n = 0 of 4) | – | – |
| | Physical abuse (n = 2 of 4) | .880 | .892 |

[a] Number of scales in each domain.
[b] Average Cronbach Alpha for the scales in the domain.

domain and two of the four physical abuse domain scales) were calculated as either a maximum, minimum, or count over a number of responses or response categories. Because these were not summative scales, internal consistencies were not calculated.

As can be seen in Table 8.2, the internal consistencies were high for most scales. There were exceptions for scales in three domains. These were the arrogant and deceitful personality domain for both the juveniles and adults, the sexualization domain for the juveniles, and the social competence domain for both the juveniles and the adults. Both the callousness and grandiosity scales in the arrogant and deceitful personality domain for both the juveniles ($\alpha$ = .598 and .623, respectively) and the adults ($\alpha$ = .426 and .419, respectively) were low. The juveniles produced low alphas for both the sexual compulsivity ($\alpha$ = .588) and sexual drive ($\alpha$ = .583) factor scales. The juveniles and the adults also both yielded low internal consistencies for juvenile employment and independence scale in the social competence domain ($\alpha$ = .562 and .632, respectively).

All summative scales were calculated by averaging participants' responses to the items that were included in the scale. Three item formats were used for the majority of the items: (a) five-point true/false format, ranging from "definitely false" (0) to "definitely true" (4); (b) five-point frequency format, ranging from "never" (0) to "very frequently [> 50 times]"; and (c) six-point temporal frequency format, ranging from "never" (0) to "almost every day" (5). Appendix A provides a brief description of the content of each of the scales assessed and the formats of the items each scale comprises.

*Table 8.3* Manovas on the factor scores and rational scales for the 13 comparison domains

| *Scale type* | *Domain* | *Wilks l* | *F* | *df* | *p* |
|---|---|---|---|---|---|
| *Factor scales* | Juvenile antisocial | .862 | 17.76 | 6, 665 | < .001 |
| | Expressive aggression | .981 | 6.42 | 2, 673 | < .01 |
| | Pervasive anger | .952 | 8.43 | 4, 673 | < .001 |
| | Sadism | .984 | 3.69 | 3, 673 | < .025 |
| | Sexualization | .963 | 8.61 | 3, 663 | < .001 |
| | Paraphilias | .976 | 4.12 | 4, 674 | < .01 |
| | Pornography exposure | .626 | 89.75 | 4, 601 | < .001 |
| | Offence planning | .977 | 2.62 | 6, 660 | < .025 |
| *Rational scales* | Social competence | .903 | 9.98 | 3, 279 | < .001 |
| | Emotional detachment | .905 | 23.66 | 3, 675 | < .001 |
| | Arrogant/deceitful | .927 | 13.21 | 4, 673 | < .001 |
| | Sexual abuse | .908 | 8.82 | 4, 348 | < .001 |
| | Physical abuse | .919 | 8.18 | 4, 373 | < .001 |

## Results

### *Overarching MANOVAs*

We compared the juvenile offenders (n = 227) to the adult offenders (n = 452) on thirty-two of the MASA factor scales from eight domains and on eighteen rationally derived scales from five domains. We first analysed each of the thirteen domains by MANOVA, and only examined the individual scale differences when the overall $F$ was significant (at least $p < .01$). The MANOVA results are presented in Table 8.3. The results for the sadism and offence planning domains did not yield overall significances on the MANOVA sufficient to meet the a priori criterion.

### *Comparisons on the factor-analytically derived scales*

Table 8.4 presents the means, standard deviations, and univariate $F$ values for the individual factor scales in the eight factor analysed domains. The univariate statistics for the sadism and offence planning domain scales are presented for inspection, even though the overall MANOVA $F$ did not reach the a priori criterion. The results of each domain will be described in turn.

*Juvenile antisocial behaviour* Consistent with the predictions from the retrospective study, juveniles scored significantly higher than adults on four of the juvenile antisocial behaviour factors (the Delinquency factor ($p < .001$); the Problems in Junior High School factor ($p < .05$); the Bully factor ($p < .001$); and the Problems in Grammar School factor ($p < .001$)). Adult offenders were higher only on the Driving Problems factor, which included such items

*Table 8.4* Juvenile versus adult sexual offenders on the factor analytic scales

| Domain | Factor scale | | Group: Juvenile sex offenders | Adult sex offenders | F |
|---|---|---|---|---|---|
| *Juvenile antisocial* | Delinquency | *M* | .592 | .447 | 10.53*** |
| | | *SD* | .547 | .551 | |
| | Problems junior high school | *M* | 1.582 | 1.392 | 5.98* |
| | | *SD* | .981 | .9394 | |
| | Bully | *M* | 1.390 | 1.007 | 33.74*** |
| | | *SD* | .857 | .787 | |
| | Driving problems | *M* | .200 | .304 | 5.98* |
| | | *SD* | .502 | .535 | |
| | Problems grammar school | *M* | 1.322 | .787 | 76.72*** |
| | | *SD* | .807 | .720 | |
| | Drug problems | *M* | .295 | .267 | .32 |
| | | *SD* | .663 | .562 | |
| *Expressive aggression* | Physical violence against women | *M* | .256 | .434 | 11.96*** |
| | | *SD* | .451 | .705 | |
| | Aggressive fantasies against women | *M* | .784 | .882 | 2.08 |
| | | *SD* | .760 | .873 | |
| *Pervasive anger* | Constant anger | *M* | 2.491 | 2.393 | 1.45 |
| | | *SD* | .969 | 1.024 | |
| | Physical fighting | *M* | 1.730 | 1.483 | 8.51** |
| | | *SD* | 1.014 | 1.060 | |
| | Fantasies of hurting | *M* | 1.139 | .829 | 13.51*** |
| | | *SD* | 1.092 | 1.007 | |
| | Cruelty to animals | *M* | .798 | .457 | 23.98*** |
| | | *SD* | .994 | .777 | |
| *Sadism* | Bondage | *M* | .516 | .595 | 1.61 |
| | | *SD* | .723 | .786 | |
| | Synergism, sex and aggression | *M* | .218 | .252 | .70 |
| | | *SD* | .428 | .524 | |
| | Sadistic fantasies | *M* | .291 | .231 | 1.74 |
| | | *SD* | .595 | .541 | |
| *Sexualization* | Sexual preoccupation | *M* | 2.024 | 2.020 | .00 |
| | | *SD* | 1.004 | 1.072 | |
| | Sexual compulsivity | *M* | 1.180 | 1.450 | 10.34*** |
| | | *SD* | .874 | 1.105 | |
| | Sexual drive | *M* | 4.420 | 4.542 | 1.19 |
| | | *SD* | 1.308 | 1.387 | |
| *Paraphilias* | Atypical | *M* | 1.022 | .839 | 6.22* |
| | | *SD* | .886 | .914 | |
| | Exhibitionism | *M* | .854 | .666 | 6.58* |
| | | *SD* | .912 | .896 | |
| | Transvestism | *M* | .794 | .488 | 15.30*** |
| | | *SD* | 1.120 | .873 | |
| | Voyeurism | *M* | 1.315 | 1.139 | 3.89* |
| | | *SD* | 1.081 | 1.106 | |

| | | | | | |
|---|---|---|---|---|---|
| *Pornography exposure* | Conventional heterosexual | *M* | .821 | 2.267 | 216.23*** |
| | | *SD* | 1.025 | 1.077 | |
| | Sadism and physical injury | *M* | .504 | .640 | 4.05* |
| | | *SD* | .733 | .730 | |
| | Adult men and children | *M* | .318 | .371 | .86 |
| | | *SD* | .505 | .638 | |
| | Family exposure | *M* | 1.469 | .949 | 34.07*** |
| | | *SD* | 1.221 | 1.027 | |
| *Offence planning* | Intimacy seeking | *M* | 1.578 | 1.563 | .03 |
| | | *SD* | 1.114 | 1.142 | |
| | Aggressive/violent fantasies | *M* | .585 | .586 | .00 |
| | | *SD* | .739 | .730 | |
| | Victim type and encounter location | *M* | 1.410 | 1.388 | .08 |
| | | *SD* | .811 | 1.044 | |
| | Sexual fantasies | *M* | 1.648 | 1.458 | 4.80* |
| | | *SD* | 1.083 | 1.047 | |
| | Eluding apprehension | *M* | 1.468 | 1.387 | .60 |
| | | *SD* | 1.284 | 1.259 | |
| | Weapons and paraphernalia | *M* | .554 | .500 | .51 |
| | | *SD* | .937 | .900 | |

* $p < .05$
** $p < .005$
*** $p < .001$

as drunk driving, driving to endanger, and driving without a licence ($p < .05$). The two groups did not differ on Drug Problems.

*Expressive aggression* Adults reported significantly more frequent ($p < .001$) physical violence toward women (e.g. beating them up, roughing them up). The two groups did not differ in their aggressive fantasies toward women.

*Pervasive anger* Juveniles reported a significantly higher frequency of Physical Fights ($p < .01$), Fantasies of Hurting ($p < .001$), and Cruelty to Animals ($p < .001$). No differences emerged in the constancy of their reported anger, although both groups reported high levels of anger.

*Sadism* No differences emerged in sadistic behaviour or fantasies. As expected, the frequencies of these behaviours and fantasies were low for both groups.

*Sexualization* Although no differences were found in Sexual Preoccupation (a measure of the pervasiveness and frequency of sexual fantasies and cognitions) and Sexual Drive (a measure of the total sexual behavioural outlet), adults reported significantly more Sexual Compulsivity (feeling compelled to do particular sexual behaviours) than the juveniles ($p < .001$).

*Paraphilias* In contrast with the sexualization results, juveniles consistently reported higher frequencies on all four paraphilia scales, which measured both fantasies and behaviours. They reported more Frotteurism and Obscene Phone Calls ($p < .05$), Exhibitionism ($p < .05$), Transvestism ($p < .001$), and Voyeurism ($p < .05$) than adult offenders.

*Pornography exposure* The pornography factors yielded strong opposing results on two factors. Juveniles acknowledged being exposed to more pornography in their family homes ($p < .001$), but the adult offenders used conventional heterosexual pornography considerably more than adolescents ($p < .001$). Adults were also exposed to violent pornography somewhat more frequently than were the juveniles ($p < .05$).

*Offence planning* Juveniles and adults were equal in all aspects of offence planning except thinking about the sexual acts that would be done in the offence, where juveniles were slightly higher ($p < .05$). The overall MANOVA *F* ratio did not reach. 01 significance, however, so this result is questionable.

*Comparisons on the rationally derived scales* Table 8.5 presents the means, standard deviations, and univariate *F* values for the individual scales in the five domains for which rationally derived scales were constructed. The results of each domain will be described in turn.

*Juvenile social competence* In the social competence domain, the results were only partially consistent with those of our earlier retrospective study. Juveniles scored significantly lower on an assessment of their job frequency and consistency and financial independence in adolescence ($p < .001$), but they were equal to adult offenders in the depth and extent of their adolescent friendships and their early dating history. Because availability of work increases with age in adolescence, the employment analyses were repeated considering only the oldest adolescents (≥ 16 years old), but the results were the same.

*Emotional detachment* In the two scales measuring deficient emotional responsivity, the juveniles showed greater deficits than the adult offenders (lack of empathy ($p < .001$) and lack of guilt ($p < .001$)). Adults, however, reported significantly less ability in perspective taking ($p < .01$), which specifically assesses looking at issues from others' point of view.

*Arrogant and deceitful personality* In the comparisons measuring aspects of the arrogant and deceitful personality style, adult offenders were higher in superficial charm and conning ($p < .001$), but juveniles were higher in measures of negative masculinity ($p < .05$). The latter variable assesses the power, dominance, risk taking, toughness, aggressiveness, honour defending, and competitiveness that characterize negative aspects of masculinity. No differences emerged on callousness or grandiosity.

*Table 8.5* Juvenile versus adult sexual offenders on the rationally derived scales

| Domain | Rational scale | | *Group* Juvenile sex offenders | Adult sex offenders | F |
|---|---|---|---|---|---|
| *Juvenile social competence* | Employment and independence | M | .604 | 1.141 | 27.84*** |
| | | SD | .696 | .882 | |
| | Friendships | M | 3.465 | 3.416 | .11 |
| | | SD | 1.290 | 1.187 | |
| | Dating | M | 2.163 | 2.240 | .26 |
| | | SD | 1.211 | 1.214 | |
| *Emotional detachment* | Lack of guilt | M | 2.125 | 1.698 | 53.34*** |
| | | SD | .727 | .715 | |
| | Lack of empathy | M | 1.507 | 1.209 | 23.66*** |
| | | SD | .776 | .760 | |
| | Poor perspective taking | M | 1.169 | 1.338 | 8.20** |
| | | SD | .683 | .744 | |
| *Arrogant/deceitful* | Callousness | M | 2.555 | 2.411 | 2.52 |
| | | SD | 1.245 | 1.041 | |
| | Charming and conning | M | 2.094 | 2.375 | 16.39*** |
| | | SD | .841 | .859 | |
| | Grandiosity | M | 2.338 | 2.377 | .37 |
| | | SD | .858 | .771 | |
| | Negative masculinity | M | 2.065 | 1.869 | 6.49* |
| | | SD | .862 | .980 | |
| *Sexual abuse* | Sexual abuse child | M | 2.362 | 2.164 | .74 |
| | Force used | SD | 1.889 | 2.057 | |
| | Sexual abuse child | M | 3.713 | 2.535 | 20.98*** |
| | Level | SD | 2.038 | 2.315 | |
| | Sexual abuse teen | M | 1.583 | 1.820 | 1.95 |
| | Force used | SD | 1.497 | 1.462 | |
| | Sexual abuse teen | M | 3.778 | 3.060 | 8.06** |
| | Level | SD | 2.013 | 2.268 | |
| *Physical/verbal abuse* | Childhood verbal abuse | M | .723 | 1.064 | 11.50*** |
| | | SD | .853 | .9557 | |
| | Adolescent verbal abuse | M | .536 | 1.004 | 24.57*** |
| | | SD | .720 | .907 | |
| | Physical abuse level | M | 2.829 | 2.931 | .50 |
| | | SD | 1.820 | 1.756 | |
| | Physical abuse | M | 2.450 | 2.705 | 4.80* |
| | Frequency | SD | 1.558 | 1.372 | |

* $p < .05$
** $p < .005$
*** $p < .001$

*Sexual abuse* Consistent with the predictions from our retrospective study, juvenile sexual offenders had experienced a higher level of sexual abuse (higher level of sexual invasiveness) in both childhood ($p < .001$) and adolescence ($p < .01$) than was experienced by adult offenders. There were, however, no differences between the two groups in the amount of force used in their sexually abusive experiences.

*Physical abuse* In contrast to sexual abuse, adult offenders experienced more verbal abuse both as children ($p < .001$) and as adolescents ($p < .001$), and a higher frequency of physical abuse ($p < .05$) than the juvenile offenders experienced.

## Discussion

The study reported in this chapter had two purposes. The first was the comparison of incarcerated juvenile sexual offenders with adult offenders to determine the similarities and differences between the two groups on critical variables related to sexual aggression. Correlative studies have demonstrated congruous patterns of relations among dimensions in the two groups (Knight and Cerce, 1999) but the absolute levels on critical variables have not been systematically evaluated. Comparability in the levels of these dimensions would provide support for exploring further the parallels between adult offenders and incarcerated juvenile sexual offenders.

The second aim was to test the hypothesis that juveniles whose sexually coercive behaviour was considered serious enough to require incarceration in special institutions might have important similarities to the adult offenders who began their sexually coercive behaviours as adolescents. Whereas juveniles with a higher potential for the persistence of their sexually coercive behaviour should be overrepresented in such select, incarcerated samples (Righthand *et al.*, 2001; Zakireh, 1999), only approximately 35 to 40 per cent of the adult sample should have been charged with a juvenile sexual crime (Knight and Prentky, 1993). As indicated in the introduction, Knight and Prentky (1993) attempted in a retrospective study of adult sexual offenders to identify characteristics of juvenile onset sexual offenders that might be candidates for predicting the persistence of sexually coercive behaviour into adulthood. Determining whether the variables that had discriminated juvenile onset adult offenders from adult onset offenders would also discriminate high-risk juvenile offenders from generic adult offenders constitutes a further test of the potential discriminatory power of these variables as markers of persistence.

The study yielded some support both for the comparability of the incarcerated juveniles to the adult offenders and for the discriminatory power of the three domains identified by Knight and Prentky (1993) – sexual abuse, juvenile antisocial behaviour, and social competence. Although the juveniles did not experience higher levels of coercion in their sexually abusive experiences than adults, their abuse was likely to be more sexually intrusive in both childhood and adolescence. That is, their sexual abuse was more likely to include penetration rather than simply exposure to sexual materials or fondling. Consistent with the prior study, incarcerated juveniles reported significantly more problems of delinquency, aggression and impulsivity in adolescence than the adults remembered. Adults only reported more problems with automotive infractions, and the two groups did not differ in teenage drug abuse. Finally, although adolescent friendships and heterosexual relationships were not significantly more problematic for the incarcerated juveniles than for the adult offenders, the juveniles did report lower levels of adolescent employment, and they achieved less financial independence than the adult offenders had as adolescents.

Several other differences between the two groups emerged, but on only a handful did the juveniles score in a less pathological direction than the adults. Juveniles disclosed more aggressive fantasies, got into more fights and were crueller to animals than adults. They were, however, less physically violent toward women than the adults, even though they did not differ in their aggressive fantasies toward women, and they acknowledged higher levels of hyper or negative masculinity, which has been found to correlate with hostility toward women (Knight and Sims-Knight, in press a; Malamuth *et al.*, 1995). Also, juveniles reported that they had experienced less verbal abuse both in childhood and adolescence than the adults, and they acknowledged a lower frequency of physical abuse.

The results in the sexual domains were mixed. Across the board juveniles disclosed more paraphiliac fantasies and behaviours, but they reported no differences in sexual preoccupation and sexual drive, and revealed less sexual compulsivity than adults. Their report of sadistic fantasies and behaviour was low and equal to the adults. They used conventional heterosexual pornography less than adults, but were exposed to more sexual materials in their family homes and in childhood. Their exposure to homosexual and child pornography equalled that of adults, and they were slightly lower in their exposure to violent pornography than adults. Juveniles also did not differ in the offence planning factors, which have been found to correlate highly with Sexual Preoccupation and Sexual Drive (Knight and Cerce, 1999).

Juveniles attributed less guilt and lower empathy to themselves than did adults. In contrast, adult offenders were higher in the manipulative behaviours of superficial charm and conning and poorer in perspective taking. The perspective taking difference is surprising, when considered in light of the normal egocentricity of adolescence (Elkind, 1967). These results could suggest what might be for adolescents the most predictive aspects of Factor 1 of the Psychopathy Checklist, which has been referred to as the callousness, unemotional factor (Frick, 1998) or as a composite of an arrogant and deceitful personality style and deficient affective experience (Cooke and Michie, 2001). In the following four sections all of the differences found in the present study are organized into related issues and then discussed in light of relevant research.

### Sexual abuse and sexual behaviour

The possibility that a history of sexual abuse may be a predictor of continuance of sexually coercive behaviour into adulthood is consistent with some other literature about sexual abuse. Burton (2000) found that his continuous offenders reported the greatest levels of sexual trauma on the Childhood Trauma Questionnaire. Moreover, sexually abusive youth who have been more severely sexually abused (i.e. more penetration) seem to commit more severe crimes (Burton *et al.*, 2002). The data in the present study also suggest that it is the seriousness of the sexual abuse that might constitute the most important risk factor.

It is clear that sexual abuse is neither a necessary nor a sufficient cause for the manifestation of sexually coercive behaviour in childhood or adolescence (Garland and Dougher, 1990). Only a proportion of males who are sexually abused become sexually abusive (Friedrich and Chaffin, 2000; Widom, 1996; Williams, 1995), and not all juvenile and adult sexual offenders have experienced sexual abuse as children or adolescents. Nonetheless, there is considerable evidence that sexual abuse plays a role as a risk factor in sexually coercive behaviour. Both adult (Graham, 1996; Langevin *et al.*, 1985; Seghorn *et al.*, 1987; Stukas-Davis, 1990) and juvenile (Becker *et al.*, 1986; Burton *et al.*, 2002; Fehrenbach *et al.*, 1986; Friedrich and Luecke, 1988; Longo, 1982; Moody and Kim, 1994) sexual offenders report a high prevalence of such abuse in their developmental histories. Sexually coercive youth were more frequently the victims of sexual abuse than nonsexually offending delinquents (Burton *et al.*, 2002). Moreover, for juveniles their sexual abusive history predicts the nature of their predatory acts (Burton, in press; DiCenso, 1992).

Isolating the specific effects of sexual abuse from other pathogenic properties of family environment, such as physical abuse, neglect and general family disruption, has remained an elusive goal because different types of childhood abuse tend to covary (Briere, 1992; Knight and Prentky, 1993; Knight and Sims-Knight, in press a). In addition, because sexual abuse is a complex phenomenon, fraught with multiple definitional, assessment and methodological problems (Haugaard, 2000; Knight and Sims-Knight, in press a; Nash *et al.*, 1993), we must be cautious in our interpretation of the immediate and long-term covariates of such abuse that have been identified.

Despite the immense complexities of sexual abuse, a convergence of findings suggests that there are identifiable sequelae to such abuse (Briere and Elliott, 1994). The most prominent immediate effects of sexual abuse include: post traumatic stress disorder (PTSD), anxiety and sexualized behaviour in preschoolers; PTSD, fear and aggression in latency age children; and depression, poor self-esteem, self-destructive behaviour and promiscuity in adolescents (Kendall-Tackett *et al.*, 1993).

Although there seems to be a consistent low order relation between sexual abuse and increased sexual fantasy and behaviour in adulthood, the link of sexual abuse to sexual fantasy and level of sexual drive in adolescence is not as clear (Knight and Sims-Knight, in press a). Hypersexuality, highly sexualized behaviour and drive, sexual deviance and promiscuity are likely to be multi-determined, involving both genetic and environmental precursors (Bailey *et al.*, 2000; Knight and Sims-Knight, in press a). Also, sexuality is clearly in its formative stages in adolescence, so the identification of consistent, cross-temporally stable sexual dispositions might not emerge until early adulthood.

Yet, some consistent patterns of differences in sexual behaviour and fantasy between juveniles and adults were evident in the present study. Despite reporting comparable levels of sexual drive and preoccupation and lower levels of sexual compulsivity, the juveniles nonetheless consistently reported higher levels of all paraphiliac fantasy and behaviour. The high incidence of paraphilias reported by the juveniles is consistent with Abel *et al.*'s (1993) finding that 42 per cent of adults report the onset of their paraphilias to be prior to age eighteen. The higher incidence of paraphilias despite comparable levels of sexual drive and preoccupation would suggest that the purported role of hypersexuality in the development of paraphilias (Kafka, 1997) is a complex one and requires the identification of additional interacting factors. Paraphilias have been found to constitute a recidivism risk factor in adult child molesters (Prentky *et al.*, 1997). Self report of paraphiliac behaviours and fantasies did not, however, differentiate juvenile onset offenders from adult onset offenders in Knight and Prentky's (1993) retrospective study. Nevertheless, the high prevalence of paraphilias in high-risk juveniles suggests that their role as a potential risk factor for persistence of adolescent sexually aggressive behaviour into adulthood should be explored further.

The lower adolescent exposure to conventional heterosexual pornography of the juvenile offenders compared to the adult offenders might reflect the increasing availability of sexual materials with age. This would be consistent with the higher level of exposure in the family of the juvenile sexual offenders, suggesting that some family members might be providing the juvenile offenders with sexual materials that they might encounter more difficulty obtaining elsewhere. Although pornography use has consistently been correlated with increased risk for sexually coercive attitudes and behaviours – especially explicit sexual acts and violent pornography (Malamuth *et al.*, 2000) – its causal role appears to be quite complex. Malamuth *et al.*'s (2000) correlational analyses strongly suggest that males with a high proclivity to sexually coercive behaviour might react to and interpret pornographic material differently, making the high use of such materials a more serious risk factor for these individuals than for individuals with a low proclivity to such aggression.

### Juvenile antisocial behaviour, impulsivity and anger/aggression

Antisocial behaviour has emerged as a recidivism risk factor in many studies of adult sexual offenders and has consequently been incorporated into many risk assessment instruments (e.g. Hanson, 2000). In a 25-year follow-up study of rapists, juvenile victimless crimes contributed to the discriminant function analysis predicting serious sexual crimes, and juvenile antisocial behaviour predicted subsequent nonsexual victim-involved crimes (Knight, 1999). In a five-year follow-up study of juvenile sexual offenders, Rassmussen (1999) found that prior nonsexual offences were associated with nonsexual recidivism, but not with sexual recidivism. Worling (2001) found that his Antisocial/Impulsive adolescent sexual offender type was more likely to be charged with subsequent violent (including sexual) or non-violent offences within six years after release. In a ten-year follow-up of adolescent sexual offenders, psychopaths, who by definition were high on antisocial behaviour, were found to have committed both more sexual and non-violent and violent offences than their non-psychopath cohorts (Gretton *et al.*, 2001). The criminal path of the psychopathic sexual offenders was more progressive, violent and generalized than their non-psychopath cohorts. It is not surprising therefore that some risk assessment indices both for adults (e.g. Epperson *et al.*, 1998) and for adolescent sexual offenders (Prentky *et al.*, 2000; Worling and Curwen, 2000) have included *juvenile* antisocial behaviour or impulsivity as a risk factor. In the present study the high-risk juvenile offenders' consistent acknowledgement of more frequent juvenile antisocial behaviour when compared with generic adult sexual offenders is consistent with these data.

In our 25-year follow-up study of rapists, pervasive anger was consistently the best predictor of both subsequent serious sexual charges and violent, nonsexual charges (Knight, 1999). That juveniles were significantly higher on three of the four pervasive anger factors suggests that this domain might predict persistence into adulthood as well as recidivism as an adult.

### Social competence

Worling's (2001) Unusual/Isolated cluster type had a significantly greater probability of recidivating in a six-year follow-up than either of his two non-pathological types, and it was indistinguishable in outcome from the Antisocial/Impulsive type adolescent sexual offenders. Unfortunately, despite its name, this type scored higher on Worling's (2001) sociability factor than a less "pathological" type with lower recidivism, the Overcontrolled/Reserved type. Consequently, it is difficult to determine the contribution of social competence per se to recidivism in this study. Kenny *et al.* (2001) found that poor social skills significantly discriminated between groups of first-time and recidivist adolescent sexual offenders, suggesting its potential prognostic value. Although Knight and Prentky (1993) found that juvenile onset sexual offenders had poorer social relations as adults than adult onset sexual offenders manifested, in the present study, no differences between juveniles and adults in social relationships in adolescence (i.e. friendships and dating) emerged. Only differences in employment and financial independence, which in adolescence might be confounded with dimensions other than social competence, were found to discriminate the juveniles. Obviously, the negotiation of social relationships is a complexly determined phenomenon (Prentky and Knight, 1991). This certainly contributes to the mixed results that have emerged. Although the data are not consistent, the tantalizing results that do exist indicate that determining what aspect of interpersonal skills and intimacy seeking (Marshall, 1989) may be relevant to the persistence of offending in juveniles is a worthy enterprise with a reasonable probability of some predictive payoff. Some data suggest that the most vulnerable group might be the loners or social isolates (Awad *et al.*, 1984; Shoor *et al.*, 1966).

### *Personality, emotional responsivity and physical abuse*

Although Factor 1 of the PCL-R (Callousness, Unemotional) has received little attention in the literature on juvenile sexual offenders, what research does exist suggests that this personality/affective factor is an important predictor in this population. Caputo *et al.* (1999) found that, consistent with the adult literature, juvenile sexual offenders had more callous and unemotional traits than other offenders. Research on adolescents indicates that this factor can be reliably measured in juveniles (Christian *et al.*, 1997; Frick, 1998). Moreover, its presence in children with significant conduct disorder problems identifies a subgroup of children with more severe behavioural problems than those with only conduct disorders (Christian *et al.*, 1997; Frick, 1998; Lynam, 1998).

Cooke and Michie (2001) have demonstrated that this factor comprises two subfactors that should be considered separately, the Arrogant and Deceitful Interpersonal Style and Defective Affective Experience. The differences in the present study are certainly consistent with Cooke and Michie's reformulation, because juveniles and adults differed in opposite directions on the two proposed subfactors. Whereas the juveniles revealed more difficulties on the components measuring Defective Affective Experience (lack of guilt and empathy), adults exceeded the juveniles on the superficial charm and conning aspect of the Arrogant and Deceitful Personality and in their poor perspective taking abilities. These data suggest that the empathy and guilt components of defective affectivity might constitute the more fertile areas to search for risk factors for juveniles. Assessment in this area is fraught with methodological conundrums (e.g. Dickie, 1998) and it has been demonstrated in adult sexual offenders that it is important to evaluate generic abilities and propensities as well as sexual-victim-specific emotional responsivity measures in assessing empathy (Marshall *et al.*, 2001). Preston and Serin's

(1999) performance-based approach seems to hold the greatest promise for developing predictive, duplicity-free measurements in this domain.

Physical abuse is grouped with the callousness, unemotional components because in the structural equation models generated both for adult and for juvenile sexual offenders physical abuse predicted the latent trait comprising components of this factor (Knight and Sims-Knight, in press a and b). This finding is consistent with the evidence supporting the hypothesis that physical abuse may encourage children to detach emotionally. Such abuse has also been found to correlate with the presence of personality disorders (Goldman *et al.*, 1992; Herman *et al.*, 1989) and with dissociation (Chu and Dill, 1990; Sandberg and Lynn, 1992). In Malamuth's (1998) recent revision of his theoretical model of sexual coercion harsh early environments, which include physical abuse, play a prominent antecedent role in sexually coercive behaviour, both potentially locking a person into short-term mating strategies and increasing the probability of both a hostile masculinity associative network and aggressive and antisocial behaviour. He cites literature supporting both hypotheses (e.g. Belsky *et al.*, 1991; Kim *et al.*, 1997).

Physical abuse plays a prominent role in the juvenile sexual offender literature. Juvenile sexual offenders have been found to have experienced more abuse than other delinquent groups (Ford and Linney, 1995; Van Ness, 1984). Likewise, Lewis *et al.* (1981) found that whereas 75 per cent of their violent adolescent *sexual* offenders had been physically abused only 29 per cent of other delinquents had experienced such abuse. Physical abuse was not, however, unique to sexual offenders. In this same study an equal percentage of violent nonsexual offenders had also been physically abused.

In our 25-five-year follow-up study of rapists the childhood physical abuse reported in archival records predicted subsequent charges for both serious sexual offences and violent non-sexual offences (Knight, 1999). The present study suggests, however, that physical abuse might not serve as a predictor of persistence of sexual offending from adolescence to adulthood, because the high-risk juveniles tested were lower on the physical/verbal abuse scales than the adult sexual offenders.

## Conclusions and limitations

The data in this chapter support the viability of generalizing models of adult sexual offenders to incarcerated, high-risk juvenile sexual offenders. The data further suggest several domains that should be explored as likely candidates for identifying those juveniles with a higher risk to continue their sexually aggressive behaviour into adulthood. The strongest candidates include being victims of childhood sexual abuse, especially more serious abuse involving penetration, juvenile antisocial behaviour and impulsivity, proclivity to pervasive anger, difficulties with anger management, the presence of frequent paraphiliac fantasies and behaviours, and various components of deficient affective responsivity. Another, less strongly supported candidate was poor social competence, where poor social skills and possibly social isolation should be studied further.

It must be stressed that the suggestion of generalizability and the proposal of persistence markers are speculative hypotheses, not corroborations. They clearly require further research and greater specification. The offenders tested here constitute a voluntary, select sample of convenience and not a random sample of all sexual offenders. Although the data were gathered under conditions of strict confidentiality and were protected by a Certificate of Confidentiality, absolutely veridical and unbiased self-report can never be completely guaranteed. It is reassuring that both juveniles and adults scored very low on the Marlowe-Crowne Social Desirability Scale, indicating low defensiveness (Saunders, 1991). Finally, it must also be emphasized that the sample of adolescents studied here were a select sample of higher risk, incarcerated offenders. These results do not apply to all juveniles who become involved in problematic sexual behaviour.

### *Author note*

This research was supported by research grants MH54263–01 from the National Institute of Mental Health and 94-IJ-CX-0049 from the National Institute of Justice. The author wishes to express his deep appreciation to the staff in the numerous institutions at which we have tested for their considerable commitment of time and energy to our research programme. I also thank all the offenders who participated in this research. Special thanks are due to David Cerce and Alison Martino for coordinating the coding of files and organizing all of our data, to Nick Fadden and Karen Fadden for help coordinating and collecting the Minnesota data, and to Karen Locke for her programming and data processing skills.

Correspondence concerning this study should be addressed to Raymond Knight, Ph.D., Department of Psychology, MS 062, Brandeis University, Waltham, Massachusetts 02454–9110. Electronic mail may be sent to Knight2@Brandeis.edu.

## APPENDIX A: FACTOR-ANALYTICALLY DERIVED SCALES

### *Juvenile antisocial behaviour*

1 *Delinquency* – This factor scale assesses instances of juvenile delinquency, including disturbing the peace, vandalism, trespassing, vagrancy, drunk-and-disorderly, larceny, stealing cars, etc. Items on this scale used

the 5-point frequency response format ("never" [0] to "very often – > 50 times" [4]). Higher scores indicate more frequent delinquent behaviour.

2 *Problems in junior high* – This factor scale assesses behavioural problems in junior high school including instances of acting out, truancy, suspension, and misbehaving in school. Items on this scale used the 5-point frequency response format ("never" [0] to "very often – > 50 times" [4]). Higher scores indicate more problems in junior high school.
3 *Fighting and assaultive behaviour (Bully)* – This factor scale assesses instances of fighting, bullying and also being picked on as a juvenile. Items on this scale used the 5-point frequency response format ("never" [0] to "very often – > 50 times" [4]). Higher scores mean more fighting and assaultive behaviour as a juvenile.
4 *Driving problems* – This motor vehicle offence scale assesses instances of motor vehicle violations (e.g. speeding, driving to endanger, etc.) as a juvenile. Items on this scale used the 5-point frequency response format ("never" [0] to "very often – > 50 times" [4]). Higher scores mean more violations as a juvenile.
5 *Problems in grammar school* – This scale assesses behavioural problems in grammar school including instances of acting out, truancy, suspension, and misbehaving in school. Items on this scale used the 5-point frequency response format ("never" [0] to "very often – > 50 times" [4]). Higher scores indicate more problems in grammar school.
6 *Drug problems* – Items on this scale assess the use and abuse of illegal substances. Items on this scale used the 5-point frequency response format ("never" [0] to "very often – > 50 times" [4]). Higher scores indicate more abuse of drugs.

### *Expressive aggression*

1 *Physical violence against women* – This factor comprises items in which the offender admits to having beaten, roughed up or physically hurt women. Items on this scale used the 5-point frequency response format ("never" [0] to "very often – > 50 times" [4]). Higher scores mean more physical violence toward women was acknowledged.
2 *Aggressive fantasies against women* – This violent fantasies involving women scale includes items that assess aggressive fantasies toward women. It includes thoughts of humiliating, frightening and beating women. Items on this scale used the 5-point frequency response format ("never" [0] to "very often – > 50 times" [4]). Higher scores mean more violent fantasies about women were acknowledged.

*Pervasive anger*

1 *Constantly angry* – This anger scale assesses instances of anger and failure to control one's temper. This scale comprises items with both true/false and temporal frequency response formats. The scale ranges from 0 to 4/5, with higher scores indicating greater and more constant anger.
2 *Physical fighting* – This physically assaultive behaviour scale assesses instances of assaultive behaviour (getting into physical fights) against both males and females. This scale comprises items with both true/false and temporal frequency response formats. The scale ranges from 0 to 4/5, with higher scores indicating more fighting.
3 *Fantasies of hurting people* – This violent fantasies scale assesses the frequency of having fantasies of hurting other people. This scale comprises items with both true/false and temporal frequency response formats. The scale ranges from 0 to 4/5, with higher scores indicating more violent fantasies.
4 *Cruelty to animals* – This scale indicates the frequency that the respondent has been cruel to animals, other than in sport (hunting). This scale comprises items with both true/false and temporal frequency response formats. The scale ranges from 0 to 4/5, with higher scores indicating more frequent cruelty to animals.

*Sadism*

1 *Bondage/restraint* – This scale includes items that involve a mixture of tying, bondage, controlling and hurting fantasies and behaviours. Items on this scale used the 5-point frequency response format ("never" [0] to "very often – > 50 times" [4]). Higher scores indicate a higher frequency of bondage/restraint fantasies or behaviours.
2 *Synergism of sex and aggression* – This scale captures what has been often referred to in the clinical literature as the combination of sexual arousal and aggression. In a number of items on this scale the respondent admits that hurting, threatening, and frightening someone increase sexual arousal and satisfaction. Items on this scale used the 5-point frequency response format ("never" [0] to "very often – > 50 times" [4]). Higher scores indicate a greater admitted linkage of sexual arousal and aggression.
3 *Sadistic fantasy* – This scale captures extreme sadistic fantasies, such as burning, strangling, cutting and whipping during sex. Items on this scale used the 5-point frequency response format ("never" [0] to "very often – > 50 times" [4]). Higher scores mean more frequent sadistic fantasies.

### Sexual preoccupation, drive, and compulsivity (sexualization)

1 *Sexual preoccupation* – This scale assesses preoccupation with sexual thoughts and fantasies. These items used both the true/false and the temporal frequency formats. The scale ranged from 0 to 4/5 with higher scores indicating greater sexual preoccupation.
2 *Sexual drive* – This scale assesses the frequency and strength of the respondent's sexual drive, or the frequency of sexual behaviour. It comprises items with multiple formats. The scale ranges from 0 to 7, with higher scores indicating a higher sexual drive.
3 *Sexual compulsivity* – This scale includes items in which the respondent characterizes himself as having to combat persistent, intrusive sexual urges that compel him to act out in a particular manner. Items on this scale used the 5-point frequency response format ("never" [0] to "very often – > 50 times" [4]). Higher scores mean more sexual compulsion.

### Paraphilias

1 *Frotteurism and obscene phone calls (atypical paraphilias)* – The scale assesses becoming sexually aroused by rubbing up against someone who does not wish such behaviour or making obscene phone calls. Items on this scale used the 5-point frequency response format ("never" [0] to "very often – > 50 times" [4]). Higher scores correspond to a greater frequency of these fantasies and behaviours.
2 *Exhibitionism* – The scale assesses exposing or fantasizing exposing one's genitals to a non-consenting person. Items on this scale used the 5-point frequency response format ("never" [0] to "very often – > 50 times" [4]). Higher scores correspond to a greater frequency of exhibitionistic fantasies and behaviours.
3 *Transvestism* – The scale assesses becoming sexually aroused by wearing the clothes of the opposite sex. Items on this scale used the 5-point frequency response format ("never" [0] to "very often – > 50 times" [4]). Higher scores correspond to a greater frequency of these fantasies and behaviours.
4 *Voyeurism* – This scale assesses fantasies and behaviours involving watching people engage in sexual activity, when they do not consent to the observation. Items on this scale used the 5-point frequency response format ("never" [0] to "very often – > 50 times" [4]). Higher scores correspond to a greater frequency of these behaviours.

### Pornography use

1 *Adult women: conventional sex* – This scale focuses on more conventional uses of pornography. The respondent is exposed to pornography as a

teen and masturbates to it as an adult. The respondent indicates that pornography is used both to relieve the urge to act out sexually and to encourage acting out sexually. These items used the temporal frequency format, ranging from "never" (0) through "every day" (5). Higher scores mean more frequent exposure to this type of sexual material.

2 *Adult women: sadism and physical injury* – This scale includes exposure to pornography that involves bondage and physical abuse. The items on this scale come from all developmental stages, starting in childhood. These items used the temporal frequency format, ranging from "never" (0) through "every day" (5). Higher scores mean more frequent exposure to this type of sexual material.

3 *Adult men and children* – Child and homosexual pornography make up this scale. This exposure starts in childhood and remains constant into adulthood. These items used the temporal frequency format, ranging from "never" (0) through "every day" (5). Higher scores mean more frequent exposure to this type of sexual material.

4 *Adult women: conventional sex within family* – This is the only scale that includes exposure to pornography by family members. The respondent indicates that he has been exposed exclusively to heterosexual material as a child, and this exposure continues on into adolescence, but does not contribute to adult sexuality. These items used the temporal frequency format, ranging from "never" (0) through "every day" (5). Higher scores mean more frequent exposure to this type of sexual material.

### *Offence planning*

1 *Intimacy-seeking fantasies* – This scale includes fantasies in which the respondent ignores the agonistic nature of coercive sexual behaviour and fantasizes about the response that his sexual overtures will elicit. Here he fantasizes about what he will say to a woman during coercive sex and what she will say and feel during the encounter. Items on this scale used the 5-point frequency response format ("never" [0] to "very often – > 50 times" [4]). Higher scores indicate more of these offence-planning fantasies.

2 *Aggressive/violent fantasies* – This scale taps the respondent's fantasies about physically harming, frightening and even killing someone during non-consensual sex. Items on this scale used the 5-point frequency response format ("never" [0] to "very often – > 50 times" [4]). Higher scores indicate more of these offence-planning fantasies.

3 *Planning an offence: victim type and encounter location* – This scale captures the respondent's forethought in seeking a particular person in a particular location for sexually coercive behaviour. Items on this scale used the 5-point frequency response format ("never" [0] to "very often – > 50 times" [4]). Higher scores indicate more of these offence planning thoughts.

4 *Sexual fantasies* – This scale includes the respondent's fantasies about what sexual acts he will perform, or have a person do to or for him during coercive sex. Items on this scale used the 5-point frequency response format ("never" [0] to "very often – > 50 times" [4]). Higher scores indicate more of these offence-planning fantasies.
5 *Eluding apprehension* – This scale taps the respondent's plans to avoid being caught after sexually coercive behaviour. Items on this scale used the 5-point frequency response format ("never" [0] to "very often – > 50 times" [4]). Higher scores indicate more of these offence-planning thoughts.
6 *Planning the offence: weapons and paraphernalia* – This scale focuses on the weapons and paraphernalia (the "rape kit") that the responder has indicated he takes with him on offences. Items on this scale used the 5-point frequency response format ("never" [0] to "very often – > 50 times" [4]). Higher scores indicate more of these offence-planning thoughts.

## RATIONALLY DERIVED SCALES

### *Social competence*

1 *Juvenile employment and independence* – This rationally derived scale assesses whether the respondent earned money and supported himself prior to incarceration, while an adolescent. Higher scores here mean greater independence; range = 0–4.
2 *Juvenile friendships* – This rationally derived scale assesses the extent and depth of interpersonal relationships that the respondent had attained in adolescence. Higher scores indicate a higher level of social relationships; range = 0–5.
3 *Juvenile dating* – This rationally derived scale assesses the frequency of dating and heterosexual socialization and the depth of heterosexual relationships attained in adolescence. Higher scores indicate a higher level of heterosexual relationships; range = 0–5.

### *Emotional detachment*

1 *Lack of guilt* – This scale measures lack of guilt and shame for negative behaviour. Items on this scale used the true/false (0–4) format, and higher scores indicate less experience of guilt or shame.
2 *Lack of empathy* – This scale measures the lack of empathy for others' misfortunes. Items on this scale used the true/false (0–4) format, and higher scores indicate less empathy.
3 *Poor perspective taking* – This scale measures difficulty with taking another's perspective and seeing both sides of a situation. Items on this

scale used the true/false (0–4) format, and higher scores indicate poorer perspective taking.

### *Arrogant and deceitful personality*

1 *Callousness* – This scale assesses the tendency to act without regard to others' feelings. Items on this scale were in the true/false (0–4) format, and higher scores indicate the higher levels of callousness.
2 *Charming and conning* – This scale measures the use of charm or deception to manipulate people to do one's bidding. Items on the scale were in the true/false (0–4) format, and higher scores indicate the presence of more aspects of this manipulativeness.
3 *Grandiosity* – This scale measures having exaggerated self-worth and entitlement. Items on the scale were in the true/false (0–4) format, and higher scores indicate greater self-aggrandizement.
4 *Negative masculinity* – This scale assesses the power, dominance, risk taking, toughness, aggressiveness, honour defending, and competitiveness that characterize negative aspects of masculinity. Items on the scale were in the true/false (0–4) format, and higher scores indicate the presence of more aspects of negative masculinity.

### *Sexual abuse in childhood and adolescence*

1 *Childhood sexual abuse, level* – This scale measures the highest level of sexual invasion achieved in childhood (≤ 12 years old) sexual abuse, ranging from no sexual abuse (0) through anal penetration (5).
2 *Childhood sexual abuse, force* – This 0 to 4 point scale measures highest amount of coercion used in childhood (≤ 12 years old) sexual abuse, ranging from no sexual abuse (0) through physical force (5).
3 *Teenage sexual abuse, level* – This scale measures the highest level of sexual invasion achieved in adolescent (13–17 years old) sexual abuse, ranging from no sexual abuse (0) through anal penetration (5).
4 *Teenage sexual abuse, force* – This 0 to 4 point scale measures highest amount of coercion used in adolescent (13–17 years old) sexual abuse, ranging from no sexual abuse (0) through physical force (5).

### *Physical abuse in childhood and adolescence*

1 *Childhood verbal abuse* – The items on this scale measure the frequency of serious verbal abuse (e.g. scare or frighten, threaten not to love) experienced in childhood (≤ 12 years old). These items used the temporal frequency format ranging from "never" (0) through "every day" (5).
2 *Adolescent verbal abuse* – The items on this scale measure the frequency of serious verbal abuse (e.g. scare or frighten, threaten not to love)

experienced in adolescence (13–17 years old). These items used the temporal frequency format ranging from "never" (0) through "every day" (5).

3 *Physical abuse, level* – This scale measures the highest level of physical abuse that was experienced in childhood or adolescence. The scale ranged from "none" (0) through "injuries requiring medical attention" (6).
4 *Physical abuse, frequency* – This scale measures the highest frequency that a caregiver was physically abusive to the offender during childhood or adolescence. The items on this scale used the temporal frequency format ranging from "never" (0) through "every day" (5).

## References

Abel, G., Osborne, C., and Twigg, D. (1993). Sexual assault through the life span: Adult offenders with juvenile histories. In H. E. Barbaree, W. L. Marshall and S. M. Hudson (eds), *The Juvenile Sex Offender*. New York: Guilford Press, pp. 104–117.

Awad, G. A., Saunders, E., and Levene, J. (1984). A clinical study of male adolescent sexual offenders. *International Journal of Offender Therapy and Comparative Criminology, 28*, 105–115.

Bailey, J. M., Kirk, K. M., Zhu, G., Dunne, M. P., and Martin, N. G. (2000). Do individual differences in sociosexuality represent genetic or environmentally contingent strategies? Evidence from the Australian twin registry. *Journal of Personality and Social Psychology, 78*, 537–545.

Barbaree, H. E., Hudson, S. M., and Seto, M. C. (1993). Sexual assault in society: The role of the juvenile offender. In H. E. Barbaree, W. L. Marshall and S. M. Hudson (eds), *The Juvenile Sex Offender*. New York: Guilford Press, pp. 1–24.

Bard, L. A., Carter, D. L., Cerce, D. D., Knight, R. A., Rosenberg, R., and Schneider, B. (1987). A descriptive study of rapists and child molesters: Developmental, clinical and criminal characteristics. *Behavioural Sciences and the Law, 5*, 203–220.

Becker, J. V., and Hunter, J. (1997). Understanding and treating child and adolescent sexual offenders. In T. H. Ollendick and R. J. Prinz (eds), *Advances in Clinical Child Psychology*, vol. 19. New York: Plenum Press, pp. 177–197.

Becker, J. V., Kaplan, M. S., Cunningham-Rathner, J., and Kavoussi, R. J. (1986). Characteristics of adolescent incest sexual perpetrators: Preliminary findings. *Journal of Family Violence, 1*, 85–97.

Belsky, J., Steinberg, L., and Draper, P. (1991). Childhood experience, interpersonal development, and reproductive strategy: An evolutionary theory of socialization. *Child Development, 62*, 647–670.

Briere, J. (1992). Methodological issues in the study of sexual abuse effects. *Journal of Consulting and Clinical Psychology, 60*, 196–203.

Briere, J. N., and Elliott, D. M. (1994). Immediate and long-term impacts of child sexual abuse. *Sexual Abuse of Children, 4*, 54–69.

Brown, E. J., Flanagan, T. J., and McLeod, M. (eds) (1984). *Sourcebook of Criminal Justice Statistics – 1983*. Washington, DC: Bureau of Justice Statistics.

Burton, D. L. (2000). Were adolescent sexual offenders children with sexual behaviour problems? *Sexual Abuse: A Journal of Research and Treatment, 12*, 37–48.

Burton, D. L. (in press). The relationship between the sexual victimization of and the subsequent sexual abuse by male adolescents. *Child and Adolescent Social Work Journal.*

Burton, D. L., Miller, D. L., and Shill, C. T. (2002). A social learning theory comparison of the sexual victimization of adolescent sexual offenders and non-sexual offending male delinquents. *Child Abuse and Neglect, 26*, 893–907.

Caputo, A. A., Frick, P. J., and Brodsky, S. L. (1999). Family violence and juvenile sex offending: The potential mediating role of psychopathic traits and negative attitudes toward women. *Criminal Justice and Behaviour, 26*, 338–356.

Christian, R. E., Frick, P. J., Hill, N. L., Tyler, L., and Frazer, D. R. (1997). Psychopathy and conduct problems in children. II: Implications for subtyping children with conduct problems. *Journal of the American Academy of Child and Adolescent Psychiatry, 36*, 233–241.

Chu, J. A., and Dill, D. L. (1990). Dissociative symptoms in relation to childhood physical and sexual abuse. *American Journal of Psychiatry, 147*, 887–892.

Cooke, D. J., and Michie, C. (2001). Refining the construct of psychopathy: Towards a hierarchical model. *Psychological Assessment, 13*, 171–188.

DiCenso, C. (1992). The adolescent sexual offender: Victim and perpetrator. In E. Viano (ed.), *Critical Issues in Victimology: International Perspectives*. Springer: New York, pp. 190–200.

Dickie, I. (1998). *An Information Processing Approach to Understanding Sympathy Deficits in Sexual Offenders*. Unpublished Master's thesis, Psychology Department, Carleton University.

Elkind, D. (1967). Egocentrism in adolescence. *Child Development, 38*, 15–27.

Epperson, D. L., Kaul, J. D, and Hesselton, D. (1998). *Final Report on the Development of the Minnesota Sex Offender Screening Tool–Revised (MnSOST-R)*. Paper presented at the 17th Annual Meeting of the Association for the Treatment of Sexual Abusers, Vancouver, British Columbia, October.

Fehrenbach, P. A., Smith, W., Monastersky, C., and Deisher, R. W. (1986). Adolescent sexual offenders: Offender and offence characteristics. *American Journal of Orthopsychiatry, 56*, 225–233.

Ford, M. E., and Linney, J. A. (1995). Comparative analysis of juvenile sexual offenders, violent homosexual offenders, and status offenders. *Journal of Interpersonal Violence, 10*, 56–70.

Frick, P. J. (1998). Callous-unemotional traits and conduct problems: A two-factor model of psychopathy in children. In D. J. Cooke, R. D. Hare and A. Forth (eds), *Psychopathy: Theory, Research, and Implications for Society*. Cordresch, the Netherlands: Kluwer Press, pp. 47–51.

Friedrich, W. N., and Chaffin, M. (2000). *Developmental-Systemic Perspectives on Children with Sexual Behavior Problems*. Paper presented at the 19th Annual Meeting of the Association for the Treatment of Sexual Abusers, San Diego, California, November.

Friedrich, W. N., and Luecke, W. J. (1988). Young school-age sexually aggressive children. *Professional Psychology Research and Practice, 19*, 155–164.

Garland, R., and Dougher, M. (1990). The abused/abuser hypothesis of child sexual abuse: A critical review of theory and research. In J. Fierman (ed.), *Pedophilia: Biosocial Dimensions*. New York: Springer-Verlag, pp. 488–509.

Goldman, S. J., D'Angelo, E. J., DeMaso, D. R., and Mezzacappa, E. (1992). Physical and sexual abuse histories among children with borderline personality disorder. *American Journal of Psychiatry, 149*, 1723–1726.

Graham, K. R. (1996). The childhood victimization of sex offenders: Underestimated issue. *International Journal of Offender Therapy and Comparative Criminology, 40*, 192–203.

Gretton, H. M., McBride, M., Hare, R. D., O'Shaughnessy, R., and Kumba, G. (2001). Psychopathy and recidivism in adolescent sex offenders. *Criminal Justice and Behaviour, 28*, 427–449.

Hanson, R. K. (2000). *Risk Assessment*. Beaverton, OR: Association for the Treatment of Sexual Abusers.

Hare, R. D., Harpur, T. J., Hakstian, A. R., Forth, A. E., Hart, S. D., and Newman, J. P. (1990). The revised Psychopathy Checklist: Reliability and factor structure. *Psychological Assessment, 2*, 338–341.

Harpur, T. J., Hakstian, A., and Hare, R. D. (1988). Factor structure of the Psychopathy Checklist. *Journal of Consulting and Clinical Psychology, 56*, 741–747.

Harpur, T. J., Hare, R. D., and Hakstian, A. (1989). Two-factor conceptualization of psychopathy: Construct validity and assessment implications. *Psychological Assessment: A Journal of Consulting and Clinical Psychology, 1*, 6–17.

Haugaard, J. (2000). The challenge of defining child sexual abuse. *American Psychologist, 55*, 1036–1039.

Herman, J. L., Perry, J. C., and van der Kolk, B. A. (1989). Childhood trauma in borderline personality disorder. *American Journal of Psychiatry, 146*, 490–495.

Johnson, G. M., and Knight, R. A. (2000). Developmental antecedents of sexual coercion in juvenile sex offenders. *Sexual Abuse: A Journal of Research and Treatment, 12*, 165–178.

Kafka, M. P. (1997). Hypersexual desire in males: An operational definition and clinical implications for males with paraphilias and paraphilia-related disorders. *Archives of Sexual Behaviour, 26*, 505–526.

Kendall-Tackett, K. A., Williams, L. M., and Finkelhor, D. (1993). Impact of sexual abuse on children: A review and synthesis of recent empirical studies. *Psychological Bulletin, 113*, 164–180.

Kenny, D. T., Keogh, T., and Seidler, K. (2001). Predictors of recidivism in Australian juvenile sex offenders: Implications for treatment. *Sexual Abuse: A Journal of Research and Treatment, 13*, 131–148.

Kim, K., Smith, P. K., and Palermiti, A. (1997). Conflict in childhood and reproductive development. *Evolution and Human Behaviour, 18*, 109–142.

Knight, R. A. (1997). *A Unified Model of Sexual Aggression: Consistencies and Differences across Noncriminal and Criminal Samples*. Paper presented at the 16th Annual Meeting of the Association for the Treatment of Sexual Abusers, Arlington, Virginia, October.

Knight, R. A. (1999). Validation of a typology for rapists. *Journal of Interpersonal Violence, 14*, 297–323.

Knight, R. A., and Cerce, D. D. (1999). Validation and revision of the Multidimensional Assessment of Sex and Aggression. *Psychologica Belgica, 39(2/3)*, 187–213.

Knight, R. A., and Prentky, R. A. (1993). Exploring the characteristics for classifying juvenile sexual offenders. In H. E. Barbaree, W. L. Marshall and S. M. Hudson (eds), *The Juvenile Sex Offender*. New York: Guilford Press, pp. 45–83.

Knight, R. A., and Sims-Knight, J. E. (in press a). The developmental antecedents of sexual coercion against women in adolescents. In R. Geffner and K. Franey (eds), *Sex Offenders: Assessment and Treatment*. New York: Haworth Press.

Knight, R. A., and Sims-Knight, J. E. (in press b). Developmental antecedents of sexual coercion against women: Testing of alternative hypotheses with structural equation modeling. In R. A. Prentky, E. Janus and M. Seto (eds), *Sexual Coercion: Understanding and Management*. New York: New York Academy of Sciences.

Knight, R. A., Prentky, R. A., and Cerce, D. (1994). The development, reliability, and validity of an inventory for the multidimensional assessment of sex and aggression. *Criminal Justice and Behaviour, 21*, 72–94.

Langevin, R., Handy, L., Hook, H., Day, D., and Russon, A. (1985). Are incestuous fathers pedophilic and aggressive? In R. Langevin (ed.), *Erotic Preference, Gender, Identity, and Aggression*. Hillsdale, NJ: Lawrence Erlbaum.

Lewis, D. O., Shanok, S. S., and Pincus, J. H. (1981). Juvenile male sexual assaulters: Psychiatric, neurological, psychoeducational, and abuse factors. In D. O. Lewis (ed.), *Vulnerabilities to Delinquency*. New York: SP Medical and Scientific Books, pp. 89–105.

Longo, R. F. (1982). Sexual learning and experience among adolescent sexual offenders. *International Journal of Offender Therapy and Comparative Criminology, 26*, 235–241.

Lynam, D. R. (1998). Early identification of the fledgling psychopath: Locating the psychopathic child in the current nomenclature. *Journal of Abnormal Psychology, 107*, 566–575.

Malamuth, N. (1998). An evolutionary-based model integrating research on the characteristics of sexually coercive men. In J. Adair, K. Dion and D. Belanger (eds), *Advances in Psychological Science*, vol. 2: *Personal, Social, and Developmental Aspects*. Hove: Psychology Press, pp. 151–184.

Malamuth, N. M., Sockloskie, R. J., Koss, M. P., and Tanaka, J. S. (1991). Characteristics of aggressors against women: Testing a model using a national sample of college students. *Journal of Consulting and Clinical Psychology, 59*, 670–681.

Malamuth, N. M., Heavey, C. L., and Linz, D. (1993). Predicting men's antisocial behaviour against women: The interaction model of sexual aggression. In G. C. Nagayama Hall, R. Hirschman, J. R. Graham and M. S. Zaragoza (eds), *Sexual Aggression: Issues in Etiology and Assessment, Treatment and Policy*. Washington, DC: Hemisphere, pp. 63–97.

Malamuth, N. M., Linz, D., Heavey, C. L., Barnes, G., and Acker, M. (1995). Using the confluence model of sexual aggression to predict men's conflict with women: A 10-year follow-up study. *Journal of Personality and Social Psychology, 69*, 353–369.

Malamuth, N. M., Addison, T., and Koss, M. (2000). Pornography and sexual aggression: Are there reliable effects and can we understand them? *Annual Review of Sex Research, 11*, 26–91.

Marshall, W. L. (1989). Intimacy, loneliness and sexual offenders. *Behaviour Research and Therapy, 27*, 491–503.

Marshall, W. L., Hamilton, K., and Fernandez, Y. (2001). Empathy deficits and cognitive distortions in child molesters. *Sexual Abuse: A Journal of Research and Treatment, 13*, 123–130.

Moody, E. B. J., and Kim, J. (1994). Personality and background characteristics of adolescent sexual offenders. *Journal of Addictions and Offender Counseling, 14*, 38–49.

Nash, M. R., Hulsey, T. L., Sexton, M. C., Harralson, T. L., and Lambert, W. (1993). Long-term sequelae of childhood sexual abuse: perceived family environment, psychopathology, and dissociation. *Journal of Consulting and Clinical Psychology, 61*, 276–283.

Prentky, R. A., and Knight, R. A. (1991). Identifying critical dimensions for discriminating among rapists. *Journal of Consulting and Clinical Psychology, 59*, 643–661.

Prentky, R. A., Knight, R. A., and Lee, A. F. S. (1997). Risk factors associated with recidivism among extrafamilial child molesters. *Journal of Consulting and Clinical Psychology, 65*, 141–149.

Prentky, R. A., Harris, B., Frizzell, K., and Righthand, S. (2000). An actuarial procedure for assessing risk with juvenile sex offenders. *Sexual Abuse: A Journal of Research and Treatment, 12*, 71–93.

Preston, D. L., and Serin, R. C. (1999). *Case File: Persistently Violent (Nonsexual) Offender Treatment Program*. Ottawa: Research Branch, Correctional Service of Canada.

Rassmussen, L. A. (1999). Factors related to recidivism among juvenile sexual offenders. *Sexual Abuse: A Journal of Research and Treatment, 11*, 69–85.

Righthand, S., Carpenter, E. M., and Prentky, R. A. (2001). *Risk Assessment in a Sample of Juveniles who have Sexually Offended: A Comparative Analysis*. Poster presented at the 20th Annual Conference of the Association for the Treatment of Sexual Abusers, San Antonio, Texas, November.

Sandberg, D. A., and Lynn, S. J. (1992). Dissociative experiences, psychopathology and adjustment, and childhood and adolescent maltreatment in female college students. *Journal of Abnormal Psychology, 101*, 391–398.

Saunders, D. G. (1991). Procedures for adjusting self-reports of violence for social desirability bias. *Journal of Interpersonal Violence, 6*, 336–344.

Seghorn, T. K., Prentky, R. A., and Boucher, R. J. (1987). Childhood sexual abuse in the lives of sexually aggressive offenders. *Journal of the American Academy of Child and Adolescent Psychiatry, 26*, 262–267.

Shoor, M., Speed, M. H., and Bartelt, C. (1966). Syndrome of the adolescent child molester. *American Journal of Psychiatry, 122*, 783–789.

Stukas-Davis, C. (1990). The Influence of Childhood Sexual Abuse and Male Sex Role Socialization on Adult Sexual Functioning. Unpublished doctoral dissertation, California School of Professional Psychology, Los Angeles.

Van Ness, S. R. (1984). Rape as instrumental violence: A study of youth offenders. *Journal of Offender Counseling, Services, and Rehabilitation, 9*, 161–170.

Weinrott, M. R. (1996). *Juvenile Sexual Aggression: A Critical Review*. Boulder: University of Colorado, Institute for Behavioral Sciences, Center for the Study and Prevention of Violence.

Widom, C. S. (1996). Childhood sexual abuse and its criminal consequences. *Society, 33*, 47–53.

Williams, L. M. (1995). *Juvenile and Adult Offending Behavior and Other Outcomes in a Cohort of Sexually Abused Boys: Twenty Years Later*. Philadelphia, PA: Joseph J. Peters Institute.

Worling, J. R. (2001). Personality-based typology of adolescent male sexual offenders: Differences in recidivism rates, victim-selection characteristics, and personal victimization histories. *Sexual Abuse: A Journal of Research and Treatment, 13*, 149–166.

Worling, J. R., and Curwen, T. (2000). *The "ERASOR" Estimate of Risk of Adolescent Sexual Offense Recidivism*, Version 1.1. Ontario: SAFE-R Program, Thistletown Regional Center.

Zakireh, B. (1999). Residential and Outpatient Adolescent Sexual and Nonsexual Offenders: History, Sexual Adjustment, Clinical, Cognitive, and Demographic Characteristics. Unpublished doctoral thesis. Psychology Department, Bryn Mawr College.

# Part III

# Intervention

Chapter 9

# Essentials of an effective treatment programme for sexually abusive adolescents

## Offence specific treatment tasks

*Bobbie Print and David O'Callaghan*

### Introduction

Young people who sexually abuse present with a range of developmental, social and interpersonal needs, and recent literature has increasingly promoted a holistic, developmentally sensitive approach to work with this group of young people (O'Callaghan, 2002; Rich, 1998; Ryan, 1999). Furthermore, the evidence base evaluating the effectiveness of interventions with young people who sexually abuse, whilst limited in its extent, also supports a holistic and multisystemic approach (Borduin *et al.*, 1990; Swenson *et al.*, 1998; Worling and Curwen, 2000). This chapter addresses some of the offence specific work frequently included in therapeutic programmes. In doing so we review some key areas of the literature pertinent to each offence specific target and then outline our current approach to clinical intervention based on our work at G-MAP (a UK service for young people who sexually abuse). In all illustrative case examples used in this chapter identifying details have been changed. We feel it is important to emphasise that the approaches described here should be considered as one component of a holistic strategy. A challenge, therefore, for services working with this group of young people is to provide a structure for assessment and intervention that encompasses the broad tapestry of an individual's developmental needs and forms connections with others in the young person's system who will be contributing to various aspects in the overall plan aimed at helping the young person develop a healthy lifestyle free from sexually abusive behaviour.

### The G-MAP programme

At G-MAP we identify six essential areas of need that should be considered for each young person who engages in sexually abusive behaviour (see Figure 9.1). Assessments are conducted to identify a young person's specific needs and assets and, where therapeutic intervention is indicated, to inform the construction of an intervention programme that usually consists of individual, group and family work. Specific targets for change are identified across each

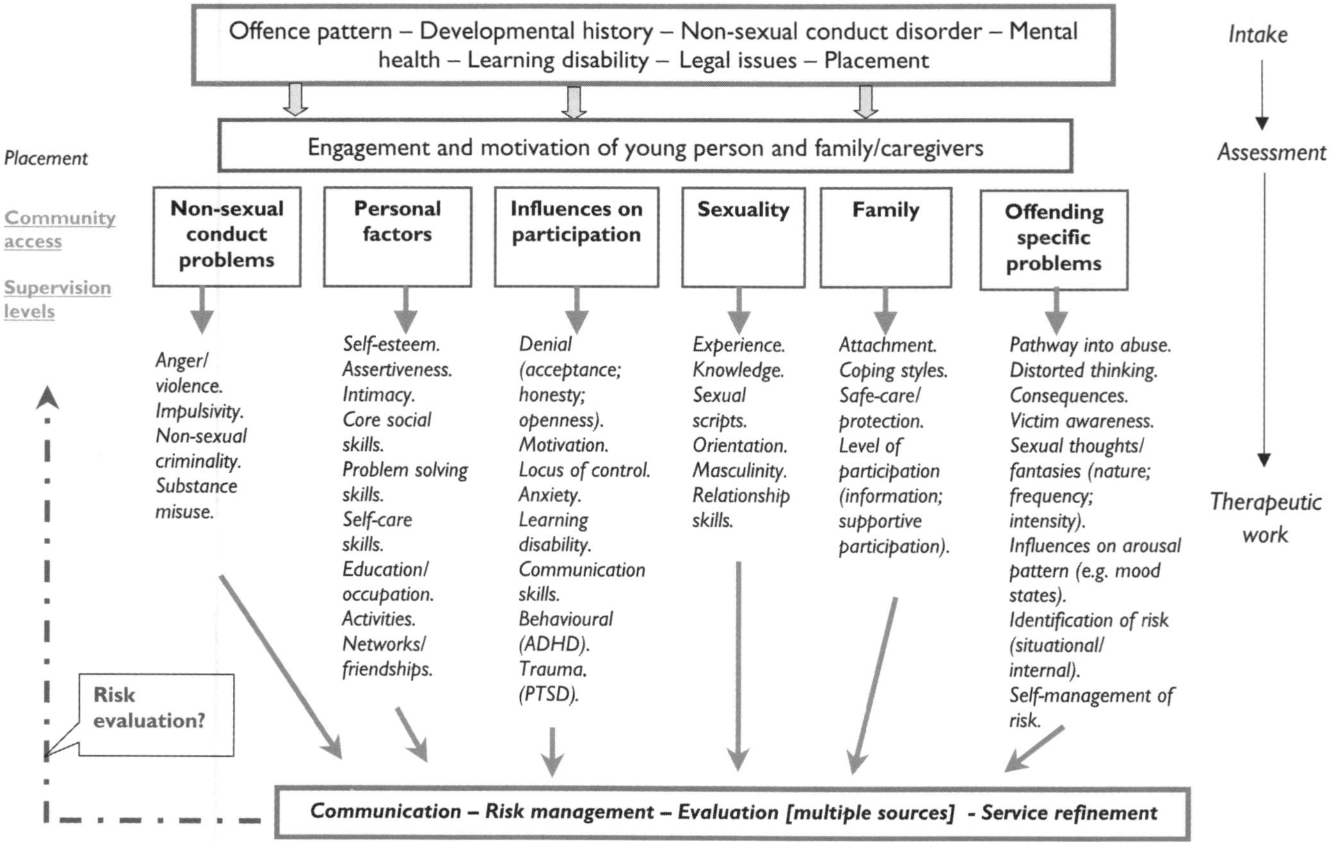


*Figure 9.1* G-MAP treatment planning model.

of the six domains included in the model and the young person's progress is reviewed and targets updated every sixteen weeks. Those involved in reviews include the young person, therapeutic staff, parents, caregivers and relevant others in the young person's support network.

As the model indicates, offence specific work constitutes one possible component within an overall programme. Elements of this area of work will undoubtedly be relevant for all young persons who require therapeutic intervention to help them address their sexually abusive behaviour. However, it may not be a primary need and it is often not the starting-point for therapeutic intervention. Clinical experience has shown that young people who have very poor self-esteem, or are otherwise psychologically vulnerable, may well become increasingly defensive or resistant when asked to consider their abusive behaviours towards others. For many young people it is therefore essential that offence specific work is carefully timed and may need to be superseded by other work on improving an individual's emotional ability to face up to their problem behaviours.

## Motivating young people to engage in treatment

Very few young people enter treatment programmes ready and eager to undertake work and achieve change. Some may recognise that they have problems that need attention and a number may even state that they want professional help in tackling the problems. Even in these cases young people are likely to find aspects of the work threatening, intrusive and demanding. A large majority are likely to demonstrate resistance at some stage. Such resistance should be understood as a defence although it may be expressed in a variety of forms ranging from total denial that there is a problem to token compliance with intervention and superficial acceptance of the need for change.

The first stage in motivating young people to engage in intervention is for those conducting the work to recognise and understand the many and significant factors that may inhibit or limit engagement and progress. These can include a fear on the young person's part that sharing information may increase the likelihood that they will: be viewed as deviant, abhorrent, sick or irredeemable; be confirmed in their own belief that they are deviant, abhorrent, sick or irredeemable; have to cope with the emotional discomfort and stress related to focusing on their negative behaviours and experiences; be subject to a negative response from the criminal justice system, the child protection system, their parents, family or the wider community. Additionally the young person may feel confused, anxious, angry or overwhelmed by the expectation that he must participate in a demanding therapeutic process. Professionals working with young people in these circumstances must accept the responsibility of anticipating, addressing and overcoming these possible blocks to engagement and progress. Whilst some young people are significantly fragile and defensive, failure to engage and motivate them should be regarded as the therapist's issue rather than an indication of the young person's dangerousness or untreatability.

A number of techniques, models and approaches have been developed in recent years to assist practitioners in motivating resistant individuals to engage in treatment. Miller and Rollnick (1991), for example, developed the model of change produced by Prochaska and DiClemente (1982), to assist those attempting to engage people with addictive behaviours. Their model is based on the premise that argumentative styles, direct confrontation of denial, or lack of engagement, is likely to increase client defensiveness and resistance. Instead they rely on theories of self-regulation and promote the use of techniques that explore client ambivalence and enhance problem recognition and the benefits of change.

Ward (2002) recently contributed a major theoretical critique of the conventional risk prevention or risk management focus of treatment work with individuals who sexually abuse. He suggested that traditional models limited the focus of work and impeded a more positive and holistic approach as individuals are seen primarily as a collection of risk variables, with treatment designed principally to address risk factors and promote relapse prevention. This limited range of issues and competencies is then seen as providing the important targets for change. In the majority of traditional programmes, therefore, little attention is given to the individual's general psychological needs and well-being. This restricted conceptualisation derives from an initial focus on risk rather than needs and goals. Ward suggests a major reappraisal and shift in emphasis such that offender rehabilitation should provide recipients with the necessary capabilities to achieve interpersonal and social goals in an acceptable manner rather than simply teaching people to reduce and manage their risk of engaging in sexually abusive behaviour.

An approach that emphasises positive goal attainment rather than the diminution of deficits or problem behaviours is not only more likely to attend to a broad range of needs and strengths but is also likely to prove more attractive and engaging to young people. Thus the holistic approaches adopted by G-MAP and promoted by Ward (2002) and Freeman-Longo (2001) (based on the attainment of "Goods Lives" and "Wellness plans" respectively) are not only likely to result in more effective change but are more likely to positively engage young people in the change process. Such an approach requires that early intervention with young people focuses on identifying realistic, achievable and meaningful life goals together with the development of strengths, resources and assets that will assist the attainment of these goals while dealing with any hurdles or obstacles (including abusive behaviours) that need to be overcome. This evaluation forms the basis of the young person's therapeutic intervention plan, and subsequent review or assessment is based on his/her progress in the necessary skill and resource attainment rather than on the traditional *sexual* offender relapse prevention model of focusing on the reduction of negative thoughts and behaviours.

In addition to fostering the development of personal goals a young person's level of motivation can also be significantly influenced by a number of external factors including the presence of a legal mandate with overt consequences for non-engagement; the attitudes of parents, caregivers and significant others; and the style and approach taken by the therapeutic workers. Each of these areas and their role as potential motivational aids is considered below.

Legal mandates may prove useful in initial engagement in that they may provide overt negative consequences to non-cooperation. Unless, however, young people are subsequently helped to develop internal motivation it is likely they will at best offer token compliance in treatment or may increasingly resent and resist the treatment process and providers. Young people entering a treatment programme are usually required to address and modify not only their abuse prone behaviours but also the thoughts and feelings that underpin the behaviours. Without a high degree of motivation young people are unlikely to truly engage in such personal and difficult change.

Progress in all forms of therapy appears to be significantly influenced by the degree of support available to the individual (McKeown, 2000). Young people engaged in treatment services for sexually abusive behaviours appear to do better if supported by either family (Sheridan *et al.*, 1998) or substitute carers (Farmer and Pollock, 1998). Other findings demonstrate similar outcomes regarding the role of interventions that target the families of problematic youth (Blechman and Vryan, 2000; Kumpfer and Alvarado, 1998).

Research has also demonstrated that a significant influence on the outcome of therapeutic work is the quality of the relationship between the therapist and client (Beech and Fordham, 1997; Marshall and Serran, 2000). The influence of this relationship on the establishment and maintenance of motivation in the client is undoubtedly a major factor that warrants particular attention and consideration.

Young people entering a treatment programme because of sexually abusive behaviours invariably have very low levels of self-esteem and high degrees of fear and shame. These are often the result of the young person's past experiences with authority figures or others with influence in their environment. Practitioners who ignore these feelings, or are not sensitive to authority and control issues in relationships, are in danger of mirroring the young person's previous experiences thereby reinforcing negative feelings and creating greater defensiveness.

Steen and Monnette (1989, p. 124) suggest that those working with young people who have sexually abused others "must recognise that they are dealing, at least initially, with people who don't want to work, who are extraordinarily resistant and hostile and at the same time weak and fragile. Change is therefore slow and in small steps." The aim therefore is to appropriately pace and develop a context for therapeutic intervention founded on respect, support and understanding and which nurtures the young person, inspires acceptance of responsibility and promotes accountable and respectful behaviour. This has to be established whilst ensuring there is no collusion with a young person's attempts to rationalise or minimise his abusive behaviour.

Ryan and Blum (1994) suggest that physical safety, nurturance and psychological safety are three overriding goals that need to be achieved in a therapeutic relationship. These can be facilitated by the use of: ongoing communication (involving setting of ground rules, honest feedback and labelling with words); empathy (the expression and validation of feelings and needs); and accountability (the validation of responsibility). In order to achieve these objectives practitioners engaging in work should aim to:

- Set realistic expectations for themselves and the young person, whilst recognising that change may be slow and difficult.
- Recognise resistant behaviours as defence or survival mechanisms.
- Be aware of their own feelings, prejudices, anxieties and preconceptions and how they may affect their presentation and responses to the young person.
- Ensure that they have sufficient access to good supervision, consultation and their own support networks.
- Offer respectful interactions based on a recognition that the young person has an identity that is much more than his abusive behaviour alone; i.e. separating behaviour from personality.
- Offer genuine interest in the young person. Acknowledge his unique set of feelings, experiences and views.
- Demonstrate appropriate sympathy and empathy.
- Avoid argument and direct confrontation.
- Develop creative methods of engaging the young person based on his individual abilities, preferences and styles.
- Identify and emphasise the young person's positive goals, assets, strengths, progress, potential and individual worthiness.
- Build the young person's esteem and avoid diminishing it.

### *Motivational methods*

Jenkins (1998) initiates work through conversations that encourage young people to explore, discover and express their preferred ways of thinking and behaving. When a young person has acted in ways that are abusive and harmful to others he is also likely to have been subjected to injustice or abuse himself. Jenkins invites the young person to explore his experiences of victimisation and unfairness, and through these he helps the young person to express his story of survival and resistance to injustice. In this manner a young person is helped to develop recognition of his positive inner values and strengths, and to identify discrepancies between these and his damaging behaviours. He is encouraged to consider why the negative behaviour occurred despite his positive qualities. For example, he may not have intended to harm others or he may have felt overwhelmed by negative feelings. This process is aimed at inviting the young person to begin to accept responsibility, not only for his past behaviour but also for determining how to ensure that his positive qualities can be enhanced to help prevent further abusive behaviours. This approach lays emphasis on a strengths rather than deficits model and encourages a young person to think in terms of dealing with restraints to positive behaviours rather than the risks of negative behaviours.

The G-MAP programme has utilised these ideas of initial engagement and developed a variety of early intervention methods and activities. One basic method is to help a young person to construct a timeline of his life. The line can be completed by means of straightforward talking and writing but can also utilise drawing, photographs, collage or in some cases transformation of the timeline into a road map, river or similar route. The young person is invited to represent on the line significant events in his life. Initially these can be simple non-threatening events such as birth, starting school, birth of siblings, holidays and significant achievements. Further details regarding personal loss, the start of puberty, friendships, experiences of abuse and other significant events can be added once rapport and trust have developed. Finally the young person is helped to identify those occasions when he has caused others to be upset or harmed.

Work on the timeline allows the practitioners to explore with the young person his understanding, feelings and thoughts regarding each of the events identified on the line. The young person's sense of justice about events, his skills and some of his inner qualities can also be identified as the process develops. The reasons for the occurrence of the abusive behaviours displayed by the young person can be viewed in the context of his experiences at the time. Consideration can also be given to which factors inhibited his positive qualities from dominating his decision making on the occasions when he behaved abusively. Projecting the timeline into the future can help the young person identify personal goals and what qualities and resources may be needed to meet these goals. It is often useful to check the timeline for accuracy and significant omissions. This can often be helped by reading case records or, with the young person's agreement, showing the line to parents, caregivers or significant others with a view to them suggesting omissions or additions. The involvement of others would also help them to see the abusive behaviour in perspective and to recognise the young person's positive qualities.

Figure 9.2 shows an example of a timeline completed with Andrew (all names and other details used in this chapter are not real), a young man referred for therapeutic work after he was convicted of the sexual abuse of his siblings. He initially presented as ambivalent, although superficially

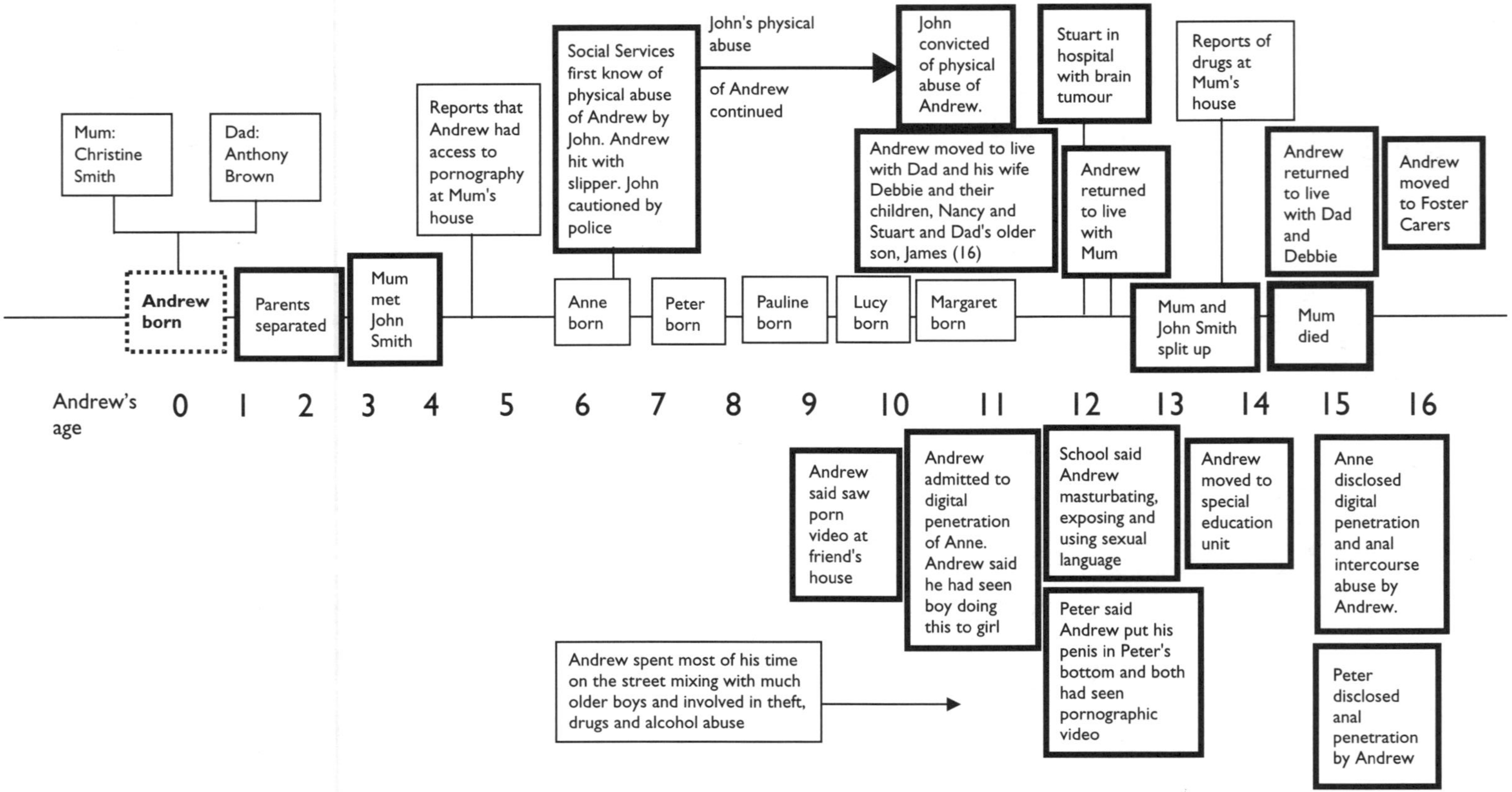


*Figure 9.2* An example of a timeline – Andrew.

compliant, and expressed a view that he did not see the point of therapeutic work as he was certain that he had learnt his lesson.

Andrew was helped to complete his timeline during the initial sixteen weeks of intervention and during this period the practitioners engaging with Andrew were able to express empathy with the painful events that Andrew had experienced and to support his sense of injustice about his step-father's behaviour towards him and his mother. They were also able to assist his recognition that unlike his step-father he was willing to work on his problems. With Andrew's assistance the practitioners helped him identify his feelings of guilt and shame and to explore how these might prevent him from facing up to his behaviour. Finally, Andrew was able to discuss his wishes for the future for himself and his siblings and how these might be achieved.

This work then enabled Andrew to identify some of the qualities that his life experiences had helped him to develop, including: strengths he had gained in coping with adversity; his wish to protect others (particularly his mother); his strong sense of justice (from the injustice he perceived with his step-father); his willingness to face up to problems (in contrast to his step-father); his ability to protect himself; his discomfort when others suffered harm; his desire to achieve successful employment (like his father); his desire to have positive, healthy intimate relationships (unlike his step-father); his desire to be well regarded by others.

On completion of his timeline Andrew had established a positive relationship with those conducting the sessions. He expressed a desire to undertake further work to help him achieve the positive goals he had identified and he identified the need to overcome his abusive behaviours as a component of this work. He considered that his inner qualities were strong enough to help him tackle some of the difficult issues he knew he would have to address. He was also keen to demonstrate, to those he thought might view him as a "lost cause", that he could successfully complete treatment.

A second motivational technique utilised on the G-MAP programme uses the concept of Old Life/New Life (adapted from Haaven *et al.*, 1990; and Mann, 2000) to help young people identify positive future goals and recognise the influence of their past experiences. Work on an individual's Old Life/New Life is usually continued and updated throughout the treatment period but is commenced early in an intervention programme. Figure 9.3 provides an example of Old Life/New Life work undertaken during the initial sixteen weeks of intervention with a young man named Aaron who was aged seventeen years and had been involved in the abuse of his natural sister and two foster siblings. He had spent most of his childhood with his foster carers (whom he described as his family) following neglect and physical and sexual abuse in his family of origin.

| Old Life | New Life |
|---|---|
| • I was bullied<br>• Hadn't got many friends<br>• I was sexually abused by my Dad<br>• I sexually abused my sisters<br>• I wasn't good at asking for help<br>• I didn't want to go to school<br>• I wasn't good at joining in<br>• I found it hard to talk to my family | • I want to be able to stick up for myself<br>• I want to build bridges with family<br>• I want to be able to have lots of friends<br>• I want to do well in exams and get a good job<br>• I want people to trust me<br>• I want to be a member of a football team<br>• I want to be able to spot a risky situation and deal with it |

General New Life goals developed for Aaron into specific target areas:

| My family | Education | Friends |
|---|---|---|
| • I have to show that I can deal with risk and can be trusted to think of others<br>• I have to be honest and prepared to talk about my feelings<br>• I have to listen to other people and show I care about their feelings<br>• I want them to recognise I have learnt from my mistakes | • I want to attend school and get exams<br>• I will have to be able to ask for help<br>• I will find my own time to catch up on school work I've missed<br>• I will find out about colleges<br>• If I don't pass exams this time I will keep studying and take them again | • I will go to college<br>• I will have to ask if I can join with things that are going on<br>• I have to be more mature and trustworthy<br>• I have to be loyal<br>• I have to stick up for myself and be myself |

*Figure 9.3* Aaron's Old Life/New Life exercise.

## Pathways into offending behaviour

A consideration of the different pathways into offending behaviour allows us to understand some of the complexity of effectively and appropriately intervening with young people with sexually abusive behaviour difficulties. O'Brien and Bera (1985) produced one of the first attempts at constructing a typology of adolescents who sexually abuse, initially identifying seven sub-types. Recently O'Brien (2000) has condensed these into three groups:

1 *Pervasive anti-social offenders* are young people with a lifestyle and world view that is predominantly criminal and supports the use of violence. O'Brien's experience is that such young people are at high risk for re-offending both sexually and non-sexually. However, traditional sexual offence specific treatment programmes are unlikely to be effective and interventions addressing criminal lifestyle are seen to be relevant.
2 *Psychosocially impaired offenders* are young people with histories of multiple abuse and complex long-standing sexual behaviour problems. *Sexual* offence specific work is relevant with this group, who additionally need to develop social and interpersonal skills.
3 *Developmental/situational offenders* are seen as young people for whom their isolated example of sexually abusive behaviour is reflective of possibly a discrete stressor or adjustment problem, e.g. the young person who engages in a single less intrusive sexual act with a younger child primarily as a result of lack of confidence and integration with peers.

Ward and Siegert (2002) have recently undertaken a comprehensive revision of the major theories exploring the emergence of abusive sexual behaviours. They posit five major pathways. Whilst these pathways are not viewed as mutually exclusive, i.e. most individuals would have deficits in more than one domain, the concept is that a particular pathway is dominant, with the exception of the fifth pathway that reflects the career pathway of individuals for whom each domain could be said to be equally relevant. The hypothesised pathways are:

1 *An intimacy deficits pathway*, where sexually abusive behaviour is viewed as primarily due to poor attachment relationships with care-givers whereby a child/young person does not develop sufficient skills and confidence that promote the formation of intimate and trusting relationships with others. This may then lead to a withdrawal from normative social interactions and a substitution of children for appropriate peer sexual and social contact.
2 *A problematic sexual scripts pathway*, where exposure to sexual abuse, particularly from multiple perpetrators or a very sexualised environment, leads to sexualised and sexually abusive behaviour. Frequently this

pathway relates to those sexualised as children who develop abusive behaviour which continues into adolescence.

3 *An emotional dysregulation pathway*, where a primary deficit concerning the ability to manage negative feelings (such as anger, frustration and sadness) promotes the development of sexually abusive behaviour. Early occurrence of abusive behaviour reflecting this pathway is likely to be associated with a co-morbid diagnosis of Attention Deficit Hyperactivity Disorder.
4 *An anti-social thinking pathway*, where a pro-criminal value system supports aggression as a viable method for securing an individual's needs for intimacy and sexual contact. Conduct Disorder is a common co-morbid diagnosis for young people whose development of sexually abusive behaviour has principally followed this particular pathway.
5 *Multiple pathways*, reflecting the developmental histories and profiles of individuals who present with severe sexual and multiple abuse histories with both sexually compulsive and general functioning problems.

In intervening therapeutically with young people who sexually abuse we need a model of practice that is relevant given the variety of pathways into sexually abusive behaviour that exist. As Rich (1998) comments, the dominant model for exploring adolescent sexual offending has been that of the Sexual Assault Cycle (Ryan, 1989). Rich's description, of how many young people find the model difficult to apply in total to their own behaviour, is consistent with the clinical experience of the present authors. This problem may be a combination of the sheer number of elements to the model and the difficulty many adolescents have in distinguishing between thoughts and feelings. Theoretically however the model provides an excellent framework for practitioners in analysing behaviours. Way and Spieker (1997) have expanded the model to provide a greater emphasis on the routes into the cycle and they identify recovery exits at each point. Ryan has recently reformulated the model as a High-Risk Cycle for a variety of repetitive dysfunctional behaviours (Ryan and Associates, 1999). These developments highlight the model's adaptability and applicability to a wide ranging group of problematic youth. However, its clinical utility in direct work with young people is more questionable, and simpler frameworks or therapeutic metaphors are needed that are accessible to most young people.

Our own approach has been to adapt Finkelhor's (1984) four stage model of sexual offending, the original components being: (1) Motivation to abuse; (2) Overcoming internal inhibitions; (3) Overcoming external inhibitions; and (4) Overcoming the resistance of the victim.

Next we consider the model's application in clinical practice with young people. It has been useful to progress through a series of stages in introducing young people to the four-step model. The emphasis is on establishing how the model provides a set of questions with which we can attempt to make better sense of behaviour that is viewed negatively or has adverse consequences. Commonly we begin with the non-sexual example of car-theft, which is particularly resonant for many young people. In doing so we introduce Finkelhor's model, illustrating how it can be used to describe the psychological process involved in car theft, as follows:

*Step One – Wanting to do it:* "Likes cars"; "Plays 'driver' on Playstation"; "Other lads in his area steal cars"; "He has gone for a ride in stolen car"; "It's a great buzz".

*Step Two – Thinking about it/Making excuse:* "Knows it's wrong"; "Thinks stealing is normal"; "People's own fault if leave them there"; "Insurance will pay"; "Won't get caught anyway"; "Doesn't matter if I do".

*Step Three – Getting a chance:* "Do it at night time or when street is quiet"; "Some cars are easier"; "Have screwdriver/sparkplug to smash window".

*Step Four – Doing it:* "Know how to start it"; "Know how to drive"; "Know rules of the road".

By using this example we are seeking to establish a number of principles in this part of the process. Chiefly these are: (a) influences on motivation are varied; (b) decision making can be in response to opportunity or subject to planning; and (c) people tend to give themselves permission or offer excuses to do things they wish to do. The next stage involves applying the four-step model to a sexually abusive scenario. One example we have devised is presented as a set of cartoons, which outline an offence in six stages (see Figure 9.4).

The individual or group is then asked to consider what further information they would need to better understand the behaviour of the character "Bill". The suggested explanatory statements offered are often reflective of the young person's own pathway into abuse. For example, common explanations include; "maybe he was just curious and wanted to find out what sex was like"; "he might not have any friends"; "someone might have done the same thing to him"; "maybe he's been watching lots of pornography". Based on our experience of the types of statements typically generated we have a set of fictional resources the individual/group can request to check out their ideas. These include (a) police reports (indicating what was on the video interview; does Bill have a computer and what's on that; have they searched his room); (b) a report from school describing how Bill gets on with other young people; (c) a Social Worker's report on an interview with parents; and (d) an extract of interview with the child who was abused, Jamie. The intervention task for the group or individual young person is to organise the information on Bill within the four-step model. That is, to construct the four steps – motivation

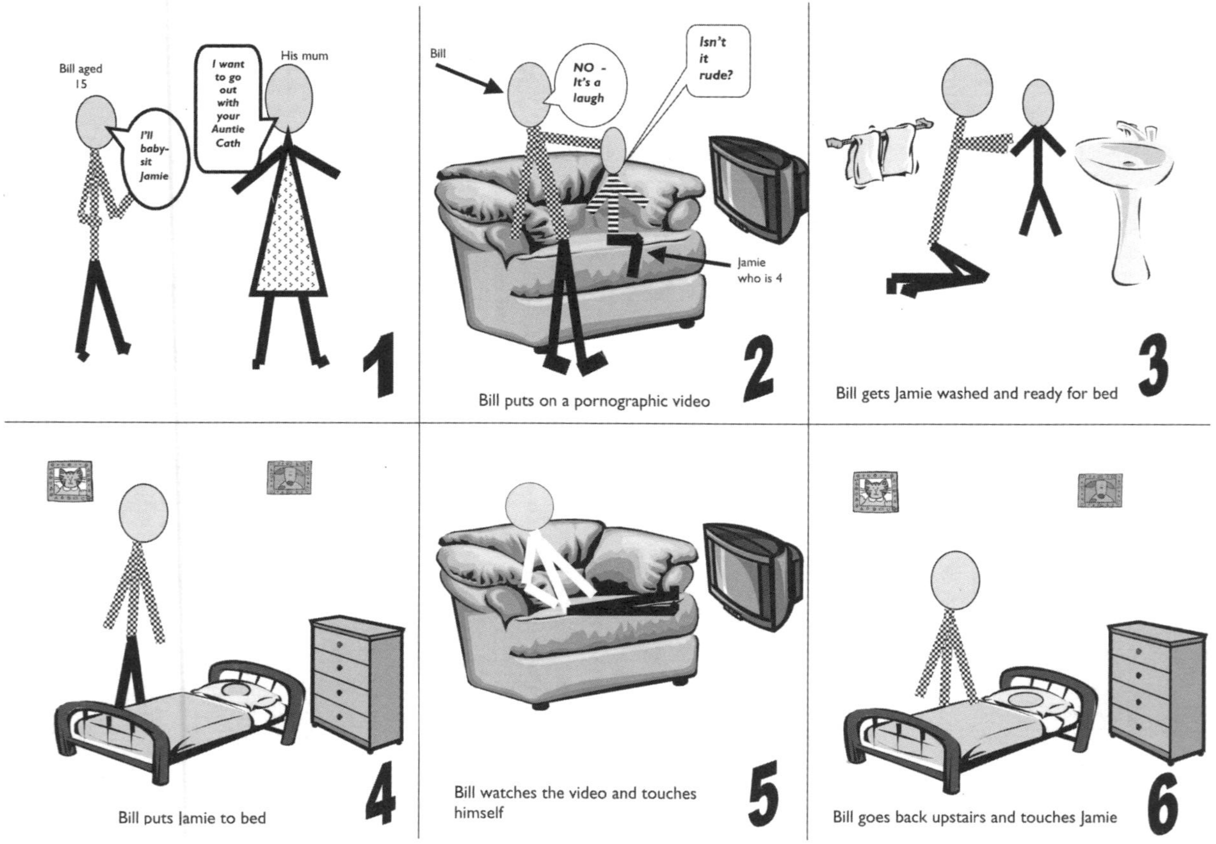


*Figure 9.4* Cartoon explaining the build-up to Bill's offence.

to abuse, overcoming internal inhibitors, overcoming external inhibitors, and overcoming the resistance of the victim – that describe Bill's behaviour.

Following this each young person has to apply the process to himself or herself. At this stage we find that young people's familiarity with the model assists them in generating information. An important difference from the car theft analogy is that when the young person is applying the model to their sexually abusive behaviour step four becomes "Getting the person to go along". From the example of Bill we will have generated ideas on how he was in a more powerful position, had been placed in authority over Jamie, and had attempted to normalise the sexual behaviour through watching the video. It is important to list more directly coercive methods, such as threat or physical force, as these will be applicable for a number of young people.

The following case study provides an example of the use of the model in practice:

### *Case study: Anthony B*

*Family Structure:*

George Bury – Father

Margaret Bury – Mother

Anthony Bury – now aged 16 years

Rebecca Bury – now aged 14 years

Anthony has been convicted of a series of specimen charges of Indecent Assault in respect of his sister Rebecca. Rebecca suffers from Cerebral Palsy and has been placed at a residential school since the age of eleven. Her early development was dominated by health problems and attempts to become more mobile. This led to Rebecca missing a great deal of schooling and contact with other children. Rebecca disclosed the abuse to a member of the care staff after returning home from a weekend visit. She said that Anthony had been "sexing" her and she was scared that she might be pregnant. The abuse had been ongoing for the last few years and was becoming progressively more intrusive.

The family are regarded by the residential school as rather cold and uncaring. Parents are openly hostile to each other and rarely take up opportunities to visit for school activities.

Anthony has been known to the local Child and Adolescent Services for many years due to an eating disorder leading to clinical obesity. This condition has been so threatening to Anthony's health that he was admitted to hospital on a number of occasions to try and control his weight. Anthony is a very isolated young man, bullied at school and rarely venturing out of the house at other times. Anthony admitted (though minimised) his abuse but when interviewed by the police stated he had been abused by an older boy at school. This allegation did not lead to a prosecution.

Anthony's use of the four-step model to organise life experiences and his thinking process around the abuse of his sister took a number of sessions. The work on his four steps provided an accessible way of organising and making connections between what, until this point, Anthony had maintained as disparate aspects of his experience (see Figure 9.5).

## Promoting empathy in young people who sexually harm

Components aimed at enhancing empathic concern for victims are a common feature of the vast majority of offence specific programmes for adults and adolescents who sexually abuse (Beckett 1999; Freeman-Longo *et al.*, 1996). This reflects a clinical assumption that empathy deficits are relevant to the perpetration of sexual aggression and that empathy enhancement has a

| Wanting to | Thinking about it/ making excuses | Getting a chance | Making the person go along |
|---|---|---|---|
| Memories of school:<br>Being bullied<br>Being abused<br>Being made fun of due to size<br><br>No friends<br><br>How it was in our family:<br>Parents' rows<br>My feelings not being noticed<br><br>What I felt most:<br>Angry | I felt like a split person:<br>Scared/guilty<br>Angry/I'll show her<br><br>I want to show her what I feel<br><br>Show the family that I am hurting<br><br>Sometimes I wondered if it was just the wrong kind of loving | Rebecca had no friends at home<br><br>Missed a lot of education when in hospital – didn't know much about sex<br><br>Mum and dad would disturb us<br><br>Leave me babysitting if they went out<br><br>Didn't talk much about anything in our family | Rebecca felt nobody would take her side in anything<br><br>Told her that *"mum and dad wanted to get rid of one of us and chose you"*<br><br>Said I would hurt or kill her if she told anyone<br><br>Sexual touching became more and more serious |

*Figure 9.5* The four factor model applied to Anthony's sexually abusive behaviour.

central role in inhibiting future abusive behaviours. Despite its virtual uniform presence in treatment programmes there appears to be a lack of specificity as to which aspect of the empathic process is relevant to sexual aggression, whether this is a consistent deficit across all groups of sexual abusers, how it is measured and what methods of intervention are potentially effective in enhancing empathy for others (Marshall *et al.*, 1999; Pithers, 1999).

### *Defining empathy*

The ability to experience and demonstrate empathic concern for others is a key element of social functioning. There is general agreement that empathy involves both cognitive and affective components. Marshall *et al.* (1995) describe a four-step model of empathy based on an information processing perspective. The first step is for an individual to accurately recognise the emotion displayed by another. Secondly, it is necessary to evaluate and interpret that emotion within the immediate context of known information (e.g. the other person has recently experienced a distressing event). Thirdly, to then experience an appropriate emotional response. Finally, to present an appropriate behavioural response. Pithers (1999) suggested that this model is too complex and of limited value as it is based on the other party to the interaction providing information from which a conclusion (emotional recognition) may be drawn. Pithers suggested that the ability to accurately anticipate another's emotional response based on an assimilation of their perspective provides a more reliable basis for promoting heightened empathic functioning.

### *Evidence of empathy deficits in sexual offenders*

Both Pithers (1999) and Marshall *et al.* (1999), in their literature reviews, conclude that there is limited evidence for generalised or global empathy deficits in those who sexually abuse. They suggest this finding may be a function of imprecise and inconsistent definitions of empathy, the limitations of currently available measures and the design methodology of studies. There is somewhat more evidence for the proposition that sexually aggressive individuals demonstrate particular deficits in empathy for their own victims or more generally for the victims of sexual assault (Beckett *et al.*, 1994; Elliott *et al.*, 1995; Hanson and Scott, 1995; Rice *et al.*, 1994; Scully, 1988). Much interest has focused on distinguishing between rapists and child molesters in terms of their specific victim empathy deficits. For example, Fernandez's work (as reviewed in Marshall *et al.*, 1999) suggested that rapists displayed the most marked empathy deficits and that child molesters are a more heterogeneous group. Ward and colleagues (Ward and Keenan, 1999; Ward *et al.*, 2000) suggested that empathy deficits in child molesters might be relatively subtle and require more sophisticated measures to identify.

The failure to respond empathetically to the distress of another may be variable both in terms of its restriction to certain individuals (i.e. victims of sexual assault) and its influence by temporal factors. Denial of the harm that behaviour causes to another, and the avoidance of self-scrutiny in order to gain gratification, may be generalised or specific to certain affective states (e.g. anger, depression) and subject to other influences such as drug or alcohol use. Johnson and Knight (2000) identified alcohol use as a key variable in their sample of adolescent sexual offenders. Pithers' (1999) research supported a view that the affective component of empathy is inhibited when individuals who sexually abuse are in an emotional state similar to that which preceded their sexual assault. The available evidence would support a view that assessments of those who sexually abuse need to identify specific empathic deficits and target treatment interventions accordingly. A focus on the management of negative affective states may be more relevant for certain groups of offenders (Nagayama Hall, 1996).

### *Empathic skills from a developmental perspective*

Positive and secure attachments are based upon empathic parenting (Erickson, 1959) within which a child's needs are accurately assessed and responded to. Ainsworth *et al.* (1978) described a continuum of attachment which has been followed by a considerable focus on the potential relationship between insecure attachments and subsequent developmental problems (Crittenden, 1995).

One explanatory mechanism relates to the "theory of mind", which refers to an individual's capacity to attribute mental states to oneself and others in an attempt to understand and explain behaviour (Gopnick and Meltzoff, 1997). Secure attachments and a positive care environment appear to provide the optimum context for children to develop an adequate theory of mind (Fongay *et al.*, 1997). Researchers have considered how failure to develop an adequate theory of mind may be related to certain behavioural outcomes. In evaluating a sample of children with Conduct Disorder, Happé and Frith (1996) suggest that such children have a skewed theory of mind that relates to negative developmental and learning experiences. This leads to a failure to accurately infer the mental and emotional states of others.

Ward *et al.* (2000) have suggested that the theory of mind concept may be useful in considering the cognitive schemas of sexual offenders. They distinguish between *framework* and *specific* theory deficits. Framework deficits are wide ranging and global and lead to a string of specific (mis)evaluations of the mental states of others. Specific deficits may reflect a lack of experience with certain kinds of interpersonal relationships or distorted learning experiences. Ward *et al.* suggest that deficits for some offenders may be state dependent and related to either affective states, psychological arousal, substance use, or the lack of motivation to apply an adequate knowledge of others' mental states given a higher motivation to offend.

Trauma is the developmental experience most commonly associated with the onset of sexually aggressive behaviour, and Ryan (1989) provided a model of how a dysfunctional response to such life events could precipitate a pattern of abusive behaviour. Latterly attention has focused on how multiple variables may mediate the impact of trauma with particular focus on how insecure attachments and inadequate care increases children's vulnerability to trauma, particularly if long-standing or repeated. Ryan (1999) suggests that such children have an internalised negative working model and consider themselves as unlovable and others as unreliable.

Ryan (1999) suggests that neglectful and abusive care profoundly affects the child's developing empathic abilities and contributes to individuals not being able to recognise their own or others' emotional needs. When considering this component with young people who have sexually harmed and who have themselves been victims of sexual abuse, it is useful to refer to the Sexual Abuse Accommodation Syndrome as initially outlined by Summitt (1983). This model outlines the potential psychological impact of sexual abuse on victims and can help to prioritise areas of need. For example, if a child has identified with their abuser as a form of psychological defence they will need to explore their own victimisation prior to having the psychological space to consider the impact on others of their own abusive behaviour (Woods, 1997).

### *Potential inhibitors in developing empathic skills*

Hanson and Scott (1995) propose a number of factors which may affect the development of empathic skills. These are: (a) an indifferent or adversarial relationship; (b) perspective taking skills; (c) how the individual copes with perceiving distress in others; (d) the ability of the individual to cope with his own emotional response.

In the UK a major evaluation of community based intervention programmes for sexually abusive adult males identified that the empathy component of certain programmes resulted in a deterioration in measured victim empathy in a significant number of offenders (Beckett *et al.*, 1994). They hypothesised that this was due to the participants being confronted with the impact of their behaviour too early in the programme and before they had achieved an adequate degree of self-esteem and emotional resilience. In considering the negative impact of confrontational approaches with those who sexually abuse, Nagayama Hall (1996) highlights the concept of *psychological reactance* (Brehm and Brehm, 1981). This is a defensive reaction to an imposition upon or the curtailment of freedom, which may be the experience of individuals who viewed a treatment initiative as being directed at how to think and feel.

### *Interventions to promote empathic responses*

Programmes for adult and adolescent sexual offenders have tended to emphasise the victim specific component of empathy and focused on empathic hindsight and foresight relative to the impact on victims of sexual assault. Ryan and Associates (1999) question whether this promotes empathy or the more limited psychological construct of sympathy. They suggest that sympathy is based on a similarity of feeling, rather than empathic concern that involves an attempt to understand the perspective and feelings of others who may be dissimilar to you.

Pithers (1999) described an empathy-enhancing component that relies on a variety of activities to attempt to assist those who have sexually abused to make links between their offences and the general experiences of sexual abuse victims. The resultant knowledge is then applied by abusers to understanding the experiences of their victims. Pithers offers one of the few specific evaluations of empathy training as a component in a treatment programme. He concluded that the intervention improved participants' ability to display cognitive empathy for victims and that this gain remained constant when the sample was retested whilst experiencing the emotional state that preceded their offence.

Freeman-Longo *et al.* (1996) provide a six-stage programme that addresses: (a) defining empathy; (b) the impact of sexual assault; (c) developing empathic skills; (d) identifying empathic states which impede empathy; (e) applying the concept of "compassionate action", i.e. a lifestyle that stresses responsible and respectful behaviours; and (f) developing a self-support system to maintain this behaviour. Marshall *et al.* (1999) describe a similar programme which they have evaluated positively but report that latterly they have produced a truncated version that treats putative "empathy deficits" as cognitive distortions.

Descriptions of this component in programmes for young sexual abusers appear to adopt an approach that parallels the adult model (Kahn, 1990; Way and Balthazor, 1990). The danger is that young people learn to replicate socially acceptable responses without an emotional response or corresponding behavioural gains. It is critical to use the supervisory network to consider whether increased empathic responses are consistently displayed and maintained during periods of stress, anger and arousal.

In the G-MAP programme specific targets are identified to evaluate the young person's capacity for empathy towards others. On a cognitive level this could include the young person completing an exercise or assignments on other individuals and their needs. Initially this might be a character from a soap opera, a well known personality/figure in the news, a character from literature or from a narrative we have created for the purpose. The next stage is to consider the young person's network and appraise the extent to which he can construct empathic accounts of the lives of others, for example, family members or caregivers, peers or others with whom he may have a significant relationship. This may then focus on specific goals whereby the young person can demonstrate empathic behaviours. Examples of this may be assisting a parent in practical tasks; vocalising thanks for acts of support; expressing sympathy regarding others' feelings; or showing sensitivity to siblings or peers over difficulties they are experiencing.

For young people who have had limited or no experiences of empathic care even such modest goals may prove extremely difficult. A lengthy period may be required during which the reality of their life experience of neglect and abuse is acknowledged and processed. In the early stages of work with young people who have such chronic histories, attempts to elicit consideration of the needs of others are likely to be met with incomprehension. Should it be possible to engage a family with such a poor care history in an allied programme of work where they are able to acknowledge the young person's early experiences and take an appropriate measure of responsibility, this can be a powerful factor in freeing the young person to consider his/her own lack of empathy for those he/she abused.

Although empathic recognition may be a cognitive process, producing the appropriate social response involves both a cognitive skill (how should I deal with this?) and the behavioural/social skills to enact it. The latter may be a more extensive developmental task for some young people than the enhancement of their recognition skills. Social skills enhancement is dependent upon opportunities to rehearse and refine skills, and suitable opportunities for doing so are likely to be influenced by considerations of risk and safe access to appropriate social environments. We have found that our service has a key role in advising other agencies when and how to take planned risks to provide young people with the opportunities to develop such social skills.

## Addressing distorted thinking

For many years treatment programmes for those who sexually abused were behaviourally based and focused on addressing deficits in anger control, social skills, expression of feelings, appropriate arousal patterns and positive attitudes towards females and children. Whilst the empirical evaluations of such programmes were generally positive in respect of short-term gains, they were less successful in the long-term maintenance of non-abusive behaviours and attitudes (Hall, 1995; Hanson *et al.*, 1993).

In recent years there has been increasing consensus that there should be a much broader understanding and treatment of abusive behaviours that must include cognitive as well as behavioural aspects of the problem. If underlying thoughts and attitudes associated with abusive behaviours remain unchanged any positive behaviour change is less likely to be maintained. This recognition has led to the development of theoretical perspectives and interventions based on the "thinking errors" approach developed by Yochelson and Samenow (1976) which suggests that an individual's "world view" determines the thoughts that influence behaviours. These developments not only help us to better understand the origins of enduring distorted thoughts but also suggest routes into addressing such cognitive aspects in treatment programmes.

### *Defining cognitive distortions*

One element of the cognitive processes commonly identified as significant in sexual offenders concerns thinking errors or cognitive distortions. These are often referred to as the beliefs that are used to rationalise sexually abusive behaviours (Hanson *et al.*, 1994; Pollack and Hashmall, 1991; Stermac and Segal, 1989). For example, "victims find sexual aggression enjoyable" or "children seek and enjoy sexual behaviour with adults". Lonsway and Fitzgerald (1994) reported that cognitive distortions regarding sexual aggression are more commonly found in males than females. Research on adult males who sexually abuse children has shown that a majority have distorted perceptions about their victims and potential victims that differentiate them from the general population (Abel *et al.*, 1984; Hayashino *et al.*, 1995). Studies of rapists, however, have shown that their beliefs are not so discernible from males in general (Burt, 1983; Malamuth, 1981; Marolla and Scully, 1986). Ward *et al.* (1997) have shown that males who sexually abuse hold diverse cognitions about their victims and that different distorted thoughts are associated with different stages of the abusive behaviour. Ward *et al.* (1998) also noted that these distortions are not necessarily associated with negative affective states or the avoidance of responsibility. Those that abuse children, for example, often have distorted beliefs that support the behaviour which they associate with positive affective states.

Beckett (1999) pointed out that whilst there is a growing literature regarding the distorted thinking of adults who sexually abuse there has been little equivalent study with adolescents. He suggested that young people who sexually abuse are less likely than adults to have entrenched distorted thoughts. Rich (1998) also suggested that the thinking errors in adolescence may be due more to developmental immaturity than to any entrenched long-term deviant beliefs. Gibbs (1996) identified that young people who demonstrate a wide range of anti-social behaviours hold an array of distorted beliefs but he expressed concern about whether these distorted thoughts constitute precursors to undesirable behaviours or serve, post offence, to minimise the offender's resultant negative feelings. The reality may be that for most who exhibit anti-social behaviours, including sexual abuse, both apply.

Gibbs and Potter (1991) suggested that distorted thoughts operate on both a primary and a secondary level. Primary distortions tend to operate consistently, influencing behaviours in most situations, whilst secondary distortions tend to be employed immediately prior to or following an anti-social act and are used specifically to reduce feelings of guilt and prevent damage to self-image. They suggest that primary distortions are those Carducci (1980) described as due to a delay, for variable reasons, in socio-moral development that result in the persistence beyond childhood of poor moral judgement and an egocentric bias. Carducci described the resultant attitude as one where an individual is intent on getting their own needs met regardless of the effects that this has on others.

Gibbs and Potter (1991) viewed secondary cognitive distortions as those that serve to support the primary distortions. They suggest that secondary distortions consist of three categories: minimising/mislabelling; assuming the worst; and blaming others. The function of these secondary categories is to minimise an offender's feelings of responsibility. Murphy (1990) identified three very similar processes in males who had sexually offended. He described these as: justifications – the process of making the behaviour morally acceptable; minimising harm or misattribution of consequences; and shifting responsibility by devaluing victims.

### *The theoretical development of distorted thinking*

Belief systems theory (Ball-Rokeach *et al.*, 1984; Rokeach, 1985; Williams, 1979) was developed to provide a framework for the understanding of self and relationships. The theory proposes that beliefs fundamentally influence cognitions, behaviours and affect, and that an individual's beliefs are determined and maintained by social and cultural contexts. Russell (1995) used this model as the basis for her study of abusive men and she found that they characteristically held beliefs about the centrality, un-connectedness, superiority and deservedness of self. She proposed that treatment should be directed at changing an individual's abusive beliefs to a respectful belief system and that this is largely achieved by the examination and confrontation of beliefs in individual and group treatment programmes.

Recent focus on the linkage between poor early attachments, sexual abuse and the development of sexually abusive behaviour (Marshall *et al.*, 2000; Ryan and Associates, 1999; Ward *et al.*, 1995) has suggested that severe attachment disorders may lead to internal working models that include negatively distorted views of self and others. These negative attitudes can be compounded by experiences of abuse and the attitudes of the abuser, for example, "a child is abused because they deserve it".

Ward and Keenan (1999), and Keenan and Ward (2000) have utilised a theory of mind perspective to also explain the development of cognitive distortions. The model suggests each individual's theory of mind or mental state (which includes desires, intentions, beliefs, emotions and perceptions) is developed from birth by virtue of his or her experiences and observations and the information they receive. It is their theory of mind that influences an individual's understanding of what others feel, think and need and that helps them to accurately identify the mental states of others. When an individual's theory of mind is developmentally disrupted or delayed, or he lacks the ability to apply his theory of mind, then distorted attributions are likely to be a consequence. So that, for example, misattribution of belief results in cognitive distortions. Ward *et al.* (2000) place emphasis on negative experiences in early childhood as having the potential to compromise the development of a theory of mind. They suggest that the nature of these detrimental experiences can impact differentially on a developing theory of mind so that some individuals may acquire permanent misattributions and distortions whilst for others their mood state may only temporarily affect their theory of mind.

### *Interventions to reduce distorted thinking*

Whilst most intervention programmes with those who sexually abuse include strategies to address cognitive distortions, very few offer detailed descriptions of methods or provide evaluations of outcomes (Murphy, 1990). The descriptions available tend to refer to the use of cognitive restructuring techniques that rely heavily on the development of "self-talk" whereby the individual learns to self-challenge his thinking, or to accept the overt confrontation of distorted thoughts by therapists or fellow group members (Beckett, 1994; Berenson, 1987; Jenkins-Hall, 1994; Steen and Monnette, 1989). The basis for such techniques appears to be an assumption that the individual who has abused is capable of recognising the feelings and thoughts of others. If his/her negative thinking is then challenged and alternative, more rational, views offered he/she will recognise the unreasonableness of his/her views and replace negative thoughts with more positive ones. If, however, cognitive distortions are the result of developmental delays and disruptions the individual may not so easily recognise the irrationality of his/her thoughts and may not have the ability to develop the perspective-taking skills necessary to adopt the new ideas offered.

Ward *et al.* (2000), Marshall *et al.* (1999) and Ryan (1999) have suggested that an individual's cognitive distortions, lack of empathy, intimacy deficits and poor social skills are all linked to developmental delays and that the nature, extent and timing of early negative experiences can lead to a variety of cognitive processing problems. It is therefore unlikely that a "one size fits all" approach to tackling these problems will be appropriate, and effective intervention, therefore, should aim to address the specific needs of the individual. Additionally, intervention that addresses an individual's abilities to accurately assess the beliefs, feelings and needs of others may result in an overall change in their empathic, social and relationship skills as well as reducing their cognitive distortions.

These developmental perspectives suggest that a variety of intervention techniques are needed, dependent on the individual's need. For example, those young people who have an array of entrenched distortions due to poor skills in recognising others' needs and feelings are likely to require considerable help to distinguish feelings and develop perspective taking skills. Others may require help to moderate mood states that increase the occurrence of specific, temporary distorted thoughts.

Our experience in G-MAP has shown that adoption of the motivational approach described above has led some young people, who recognise their "inner positive qualities", to question for themselves distorted thoughts that do not concur with these qualities. Work on timelines and biographies has helped them identify how views and beliefs may have developed and in some instances how these can be associated with particular moods or situations.

For example, Andrew, whose timeline is shown in Figure 9.2, was able to identify during this work that he had developed a view in early childhood that it was "better to get them before they got you". His experiences of abuse and lack of protection led him to a view that no one could be trusted, that it was better to be an abuser than a victim, and that those who were abused were to blame because they had not learnt to protect themselves. He was helped to recognise these beliefs as understandable given his experiences but also encouraged to consider how these views might vary from those based on his "inner qualities" perspective. One of the exercises used to help this process was an exercise developed from the work on schemata developed by Mann and Schofield (1999). This involved the construction of two pairs of different coloured cardboard glasses and attributing to one pair the abuse-supportive view of the world Andrew developed in childhood, and to the other pair, the "inner qualities" view of the world. Andrew was then asked to respond to case studies and role-play scenarios whilst wearing one or other of the pairs of glasses. In this way he was helped to recognise the different perceptions each view brought about and he was able to rehearse and refine his perspective-taking skills using the positive qualities viewpoint. Andrew was also, over time, able to recognise how his choice of "glasses" (or viewpoint) in everyday life was often affected by the mood he was in at the time. When he felt insecure, threatened or rejected, for example, his ability to see the world through the "positive qualities glasses" could be overwhelmed by reversion to his long held use of the "abuse prone glasses". This understanding resulted in Andrew recognising that he could change his way of thinking during times of stress but that this required effort, and the more he rehearsed and used his positive view the more easily accessible it would be in negative mood states.

It has become increasingly apparent in our work with young people that changing thoughts and behaviours is for most a difficult, painful and lengthy process. The process is most effective when young people are motivated to change, actively supported and provided with opportunities to rehearse change. These circumstances generally require a therapeutic style that is supportive and guiding so that the benefits of change are identified and the tools to enable change are constructed, their use explained and their usage supported and modified as necessary. Such an approach does not embrace the directly confrontational techniques that have often been employed in addressing cognitive distortions whereby a young person is overtly challenged to explain and defend such views in the hope that they will recognise them to be irrational. We have, however, recognised that a safe group-work environment can offer an important opportunity for young people to explore views and beliefs with peers.

## Problematic sexual interests

Although there have been numerous studies and discussions on the role that inappropriate sexual thoughts play in the occurrence and maintenance of sexually aggressive behaviours there have been few attempts to define what constitutes "offence prone" or deviant sexual thoughts.

Fisher and McGregor (1997) suggested the following are features of *appropriate* fantasy: full consent; equal power relationship; mutual agreement to the activity; positive emotions; absence of coercion; and the focus of the fantasy should not be someone whom the adolescent is angry with or dislikes. For adolescents who demonstrate evident sexual interest in children or in whom self-report or other evidence identifies predatory sexual thoughts involving coercion or force, this area should be considered an important target for further assessment and decision making concerning intervention.

### *The relevance of deviant sexual arousal*

The concept that repeated sexually abusive behaviours are supported and reinforced by a deviant pattern of sexual arousal and fantasy was an influential concept in the development of interventions with sexual aggressors. Arguments supporting intervention with adolescents who sexually abused was advocated on the basis that they may be developing fixed patterns of sexual interests, which, unless addressed, would continue on into adulthood. The work of Abel *et al.* (1993) was highly significant in informing this perspective. The relevance of deviant sexual arousal is however debated even within the adult field. Langevin *et al.* (1998) administered written questionnaires to 201 male adult sexual offenders, finding that one-third self-reported having experienced deviant sexual fantasies; this appeared a significant factor, particularly for men who had abused non-related boys. Marshall *et al.* (1991) found that approximately half of the male child molesters they interviewed identified deviant fantasies but only one-fifth stated these fantasies were present in adolescence prior to their first offence. In reviewing the available data on the sexual preference hypotheses, Marshall *et al.* (1999) concluded that there was inconsistent evidence that deviant sexual fantasy was a significant feature for the majority of sexual offenders.

Hunter and Becker (1994) concluded that arousal patterns in adolescents were likely to be more variable than in adults and that even less inference should be drawn from exhibited behaviours as to their underlying arousal patterns. For example, it cannot be assumed that all adolescents who sexually abuse children have a primary sexual interest in children.

### ***Are sexual interests associated with risk?***

Hanson and Bussiere's (1998) meta-analytic study did identify offence related sexual preferences as predicting future sexual re-offence. Hudson *et al.* (2002) found a positive association between deviant sexual interests, measured via psychometric testing, and recidivism. However, there is a need to be cautious about attempting to identify sexual arousal patterns during assessment. Swaffer *et al.* (2000) found a significant increase in the number of adult sexual offenders who acknowledged deviant fantasies *post*-participation in a treatment programme as opposed to those who did so at the assessment/intake stage.

Prentky *et al.* (2000) attempted to find factors that positively correlated with re-offence risk in a follow-up study of ninety-six adolescents who had sexually offended. Four potential domains were identified. However, of these the Sexual Drive/Preoccupation domain was not significantly associated with re-offence risk, while an Impulsive/Anti-Social Behaviour domain was. In contrast Worling and Curwen (2000) found that a self-report of sexual interest in children was a predictive factor of subsequent sexual recidivism in their sample of fifty-eight adolescents who had a follow-up period of between two and ten years. Butz and Spaccarelli (1999) identified a significant relationship between the degree of force used in an abusive act and the degree of sexual assault fantasy, predatory behaviour, greater preoccupation with children and more general deviant sexual interests. They suggested that use of physical force as an offence characteristic in sub-typing adolescent sexual offenders may be a more applicable criterion than that of a model primarily differentiating between child molesters and rapists.

### ***Developmental factors associated with deviant sexual arousal***

Summarising a number of research studies undertaken by their team, Hunter and Becker (1994) concluded that there was a significant relationship between a history of sexual victimisation; offence pattern (more male children, more victims overall); and a more deviant/offence prone erectile response measured via penile plethysmography.

Burton (2000) compared three groups of young people. These were (1) adolescents who exhibited sexually aggressive behaviours before the age of twelve and had ceased to display such behaviour; (2) adolescents who had initiated sexually aggressive behaviours after the age of twelve; and (3) adolescents whose sexual behaviour had begun before the age of twelve and continued on into later adolescence. He found that of these the third group presented with complex abusive behavioural patterns and were significantly more likely to have experienced sexual victimisation themselves.

Johnson and Knight (2000) applied Malamuth's Developmental Model of

Sexually Aggressive Behaviour (Malamuth, 1993) to a group of 122 adolescents who had sexually abused. They found that a history of sexual victimisation was predictive of a higher level of sexual compulsivity measured by an instrument they developed (the Multidimensional Assessment of Sex and Aggression – MASA). The study also identified that a domain they termed 'Misogynistic Fantasies' had a significant relationship to the degree of sexual coercion expressed by the individual. Cooper *et al.* (1996) using several measures studied a sample of 300 sexually aggressive adolescents, with and without histories of physical or sexual abuse. They concluded that youths with a history of sexual abuse appeared more likely to develop deviant sexual arousal patterns. In her paper on young people who present sadistic and violent behaviour, Bailey (1997) suggests fantasy should be a significant focus of investigation and that young people in this group often have extreme histories of traumatic victimisation.

### *Interventions with young people who present problematic sexual arousal*

Fisher and McGregor (1997) undertook a detailed review of behavioural methods for reducing deviant arousal in adolescents and suggested several reasons why these approaches are infrequently integrated into programmes working with sexually abusive adolescents. These were as follows:

- The general lack of understanding of the role deviant arousal may play in sexual offending.
- Many of the techniques require considerable co-operation and honesty from a young person as well as support from the family or caregivers.
- Some of the procedures involve the use of sexually explicit materials or visual stimuli and that this may raise ethical problems for clinicians.
- Many fantasy modification techniques are invasive and intrusive and it may be difficult for the young person to give informed consent.
- Given the lack of phallometric assessment for adolescents within the UK, British clinicians generally rely primarily on the adolescent's self-report.
- Much of the therapeutic work with adolescents in the UK is undertaken by practitioners who may not have an appropriate level of understanding of the psychological processes and methods to be applied.
- Interventions with adolescents have relied primarily on groupwork as a format to deliver treatment, and a group is an inappropriate context in which to undertake work on deviant fantasy.

Hunter and Lexier (1998) note that clinical findings as to the effectiveness of any arousal conditioning approach are confounded by the fact that such interventions are generally part of a much broader programme and it is difficult to isolate the treatment effect of this single element. They conclude that at present we have little reliable data as to utility or as to the types of adolescents for whom such interventions should be considered. Nagayama Hall (1996) concluded that there is little evidence in support of behavioural methods being used as a primary intervention but they may have some value as an intermediate risk management strategy, suggesting a more effective intervention target may be the management of the negative affective states associated with sexual arousal.

For a proportion of young people, where there is self-report and external evidence that deviant sexual arousal is a major driving force in their offence behaviour, there may be an argument in offering the development of thought stopping techniques. The use of intrusive procedures with young people needs to be approached with caution and we have found the following criteria to be relevant:

- The young person experiences the arousal as problematic and is motivated to work on this difficulty.
- Experience would support a view of the young person as open and communicative about their sexual drives and interests.
- The pattern of deviant sexual fantasy is reasonably distinct and consistent.
- The young person is supervised and receives considerable support from caregivers.

In such circumstances there appear to be a couple of techniques that are applicable and helpful to this small proportion of adolescents. Weinrott *et al.* (1997) provide one of the few attempts to empirically validate a behavioural treatment approach to modifying deviant sexual preferences in adolescents who sexually abuse. Their study focused entirely upon adolescents who had sexually victimised children. The intervention applied was termed "Vicarious Sensitisation", a behaviourally based procedure with several elements. The primary intervention, aimed at inhibiting deviant sexual arousal, involved a series of aversive vignettes. These were scripted by the clinical team, performed by actors and videotaped. The vignettes explored the legal, social, physical and emotional consequences of further sexual offending. The test group was subject to twenty-five sessions of the intervention twice weekly for three months. The team concluded that vicarious sensitisation reduced arousal to pre-pubescent girls but that patterns of arousal to same-sex victims was more difficult to interpret. The young people were also given a wallet card with a summary of all the aversive scenarios for reference. The participants and their parents reported high levels of satisfaction with the intervention. This latter comment may suggest that a particularly useful effect of such methods is that of providing the young person with a sense of hope and self-actualisation. Other conclusions from the study were that a significant minority of subjects showed no change following vicarious sensitisation and, in general, adolescents become more highly aroused more quickly and to a wider range of stimuli than do adults.

A technique that may have more practical application in the context of most services working with adolescents is that of Verbal Satiation (Laws, 1995). The principal is similar to that of masturbatory satiation though it avoids certain of the ethical concerns regarding the use of that technique with young people. The individual records his deviant fantasy onto tape for a directed period (no less than 30 minutes) at set times over the course of the week. Our clinical experience reflects Laws' description in that the individual becomes bored with the previously powerful fantasy over a period of weeks and begins to employ other fantasy imagery at other times. However, if the individual is honest in their self-report, the new fantasy may then need to become the target for further intervention. We have found that the period it takes for young people to become bored with the new fantasy material is significantly shorter than at the outset of the process. The practicalities of employing this technique (how and where is the young person going to use a tape recorder) and the substantial clinician time involved in reviewing the tapes mean that it is only applicable with the most motivated clients who experience aspects of their sexual arousal as highly problematic.

An allied issue is whether the young person has non-problematic/appropriate sexual interests to replace the targeted inappropriate thoughts. Prior to targeting problematic areas of sexual interest it is important to establish clarity over appropriate sexual responses (see Fisher and McGregor above). In our clinical practice we have found it important to establish with the young person a mutually understood concept of what are acceptable and unacceptable sexual thoughts. This should be built up slowly using a language and possibly imagery (non-sexually explicit photographs and drawings) that are meaningful to the young person. This can then lead to consideration, with the young person, of the extent to which he may experience risky or inappropriate sexual thoughts and what external influences there may be upon these.

When employing aversive imagery and scenarios, young people need to be closely involved in the production of these so that they are as individualised and as salient as possible. For example, some young people may find imagining the response of people in the immediate environment to an offence (public anger) a powerful image if they have a history of offending in the community. For other young people the imagined reaction of family (anger, distress, rejection) to re-offending has an equally important impact. Images such as prison may have a salient impact for some adolescents.

To monitor sexual arousal and masturbation patterns we have designed daily diary sheets employing language or symbols agreed upon with the young person. We have found that such techniques can be applicable to young people and are most likely to be viable with those most highly motivated and in highly supportive care environments. Arousal management may be important for individuals to achieve a sense of control and to start to take responsibility for their behaviour. It is important to assist the development of effective means of coping with situational stimuli. Strategies should be designed to aid retention and composed of broad rules that are not too specific and therefore adaptable to a variety of situations. It is important to develop honesty and realism as key concepts. Self-reporting of deviant arousal should not be seen by individuals as a failure but rather a sign of commitment to self-management.

## Effective general self-management

With many individuals more general, effective self-management might be a more achievable goal than the elimination of deviant sexual arousal. A simple but effective framework we have adapted towards this end in the G-MAP programme is that of developing a set of thinking skills known as ACE (Avoid – Control – Escape). Young people are introduced to the strategy as follows:

- *Avoid* is the skill used to think about something that may happen in the future and to decide whether it might be safer to choose not to take part, go to, or join in with the anticipated event.
- *Control* is the skill used to think about something that may happen or is already happening. Control involves making a choice to take part in, go to, or join in with something because it can be made safe (for example, ensuring that you will not be on your own with someone).
- *Escape* is the skill that is usually used in a situation that is happening when control is not possible. It is knowing how to safely get out of a situation that cannot be controlled.

Everyday examples, such as the ones below, are presented, and the young person is asked how ACE choices could help them to manage each situation safely.

- *John is out with his mates for the evening. One of them suggests that they nick a car and go joyriding.*
- *Bill's girlfriend wants to have sexual intercourse but Bill has no condoms and the girlfriend has no available form of contraception.*
- *Ted is feeling unwell but has a job interview to go to.*
- *Jim has heard that Steve is threatening to thump him because he is going out with Steve's ex-girlfriend. Jim has tickets for a club but knows that Steve is likely to be there.*
- *Dan is out with a mate who gets into an argument with another lad.*

The young person then re-visits examples of their own offending behaviour and applies the ACE model to work out how they could have managed those situations safely. We teach the relevance of ACE skills to self-management of risk (relapse prevention) by rehearsing ACE responses to potentially risky situations relevant for the young person now or in the near future. Typical examples of risky situations rehearsed include:

- *You are walking along a canal path and a woman on her own walks past.*
- *A neighbour asks you to baby-sit.*
- *You are at home and one of your young cousins comes round with your Auntie.*
- *You are on the computer and are tempted to go to sex sites on the Internet.*
- *A young child is outside on the street and asks you to play with them.*
- *You are at the home of a friend who has a child and the child asks if you will put them to bed and read them a story.*

Finally, the young person completes an eco-map of helpers and supporters and indicates: how much each person knows about the abusive behaviour; what type of help and support they provide; and whether the person concerned knows that their continued help is expected by the young person. The emphasis of the ACE approach is not to assume that the young person will respond in a deviant manner to all potentially risky situations but to help him/her to establish clear strategies for the self-management of those situations.

## Conclusions

This chapter has attempted to provide an overview of some of the current research and clinical practice in relation to offence specific interventions. Over the last five years there has been increasing consensus that this work should be encompassed within a holistic approach that includes the involvement of families, the promotion of positive goals and the development of social and emotional competence. There is significant overlap with this current view and the development of thinking in work with adult *sexual* offenders (Hanson *et al.*, 2002). As research and theoretical thinking develops over the next five years this trend may well extend so that the intervention focus on offence specific work with some young people who sexually harm becomes increasingly secondary to life skills development. At present, however, best practice would suggest the integration of offence specific work within a holistic and developmental framework.

## References

Abel, G., Becker, J., and Cunningham-Rathner, J. (1984). Complications, consent and cognitions in sex between children and adults. *International Journal of Law and Psychiatry, 7*, 89–103.

Abel, G., Osborn, C., and Twigg, D. (1993). Sexual assault through the life span: Adult offenders with childhood histories. In H. Barbaree, W. L. Marshall and S. Hudson (eds), *The Juvenile Sex Offender*. New York: Guilford Press.

Ainsworth, M. D., Blehar, M. C., Walters, E., and Wall, S. (1978). *Patterns of Attachment: A Psychological Study of the Strange Situation*. Hillsdale, NJ: Lawrence Erlbaum.

Bailey, S. (1997). Sadistic and violent acts in the young. *Child Psychology and Psychiatry Review, 2*, 92–102.

Ball-Rokeach, S. J., Rokeach, M., and Grube, J. W. (1984). *The Great American Values Test: Influencing Behaviour and Belief Through Television*. New York: Free Press.

Becker, J. V., and Kaplan, M. S. (1988). The assessment of adolescent sexual offenders. *Advances in Behavioral Assessment of Children and Families, 4*, 97–118.

Beckett, R. (1994) Assessment of sex offenders. In T. Morrison, M. Erooga and R. Beckett (eds), *Sexual Offending Against Children: Assessment and Treatment of Male Abusers*. London: Routledge.

Beckett, R. (1999) Evaluation of adolescent sexual abusers. In M. Erooga and H. Masson (eds), *Children and Young People who Sexually Abuse Others: Challenges and Responses*. London: Routledge.

Beckett, R. C., Beech, A., Fisher, D., and Fordham, A. S. (1994). *Community-Based Treatment for Sex Offenders: An Evaluation of Seven Treatment Programmes*. London: Home Office.

Beech, A., and Fordham, A. S. (1997). Therapeutic climate of sex offender treatment programmes. *Sexual Abuse: A Journal of Research and Treatment, 9*, 219–236.

Beech, A., Friendship, C., Erikson, M., and Hanson, R. K. (2002). The relationship between static and dynamic risk factors in a sample of U.K. child abusers. *Sexual Abuse: A Journal of Research and Treatment, 14(2)*, 155–167.

Berenson, D. (1987). Choice, thinking, and responsibility: Implications for treatment. *Interchange*. Denver, Colorado: Kempe National Center.

Blechman, E. A., and Vryan, K. D. (2000). Pro-social family therapy: A manual for preventive intervention for juvenile offenders. *Aggression and Violent Behaviour, 5(4)*, 343–378.

Borduin, C., Hengeller, S., Blaske, D., and Stein, R. (1990). Multisystemic treatment of adolescent sex offenders. *International Journal of Offender Therapy and Comparative Criminology, 34*, 105–113.

Brehm, S., and Brehm, J. W. (1981). *Psychological Reactance: A Theory of Freedom and Control*. New York: Academic Press.

Burt, M. R. (1983). Justifying personal violence: A comparison of rapists and the general public. *Victimology: An International Journal, 8*, 131–150.

Burton, D. L. (2000). Were adolescent sexual offenders children with sexual behavior problems? *Sexual Abuse: A Journal of Research and Treatment, 12*, 37–48.

Butz, C., and Spaccarelli, S. (1999). Use of physical force as an offense characteristic in subtyping juvenile sexual offenders. *Sexual Abuse: A Journal of Research and Treatment, 11*, 217–222.

Carducci, D. J. (1980). Positive peer culture and assertiveness training: Complementary modalities for dealing with disturbed and disturbing adolescents in the classroom. *Behavioural Disorders, 5*, 156–162.

Cooper, C. L., Murphy, W. D., and Haynes, M. R. (1996). Characteristics of abused and non-abused adolescent sexual offenders. *Sexual Abuse: A Journal of Research and Treatment, 8(2)*, 106–119.

Crittenden, P. M. (1995). Attachment and psychopathology. In S. Goldberg, R. Muir and J. Kerr (eds), *Attachment Theory: Social, Developmental, and Clinical Perspectives*. Hillsdale, NJ: Analytic Press.

Elliott, M., Brown, K., and Kilcoyne, J. (1995). Child sexual abuse prevention: What offenders tell us. *Child Abuse and Neglect, 18*, 579–594.

Erickson, E. (1959). *Identity and the Life Cycle*. New York: Norton.

Farmer, E., and Pollock, S. (1998). *Sexually Abused and Abusing Children in Substitute Care*. London: Wiley.

Finkelhor, D. (1984). *Child Sexual Abuse: New Theory and Research*. New York: Free Press.

Fisher, D., and McGregor, G. (1997). Behavioural treatment techniques. In M. S. Hoghughi, S. R. Bhate and F. Graham (eds), *Working with Sexually Abusive Adolescents*. London: Sage.

Fongay, P., Redfern, S., and Charman, T. (1997). The relationship between belief–desire reasoning and a projective measure of attachment security (SAT). *British Journal of Developmental Psychology, 15*, 51–61.

Freeman-Longo, R. E. (2001). *Paths to Wellness: A Holistic Approach and Guide to Personal Recovery*. Holyoke, MA: Neari Press.

Freeman-Longo, R. E., Bird, S., Stevenson, W., and Fiske, J. (1995). *1994 Nationwide Survey of Treatment Programmes and Models Serving Abuse-Reactive Children and Adolescents and Adult Sex Offenders*. Burlington, VT: Safer Society Press.

Freeman-Longo, R. E., Bays, L., and Bear, E. (1996). *Empathy and Compassionate Action: Issues and Exercises – A Guided Workbook for Clients in Treatment*. Burlington, VT: Safer Society Press.

Gibbs, J. C. (1996). Sociomoral Group Treatment for Young Offenders. In C. R. Hollin and K. Howells (eds), *Clinical Approaches to Working with Young Offenders*. Chichester: Wiley and Sons.

Gibbs, J. C., and Potter, G. (1991). *Aggression Replacement Training in the Context of Positive Peer Culture*. Paper presented at the meeting of the Ohio Council for Children with Behavioral Disorders, Columbus, Ohio.

Gopnick, A., and Meltzoff, A. N. (1997). *Words, Thoughts and Theories*, Cambridge, MA: MIT Press.

Haaven, J., Little, R., and Petre-Miller, D. (1990). *Treating Learning Disabled Sex Offenders: A Model Residential Programme*. Orwell, VT: Safer Society Press.

Hall, G. C. N. (1995). Sexual offender recidivism revisited: A meta-analysis of recent treatment studies. *Journal of Consulting and Clinical Psychology, 63*, 802–809.

Hanson, R. K., and Bussiere, M. T. (1998). Predicting relapse: A meta-analysis of sexual offender recidivism studies. *Journal of Consulting and Clinical Psychology, 66*, 348–362.

Hanson, R. K., and Scott, H. (1995). Assessing perspective-taking among sexual offenders, nonsexual criminals, and non-offenders. *Sexual Abuse: A Journal of Research and Treatment, 7*, 259–277.

Hanson, R. K., Steffy, R. A., and Gauthier, R. (1993). Long-term recidivism of child molesters. *Journal of Consulting and Clinical Psychology, 61(4)*, 646–652.

Hanson, R. K., Gizzarelli, R., and Scott, H. (1994). The attitudes of incest offenders:

Sexual entitlement and acceptance of sex with children. *Criminal Justice and Behaviour, 21*, 187–202.

Hanson, R. K., Gordon, A., Harris, A. J. R., Marques, J. K., Murphy, W., Quinsey, V. L., and Seto, M. C. (2002). First report of the Collaborative Outcome Data Project on the effectiveness of psychological treatment for sexual offenders. *Sexual Abuse: A Journal of Research and Treatment, 14(2)*, 169–194.

Happé, F., and Frith, U. (1996). Theory of mind and social impairment in children with conduct disorder. *British Journal of Developmental Psychology, 14*, 385–398.

Hayashino, D. S., Wurtele, S. K., and Klebe, K. J. (1995). Child molesters: An examination of cognitive factors. *Journal of Interpersonal Violence, 10*, 106–116.

Hudson, S., Wales, D. S., Bakker, L., and Ward, T. (2002). Dynamic risk factors: The Kia Marama evaluation. *Sexual Abuse: A Journal of Research and Treatment, 12(2)*, 103–119.

Hunter, J. A., and Becker, J. (1994). The role of deviant arousal in juvenile sexual offending: Etiology, evaluation and treatment. *Criminal Justice and Behaviour, 21*, 132–149.

Hunter, J. A., and Lexier, L. J. (1998). Ethical and legal issues in the assessment and treatment of juvenile sex offenders. *Child Maltreatment, 3(4)*, 339–348.

Jenkins, A. (1998). Invitations to responsibility: engaging adolescents and young men who have sexually abused. In W. Marshall, Y. Fernandez, S. Hudson and T. Ward (eds), *Sourcebook of Treatment Programmes for Sexual Offenders*. New York: Plenum.

Jenkins-Hall, K. D. (1994). Outpatient treatment in child molesters: Motivational factors and outcome. In N. Pallone (ed.), *Young Victims, Young Offenders: Current Issues in Policy and Treatment*. New York: Hawthorne Press, pp. 139–150.

Johnson, G. M., and Knight, R. A. (2000). Developmental antecedents of sexual coercion in juvenile sexual offenders. *Sexual Abuse: A Journal of Research and Treatment, 12(3)*, 165–178.

Kahn, T. J. (1990). *Pathways: A Guided Workbook for Youth Beginning Treatment*. Orwell, VT: Safer Society Press.

Keenan, T., and Ward, T. (2000). A theory of mind perspective on cognitive, affective, and intimacy deficits in child sexual offenders. *Sexual Abuse: A Journal of Research and Treatment, 12*, 49–60.

Kumpfer, K. L., and Alvarado, D. R. (1998). Effective family strengthening interventions. *Juvenile Justice Bulletin* (NCJ 171121), November. US Department of Justice, Office of Juvenile Justice and Delinquency Prevention.

Langevin, R., Laing, R. A., and Curnoe, S. (1998). The prevalence of sex offenders with deviant fantasies. *Journal of Interpersonal Violence, 13(3)*, 315–327.

Laws, R. (1995). Verbal satiation: Notes on procedure with speculations on its mechanism of effect. *Sexual Abuse: A Journal of Research and Treatment, 7(2)*, 155–165.

Lonsway, K. A., and Fitzgerald, L. F. (1994). Rape myths: In review. *Psychology of Woman Quarterly, 18*, 133–164.

McKeown, K. (2000). *A Guide to What Works in Family Support Services for Vulnerable Families*. Dublin: Social and Economic Research Council, Department of Health and Children.

Malamuth, N. M. (1981). Rape proclivity among males. *Journal of Social Issues, 37*, 138–157.

Malamuth, N. M. (1993). Pornography's impact on male adolescents. *Adolescent Medicine, 4(3)*, 563–576.

Mann, R. E. (2000). Managing resistance and rebellion in relapse prevention intervention. In D. R. Laws, S. M. Hudson and T. Ward (eds), *Remaking Relapse Prevention with Sex Offenders: A Sourcebook*. Thousand Oaks, CA: Sage.

Mann, R., and Schofield, C. (1999). *Working with Sex Offender Schemata*. Seminar presentation at National Organisation for the Treatment of Abusers (NOTA) Conference, Glasgow.

Marolla, J., and Scully, D. (1986). Attitudes towards women, violence and rape: A comparison of convicted rapists and other felons. *Deviant Behaviour, 7*, 337–355.

Marshall, W. L., and Serran, G. (2000). Improving the effectiveness of sexual offender treatment. *Trauma, Violence, and Abuse: A Review Journal, 1*, 203–222.

Marshall, W. L., Barbaree, H. E., and Eccles, A. (1991). Early onset and deviant sexuality in child molesters. *Journal of Interpersonal Violence, 6(3)*, 323–336.

Marshall, W. L., Hudson, S. M., Jones, R., and Fernandez, Y. M. (1995). Empathy in sex offenders. *Clinical Psychology Review, 15*, 99–113.

Marshall, W. L., Anderson, D., and Fernandez, Y. M. (1999). *Cognitive Behavioural Treatment of Sexual Offenders*. Chichester: John Wiley.

Marshall, W. L., Serran, G. S., and Cortoni, F. A. (2000). Childhood attachments, sexual abuse, and their relationship to adult coping in child molesters. *Sexual Abuse: A Journal of Research and Treatment, 12*, 17–26.

Miller, W. R., and Rollnick, S. (1991). *Motivational Interviewing: Preparing People to Change Addictive Behavior*. New York: Guilford Press.

Murphy, W. D. (1990). Assessment and modification of cognitive distortions in sex offenders. In W. L. Marshall, D. R. Laws and H. E. Barbaree (eds), *Handbook of Sexual Assault: Issues, Theories and Treatment of the Offender*. New York: Plenum Press.

Nagayama Hall, G. C. (1996). *Theory-based Assessment, Treatment, and Prevention of Sexual Aggression*. New York: Oxford University Press.

O'Brien, M. (2000). *A Typology of Adolescent Sexual Offender*. Paper presented to Positive Outcomes Conference, Manchester, UK, June.

O'Brien, M., and Bera, W. (1985). *The PHASE Typology*. Minneapolis, MN: Program for Healthy Adolescent Sexual Expression.

O'Callaghan, D. (2002). Providing a research informed service for young people who sexually harm others. In M. Calder (ed.), *Young People who Sexually Abuse: Building an Evidence Base for Your Practice*. Brighton: Russell House.

Pithers, W. D. (1999). Relapse prevention with sexual aggressors: A method for maintaining therapeutic gain and enhancing external supervision. In W. L. Marshall, D. R. Laws and H. E. Barbaree (eds), *Handbook of Sexual Assault: Issues, Theories and Treatment of the Offender*. New York: Plenum.

Pollack, N. L., and Hashmall, J. M. (1991). The excuses of child molesters. *Behavioural Sciences and the Law, 9*, 53–59.

Prentky, R., Harris, B., Frizzell, K., and Righthand, S. (2000). An actuarial procedure for assessing risk with juvenile sex offenders. *Sexual Abuse: A Journal of Research and Treatment, 12(2)*, 71–93.

Prochaska, J., and DiClemente, C. (1982). Transtheoretical therapy: Toward a more integrative model of change. *Psychotherapy: Theory, Research and Practice, 19(3)*, 276–278.

Rasmussen, L. A. (1999). Factors related to recidivism among juvenile sexual offenders. *Sexual Abuse: A Journal of Research and Treatment, 2*, 69–85.

Rice, M. E., Chaplin, T. C., Harris, G. T., and Coutts, J. (1994). Empathy for the victim and sexual arousal among rapists and nonrapists. *Journal of Interpersonal Violence, 9*, 435–449.

Rich, S. A. (1998). A developmental approach to the treatment of adolescent sexual offenders. *Irish Journal of Psychology, 19*, 102–118.

Rokeach, M. (1985). Inducing change and stability in belief systems and personality structures. *Journal of Social Issues, 41*, 153–171.

Russell, M. N. (1995). *Confronting Abusive Beliefs: Group Treatment for Abusive Men*. Thousand Oaks, CA: Sage.

Ryan, G. (1989). Victim to victimizer: Rethinking victim treatment. *Journal of Interpersonal Violence, 4*, 325–341.

Ryan, G. (1999). Treatment of sexually abusive youth: The evolving consensus. *Journal of Interpersonal Violence, 14*, 422–436.

Ryan, G., and Blum, J. (1994). *Childhood Sexuality: A Guide for Parents*. Denver: Kempe Center.

Ryan, G., and Associates (1999). *Web of Meaning: A Developmental-Contextual Approach in Sexual Abuse Treatment*. Brandon, VT: Safer Society Press.

Scully, D. (1988). Convicted rapists' perceptions of self and victim: Role taking and emotions. *Gender and Society, 2*, 200–213.

Sheridan, A., McKeown, K., Cherry, J., Donohoe, E., McGrath, K., O'Reilly, K., Phelan, S., and Tallon, M. (1998). Perspectives on treatment outcome in adolescent sexual offending: A study of a community-based treatment programme. *Irish Journal of Psychology, 19(1)*, 168–180.

Steen, C., and Monnette, B. (1989). *Treating Adolescent Sex Offenders in the Community*. Springfield, IL: Thomas Books.

Stermac, L. E., and Segal, Z. V. (1989). Adult sexual contact with children: An examination of the cognitive factors. *Behaviour Therapy, 20*, 573–584.

Summitt, R. (1983). The child sexual abuse accommodation syndrome. *Child Abuse and Neglect, 7*, 177–193.

Swaffer, T., Hollin, C., Beech, A., Beckett, R., and Fisher, D. (2000). An exploration of child sexual abusers' sexual fantasies before and after treatment. *Sexual Abuse: A Journal of Research and Treatment, 12*, 61–68.

Swenson, C. C., Hengeller, S. W., Schoemwald, S. K., Kaufman, K. L., and Randall, J. (1998). Changing the social ecologies of adolescent sexual offenders: Implications of the success of multisystemic therapy in treating serious anti-social behaviour in adolescents. *Child Maltreatment, 3(4)*, 330–338.

Ward, T. (2002). Good lives and the rehabilitation of sexual offenders. In T. Ward, D. R. Laws and S. M. Hudson (eds), *Sexual Deviance: Issues and Controversies*. Thousand Oaks, CA: Sage.

Ward, T., and Keenan, T. (1999). Child molesters' implicit theories. *Journal of Interpersonal Violence, 14*, 821–838.

Ward, T., and Siegert, R. J. (2002). Towards a comprehensive theory of child sexual abuse: A theory knitting perspective. *Psychology, Crime and Law, 8*, 319–351.

Ward, T., Hudson, S., Marshall, W. L., and Siegert, R. (1995). Attachment style in sex offenders: A preliminary study. *Journal of Sex Research, 33*, 17–26.

Ward, T., Hudson, S., Johnston, L., and Marshall, W. L. (1997). Cognitive distortions in sex offenders: An integrative review. *Clinical Psychology Review, 17*, 479–507.

Ward, T., Fon, C., Hudson, S., and McCormack, J. (1998). Classification of cognition in sex offenders: A descriptive model. *Journal of Interpersonal Violence, 13*, 129–155.

Ward, T., Keenan, T., and Hudson, S. M. (2000). Understanding cognitive, affective and intimacy deficits in sexual offenders: A developmental perspective. *Aggression and Violent Behaviour, 5*, 41–62.

Way, I., and Balthazor, T. (1990). *Manual for Structured Group Treatment of Adolescent Sex Offenders*. Notre dame, IN: Jalice.

Way, I. F., and Spieker, S. D. (1997). *The Cycle of Offense: A Framework for Treating Adolescent Sexual Offenders*. Notre dame, IN: Jalice.

Weinrott, M. R., Riggan, M., and Frothingham, S. (1997). Reducing deviant arousal in juvenile sex offenders using vicarious sensation. *Journal of Interpersonal Violence, 12*, 704–728.

Williams, R. M. (1979). Change and stability in values and value systems. A sociological perspective. In M. Rokeach (ed.), *Understanding Human Values: Individual and Societal*. New York: Free Press.

Woods, J. (1997). Breaking the cycle of abuse and abusing: Individual psychotherapy for juvenile sex offenders. *Clinical Child Psychology and Psychiatry, 2*, 379–392.

Worling, J. R., and Curwen, T. (2000). Adolescent sexual offenders recidivism: Success of specialized treatment and implications for risk prediction. *Child Abuse and Neglect, 24(7)*, 965–982.

Yochelson, S., and Samenow, S. (1976). *The Criminal Personality*, vol. 1. Northvale, NJ: Aronson.

Chapter 10

# Essentials of a good intervention programme for sexually abusive juveniles

## Offence related treatment tasks

*James R. Worling*

### Offence related versus offence specific treatment

Like many clinicians, I work with adolescents who offend sexually, in a holistic fashion within a comprehensive treatment programme. Our assessment process is designed to highlight unique strengths and weaknesses with respect to a wide variety of issues such as social orientation, sexual fantasy, family communication, affective expression, sexual attitudes, and so on. As such, it initially felt somewhat arbitrary to separate those treatment targets that are "offence specific" from those that are "offence related". While it is clear that treatment aimed at reducing an adolescent's deviant sexual arousal is clearly in the "offence specific" category, it becomes less clear when the treatment target is enhancing nonsexual affective expression; especially when an individual's sexual offences are closely tied to an inability to cope effectively with negative affect such as increased anger or boredom. In cases such as this, therefore, cognitive-behavioural treatment aimed at assisting the adolescent to cope with negative affect is crucial (and directly related one could argue) to the reduction of risk of sexual assault recidivism. For the purposes of this chapter, however, "offence related" treatment tasks are those that do not involve reference to sexual offending specifically. Furthermore, although family interventions are surely essential ingredients of offence related treatment, these are discussed in significant detail elsewhere in this volume. There are any number of sexual offence related treatment goals depending on the unique needs and strengths of each adolescent and his or her family. The offence related treatment goals addressed in this chapter are those most frequently noted in the literature as essential. These include social skills, romantic relationships/sexual education, anger expression/control, impulse control, and prior victimisation.

Much of traditional, specific-specific treatment for adolescents is aimed at reducing deviant sexual thoughts, behaviours and attitudes. Of course, good treatment does not focus solely on the removal of problem behaviours, cognitions or attitudes; rather, good treatment also includes the support of positive alternatives. As one goal of specific-specific treatment is to provide the adolescents with the tools they can use to form healthy sexual relationships in the future, it is important to address any social skills deficits, significant difficulties coping with anger, heightened impulsivity, deficits in knowledge regarding human sexuality, and any post-traumatic stress from childhood abusive experiences.

As is true for much of the specific-specific treatment described in this volume, most empirical support with respect to these offence related interventions comes from authors employing cognitive-behavioural interventions. Cognitive-behavioural treatment is not a unitary intervention; rather, it consists of a variety of related strategies such as operant conditioning, role playing, modelling, homework assignments, and education regarding social skills, problem solving and affective expression. The various theoretical orientations that joined to form cognitive-behavioural approaches include cognitive therapy, behaviour modification, and rational-emotive therapy. Cognitive-behavioural treatment requires that the therapist collaborate with the client to develop and practise new skills, and to teach the client alternative coping strategies to intervene in dysfunctional thought–affect–behaviour patterns.

## Social skills

Social competency involves a diverse and complex array of interpersonal and intra-personal skills such as interpreting verbal and nonverbal cues, regulating affect, gauging intention, active listening, and encouraging reciprocity. Given the importance of social competency in day-to-day living for adolescents, social skill deficits impact negatively on virtually all areas of functioning, and they are particularly evident with respect to the deleterious influence on self-esteem, academic achievement and family and peer relationships. Providing treatment for social skills deficits is obviously critical to sexual offence risk reduction as the adolescent will require the skills and confidence necessary to form healthy intimate relationships in the future.

One of the most prevalent clinical assumptions regarding adolescents who offend sexually is that they *all* demonstrate poor social skills, and that this factor has significant aetiological importance with respect to their offending behaviours. While some adolescents who commit sexual offences demonstrate low social competency, it is important to stress that adolescents who offend sexually are heterogeneous with respect to social prowess. Indeed, each adolescent who commits a sexual offence is a unique individual with distinctive strengths, deficits and background characteristics.

Despite individual uniqueness, however, there are clusters or subgroups of adolescents who offend sexually who share some similarities and treatment needs. With respect to social orientation, for example, Smith *et al.* (1987) and Worling (2001) both identified four subgroups of adolescents who varied with respect to interpersonal orientation. In both investigations, two relatively "healthy" personality-based groups were identified: one group of emotionally over-controlled and socially reserved adolescents and one group of confident and outgoing adolescents who are prone to occasional aggression towards others. Similarly, two more pathological groups were identified in each study: one group of antisocial and impulsive teenagers and one group of emotionally disturbed and socially awkward adolescents. Given the diversity with respect to social competencies, these four groups would likely benefit from remediation in different skills.

There are a number of commercially available treatment packages for teaching adolescents social skills, and several of these approaches have been validated empirically. Two of the more popular empirically-based programmes are *Asset* (Hazel *et al.*, 1996) and *Skillstreaming the Adolescent* (Goldstein and McGinnis, 1997). Both treatment packages are exceptionally well-designed in that specific goals, exercises and homework activities are presented for each educational goal. Both interventions involve the use of modelling, role-playing, participant discussion and feedback, and homework assignments to assist generalisation of new skills beyond the therapy setting. In their *Skillstreaming* manual, Goldstein and McGinnis (1997) have broken down each social skill into a number of concrete steps that can be taught, modelled and practised. For example, the steps outlined for "using self-control" include teaching the adolescent to (1) tune in to body language that may indicate an impending loss of control; (2) consider external events and/or internal thoughts that may have led to this sensation; (3) think of the methods (also taught separately) that could be used to encourage self-control, such as relaxation, escape from the situation, counting to 10; and (4) selecting the best method for self-control.

Specific social skills from the *Skillstreaming* programme can be taught to adolescents who sexually offend depending, of course, on clinical need. For example, adolescents who are more antisocial and impulsive would likely benefit from intensive instruction on the set of nine social skills categorised as "alternatives to aggression". These include skills labelled as "using self-control", "keeping out of fights" and "avoiding trouble with others". The emotionally over-controlled and shy adolescents, on the other hand, do not share the delinquent attitudes or interpersonal orientation of the antisocial and impulsive adolescents. More specifically, the over-controlled adolescents endorse prosocial attitudes, they are cautious to interact with others, and they tend to keep their feelings to themselves. Unlike the antisocial adolescents described above, these adolescents will need to work on the outward expression of affect and the ability to take risks to form social relationships. Using the Goldstein and McGinnis (1997) manual, these adolescents would likely benefit from instruction in skills labelled as "joining in", "expressing your feelings" and "standing up for your rights".

The development and maintenance of an intimate sexual relationship with a consenting peer may be particularly problematic for the socially awkward and isolated adolescents given their significant social deficits. Goldstein and

McGinnis (1997) outline behavioural instruction in a number of basic, or "beginning", social skills that would likely be helpful for this group such as "listening", "starting a conversation", "asking a question", and "introducing yourself". In direct contrast, adolescents in the outgoing-yet-aggressive group have much better-developed social skills, and they would not benefit from intensive remedial instruction in basic social skills. Successful interventions with this group would require that their sometimes aggressive and self-centred orientation be targeted specifically. Social skills described by Goldstein and McGinnis (1997) that could be helpful for this group include "sharing something", "understanding the feelings of others", and "being a good sport".

Although most treatment-outcome research with adolescents who sexually offend has been focused on criminal recidivism (see Worling and Curwen, 2000, for a review), there has been one study focused on the acquisition of social skills. Graves *et al.* (1992) used the Asset Program and found that, relative to a comparison group, the adolescents who received formal instruction in social skills made significant gains. The authors also found that self-esteem increased significantly for the treatment group; particularly with respect to perceived popularity with peers and perceived physical attractiveness.

There has been some recent debate regarding the appropriateness of placing adolescents who offend sexually in groups given that association with delinquent peers tends to be one of the most robust predictors of later criminal involvement (Loeber, 1990). Of course, group therapy will be contraindicated for some adolescents; particularly those adolescents who have difficulty curbing their sexual arousal during discussion of offence specific interventions. On the other hand, however, groups can provide an excellent forum for teaching, modelling and practising prosocial skills for adolescents who offend sexually. The adolescents' developmental need to form close associations with peers, for example, lends itself naturally to group therapy, and adolescent peer pressure is a powerful vehicle for encouraging participation, practice and compliance with homework tasks. There is also a better chance of generalisation beyond the therapy room when social skills are being modelled and critiqued by peers as opposed to adult therapists.

It goes without saying that community-based group treatment, in isolation, is not likely to lead to successful social skill acquisition and generalisation; particularly when the deficits are considerable. Homework assignments can be helpful to generalise treatment gains, and the commercially available packages contain a number of suggested homework exercises for each skill area. In cases where the adolescent requires more intensive social skills training, however, we have found it useful to enlist the support and expertise of other community agencies that offer enhanced social skills group treatment (not sexual offence specific) and/or individual contract workers who can spend several hours each week in the community with the adolescent building upon the gains made in treatment. Wherever possible, we also support the adolescent's involvement in structured and supervised social activities, such as participation on sports teams. This form of peer involvement allows for more opportunities to practise and generalise social skills, provides further opportunity for social interaction and friendships, and assists the adolescent to form new recreational interests. Social skill acquisition is also enhanced when individuals from the adolescent's place of residence are actively involved in treatment. Whether working together with parents or staff from a residential setting, it is critical to ensure that these individuals are aware of the treatment goals and expectations. Good communication is also important to ensure that the adolescent is actively practising the assigned tasks to foster generalisation.

## Human sexuality education and romantic relationships

Although some clinicians have commented that adolescents who offend sexually have a poor fund of knowledge regarding human sexuality, it is important to note that (1) low sexual knowledge is certainly not unique to those adolescents who commit sexual offences and (2) limited sexual knowledge does not lead directly to the commission of a sexual offence by an adolescent. While inaccurate information about human sexuality is not the cause of offending behaviours, the amelioration of knowledge deficits is important for *all* adolescents in the formation and maintenance of future sexual relationships. Some adolescents will have developed particularly distorted beliefs and attitudes about sexuality as a result of their sexual offence behaviours. Similarly, some adolescents who are survivors of childhood sexual abuse will have developed unusual thoughts and beliefs about sex as a result of their victimisation experiences. Specific educational topics to be taught and discussed with respect to human sexuality include human physiology, reproduction and sexually transmitted diseases.

Of course, it is essential for clinicians to go beyond the basic "plumbing" in their education regarding human sexuality. Most social skills training programmes (discussed above) focus on a variety of aspects of interpersonal relationships; however, very few of the commercially available treatment manuals address issues related to romantic relationships. If the goal of treatment for adolescent sexual offenders is to assist them to form romantic relationships in the future, skills training must also address the development of healthy attitudes towards dating and relationships. Specific issues to be addressed include basic dating skills (e.g. making dates, choosing dating activities, coping with possible rejection) sexual decision making, sexual values, the consent process, and the interplay between sex, love and intimacy.

In addition to the direct benefit of having more accurate knowledge and prosocial sexual attitudes, human sexuality education provides additional benefits with respect to treatment for the adolescent who has offended sexually. For example, good sexual education can provide clients with a common language for sexual offence specific treatment and relapse prevention. In the interest of time, it is often tempting to assume that a particular adolescent knows what terms like "intercourse" and "masturbation" mean and to proceed with offence specific treatment. Education and discussion regarding human sexuality is important for the parents of adolescents as well, especially when they are being asked to assist with the formation and monitoring of relapse prevention plans or to support their adolescent to deal with issues from childhood sexual victimisation experiences. Another benefit of human sexuality education is that well-presented information regarding sexually transmitted diseases can assist adolescents when they begin covert sensitisation. Specifically, many adolescents have used vivid descriptions of symptoms of various venereal diseases when devising their punishment scripts to be used to covertly punish deviant sexual fantasies. Finally, education and discussion regarding sexual orientation can also be extremely helpful for those adolescents who have experienced same-sex childhood sexual victimisation, or who committed sexual offences against same-sex children or peers, and are struggling with questions about their own sexual orientation.

A favourite activity (for both clinicians and adolescents) for addressing both sexual attitudes and knowledge is the "Sexual Pursuit Game", mentioned briefly by Steen and Monnette (1989). This activity can be used in group, family or individual treatment, and questions can be tailored to meet specific treatment or educational needs. When used in group treatment, we have found it most productive to have adolescents work in teams of two or three members. This also increases opportunities for social-skills practice in smaller groups. For this game, we typically have five categories of questions, and the adolescents roll a die to determine which category the question will be from (1 = *sexual offending*, 2 = *health*, 3 = *dating*, 4 = *myths*, 5 = *human physiology*, and 6 = *miss a turn*). Some of the questions are multiple choice (e.g. "What percentage of adolescents who have committed a sexual offence were abused sexually as children? (a) 0% (b) 10% (c) 45% (d) 90%"); whereas others are true/false (e.g. "If a date goes to your house on your first date, that means that they want to have sex"). When the group or family is involved, we have also included some open-ended questions, such as "How do you know when someone is consenting to have sex with you?" In these instances, players from the opposing team(s) determine whether the answer is acceptable. We have found that this game format is an excellent way to address a number of issues related to both offence related and offence specific treatment. Rather than simply racing through the questions, however, the best aspect of this game is the discussion that follows each question.

Another exercise that is useful for introducing a number of topics regarding sexual knowledge and dating attitudes is a variation of the "Sexual Myth Game" described initially by Steen and Monnette (1989). We divide our group into two teams (one could use this exercise with families as well), and we give each team about forty true/false statements on strips of paper together with two containers: one container labelled "true" and the other labelled "false". When we use this exercise for addressing sexual attitudes, example items include "Jealousy is a sign of love"; "If your date lets you kiss them, it means that it is OK to touch them sexually"; and "Honesty is important in a dating relationship". We have also used this game successfully to address information regarding human sexuality with true/false questions such as "The changes at puberty happen sooner for boys than for girls"; "Alcohol does not affect the developing foetus"; and "A condom can be used only once". To play the game, the group leaders tell the teams to sort through the slips of paper as quickly as possible, and to make a group decision as to whether each statement is generally true or false and to place each paper into the appropriate container. Although the sorting aspect of the game goes quickly, lengthy and meaningful group discussions take place when the groups review and justify their decisions. Of course, these discussions provide an opportunity for group leaders to provide education and to assess individual and group deficits regarding knowledge and attitudes.

Videos can also be powerful tools when addressing sexual attitudes with adolescents, and they provide a welcome break from didactic instruction. Canadian productions such as *Love Taps* (Torrence and O'Donoghue, 1996) and *Unsuitable Actions* (Krepakevich *et al.*, 1997) have been designed specifically for teenagers to deal with issues of sexual harassment, possessiveness and jealousy in intimate relationships. It is important to note, however, that videos such as these quickly become outdated given the rapid changes in adolescent style, fashion and language, and regional dialects in some productions limit their acceptance to adolescents in a variety of jurisdictions. One way to avoid film critiques and to encourage active listening is to assign specific tasks to the adolescents to engage in while viewing the films. For example, in a vignette that depicts a female victim of harassment talking with a friend, adolescents can be asked to write a list of impact issues (thoughts, feelings and behaviours) for victims of sexual harassment. Alternatively, while watching a vignette depicting an aggressive teen on a first date, adolescents can be asked to stop the tape at the first occurrence of the use of pressure or intimidation.

Given the adolescents' reluctance to admit that there may be something about human sexuality that they do not already know, we have also had some success with an anonymous suggestion box in which the adolescents and therapists (or family members) can place questions about human sexuality. One of the most efficacious interventions regarding human sexuality education has been to invite a nurse from our local department of health. There are a number of health care nurses in the community who have developed an excellent curriculum for teaching many aspects of human sexuality within junior and senior high schools. Nurses in our community have a number of modules available on topics such as sexually transmitted diseases, birth control and dating.

Although much of the treatment manual for adolescents who sexually offend written by Way and Balthazor (1990) is focused on sexual offence specific exercises, there are a number of excellent exercises regarding other treatment issues. For example, the manual outlines an exercise regarding sexual orientation that begins with a brief true/false questionnaire for the adolescent regarding attitudes and concerns about gay and lesbian individuals (e.g. "A teen male who molested a male child must be gay"). This exercise can be very useful in family, individual or group sessions. Another exercise relates to physical intimacy between males and the role of physical touch. Once again, there is an initial homework exercise that is used for later discussion of physical touch, physical intimacy and the differences between sex, affection and aggression. For example, adolescents are asked to list examples of when males would hug, and they are also asked to rate whether or not this is acceptable.

Another resource that is extremely useful for teaching human sexuality is the three-book series by Kieren (1988) called *Growing Through Knowing: Issues in Sexuality*. Although some of the photographs will be dated now, most of the pictures in the books are hand drawings, and the author provides a number of quizzes, checklists and exercises that are written specifically for teens. Kieren addresses a wide variety of topics including coping with pubertal changes, sexual health issues, sex roles, sexual decision making, pregnancy and the expression of love and physical intimacy. Throughout the workbooks, Kieren has also included specific question and answer test boxes outlining questions that adolescents typically ask, such as "Can a female get pregnant if she has intercourse before she ovulates?"; "What is a wet dream?" Furthermore, the language used in these workbooks makes them particularly valuable to look up answers, together with the young person, when I am unsure of a response (which is often). This is one of the more valuable therapeutic exercises in that it is helpful to model the fact that one cannot possibly ever know everything about sex.

When looking at dating behaviours, it can be really helpful to break down some of the early dating skills into smaller steps for instruction, modelling, and practice – as has been done in the social skills programmes outlined briefly above. For example, dating skills for instruction could include: (1) how to look for a potential date; (2) asking a person for a date; (3) coping with possible rejection/acceptance; (4) selecting activities for a date; (5) communicating during the date; (6) terminating a date; and (7) following up from a first date. It is critical to stress, however, that clinicians should not assume that all adolescents who have offended sexually are heterosexual: a practice that is often adopted when discussing dating with adolescent males. Talking about "dating girls" within a group of adolescent males who offended sexually could be potentially very harmful for any males who are gay or questioning their sexual orientation, and the potential negative impact on their self-esteem and personal identity is considerable.

Another issue related to homophobic attitudes is that it is often very difficult for a group of adolescent males to role play dating skills with each other within the group context. Indeed, some adolescent males will not be able to role play with a male therapist in individual therapy either. To avoid this dilemma, we have had some success when adolescent males role play dating skills with the female group co-therapist.

Although there is very little research regarding the outcome of interventions for enhancing sexual knowledge/attitudes for adolescents who have offended sexually, Kaplan *et al.* (1991) found that one group session focused on sexual knowledge did not lead to reliable increases in sexual knowledge. It has been my experience that it takes many sessions and homework assignments to address deficits in the area of sexual knowledge, sexual attitudes and romantic-relationship skills. Furthermore, as in the case of the other treatment targets discussed in this chapter, it is important to ensure that there is concomitant work with families and staff at residential settings to ensure that positive changes are generalised beyond the therapy setting. In addition to including these individuals in sexual education exercises with the adolescents, it is also good practice to ensure that some of the homework assignments require the adolescent to involve residential staff and/or parents.

## Anger expression and control

"Anger management" is frequently listed as an important area of therapeutic focus for adolescents who offend sexually. Although it is seldom explicitly stated, this is presumably based on the assumption that much of sexual offending is closely tied to the expression of anger – or more precisely, the under-controlled expression of anger. While poorly controlled anger certainly receives a lot of attention because of the aggressive behaviours that often result, it is important to recall that some adolescents who sexually offend are emotionally over-controlled, and they have tremendous difficulty expressing negative affect such as anger (Worling, 2001). Regardless of the degree of emotional over- or under-control, however, anger is frequently listed as an emotion that immediately precedes sexual offences for adolescents (e.g. Steen and Monnette, 1989; Way and Balthazor, 1990). Furthermore, Hanson and Harris (2000) suggested that an increase in anger is a significant risk factor for adult sexual offence recidivism.

There is considerable empirical support for the use of cognitive-behavioural strategies when addressing anger control problems with adolescents and adults (Beck and Fernandez, 1998). The cognitive-behavioural model of anger that underlies most treatment manuals is based on the pioneering work of Novaco (1975). Briefly, Novaco posited that anger results from a combination of physiological arousal caused by an aversive event and the individual's cognitive labelling of that arousal as anger. Adolescents who have difficulty expressing or controlling anger, therefore, may have deficits with respect to their ability to recognise, process and label physiological reactions or environmental events or "triggers". Adolescents who are typically aggressive often assume that others are being angry with them, despite contrary evidence, or they tend to selectively attend to hostile environmental cues (Dodge *et al.* 1990). Conversely, adolescents who are over-controlled in the expression of their anger often expend considerable energy avoiding internal and environmental anger cues and they prevent the outward expression of anger wherever possible (Spielberger, 1999). Although virtually all anger-treatment programmes for adolescents are designed for those adolescents who lack anger controls, the over-control of hostility can also result in difficulties such as passivity, withdrawal, depression and the inability to react assertively (Spielberger, 1999). Emotionally over-controlled adolescents do benefit, however, from many of the exercises that have been designed for overtly aggressive youth; particularly assertiveness training.

One of the more popular cognitive-behavioural treatment manuals for assisting children and adolescents to cope more effectively with anger is called *Keeping Your Cool* (Nelson and Finch, 1996). The treatment exercises in this programme can be used in either group or individual contexts, and they are organised around five empirically supported interventions. Furthermore, an important part of this treatment package is to teach adolescents to recognise their unique anger triggers and the cognition–affect–behaviour links that lead to problems with anger expression.

The first skill in the *Keeping Your Cool* workbook is self-instruction, or "self-talk", which is based on self-instructional training for impulsive children developed by Michenbaum and Goodman (1971, discussed in more detail below regarding Impulse Control). Essentially, adolescents are taught to engage in covert (i.e. silent) anger-reducing self-verbalisations (e.g. "take a deep breath"; "I can wait it out") to stop the cognitive–affective–behavioural chain that typically leads them to respond aggressively. The second intervention in this package involves teaching the adolescents progressive muscle relaxation. In addition to coaching adolescents to employ relaxation techniques to avoid aggression, the relaxation training component can also provide an opportunity for the adolescents to more closely examine and reinterpret physiological cues such as muscle tension. The third treatment component is teaching adolescents general problem-solving skills, as it has been found that many aggressive children tend to lack a repertoire of solutions and they often respond to many interpersonal situations with anger. The problem-solving approach taken by Nelson and Finch (1996) is broken into five steps for instruction:

1 Stop (identify the problem);
2 Think (brainstorm possible solutions);

3 Evaluate (identify the best solution);
4 Act (try it out);
5 React (evaluate your solution).

The fourth intervention involves assertiveness training. Adolescents are first taught to distinguish among aggressive, passive and assertive behavioural responses. In our groups (and with families), we have had a lot of success using a game for this exercise in which a member of one team selects (a) a role-play card (e.g. "You disagree with your teacher on your mark on a geography project") and (b) one card labelled either "passive", "aggressive" or "assertive". The adolescent then acts out the scenario and his or her teammates must decided whether the response is passive, aggressive or assertive. After learning to differentiate passive/aggressive/assertive responses, they are then taught to identify the specific irrational thoughts that support their non-assertive behaviours. Over-controlled adolescents, for example, often assume that others will reject them if they express their anger assertively. The fifth intervention is to teach adolescents to think of something humorous to interrupt their aggressive response to feeling angry. Although the authors note that there is little supporting research regarding the use of humour, it is assumed that humour elicits emotional reactions that are incompatible with anger.

As in the case of the other cognitive-behavioural interventions, homework assignments are an integral component of treatment so that gains are generalised beyond the therapy room. It is especially important to ensure that those adults with whom the adolescent is living are included in the treatment planning so they can support the adolescent to practise new anger-expression skills. For example, parents and/or residential staff will have to be aware of homework instructions for an over-controlled adolescent to express his or her anger more assertively. Without adult awareness and participation, the adolescent may be punished for expressing anger in the residence. Once the adolescent has mastered new strategies in role-play situations in treatment, homework assignments can include having staff and/or parents subtly "provoke" minimal anger with the adolescent (in a planned and therapist-directed fashion) and then record the adolescent's coping responses for discussion in treatment. It may also be the case that one or both parents have some difficulty with anger expression, and they may benefit from some of the cognitive-behavioural intervention and practice strategies as well.

Another popular treatment manual for reducing aggression and enhancing anger control for adolescents is the *Aggression Replacement Training* programme by Goldstein *et al.* (1998). Although there are several components to this programme, including "Skillstreaming" (discussed previously) and moral-reasoning training, the exercises related to anger control training are particularly useful for addressing anger control/expression problems with adolescents. Goldstein *et al.* (1998) outline an exceptionally well-designed ten-week programme for anger control training that includes teaching adolescents to identify their internal and external anger triggers; the development of alternative coping skills such as deep breathing, counting backwards and using pleasant imagery; and instruction and practice for the adolescents to engage in active self-evaluation and self-reward. As in the case of "Skill-streaming", this programme utilises role plays, modelling and homework assignments to teach new skills, and each of the ten sessions are quite detailed with respect to specific therapeutic goals and exercises.

Although anger is frequently the emotion that is targeted for interventions with adolescents who offend sexually, it will be important to assess other potential affective difficulties such as depression and anxiety. In a recent study of juvenile delinquents, Howell *et al.* (1997) found that negative affect can be a critical immediate precursor to criminal recidivism. In addition to perceived anger, the authors found that negative affect commonly identified by the adolescents included depression, rejection by parents and friends, hopelessness, and isolation. It is often equally important, therefore, to provide cognitive-behavioural treatment for depression. For excellent descriptions of treatment approaches for adolescent depression, see Rehm and Sharp (1996) and Stark *et al.* (2000).

## Impulse control

Although many adolescents initially state that their offences "just happened", there is always *some* planning with respect to the commission of a sexual offence. For example, most adolescents will acknowledge that they did not commit their sexual offences in front of their parents, that they did not always sexually assault the first person whom they saw when they woke up, and that they did not typically commit their offences in a prominent public place. After some discussion, therefore, adolescents will be able to acknowledge that there were at least some cognitive processes regarding victim and location selection, for example. Unfortunately, parents also support the view that their child's sexual offences "just happened", as they often believe that even some premeditation is synonymous with heightened risk and the entrenchment of sexual deviance. Contrary to this assumption, however, is the fact that juvenile offenders who are highly impulsive are at elevated risk of continued involvement with the legal system; particularly for nonsexual offences (Lipsey and Derzon, 1998; Loeber, 1990; Worling, 2001). There is also some evidence to suggest that heightened impulsivity is predictive of sexual reoffending as well (Hanson, 2000; Worling and Curwen, 2001). In addition to increased risk of continued involvement with the legal system, impulsivity is also related to a host of additional problems for adolescents, such as learning difficulties, peer rejection, aggression, risk-taking behaviours, and problematic parent–child relationships (Kendall and Braswell, 1993). It is critical, therefore, for the adolescent to reduce heightened impulsivity, if present.

Kendall and Braswell (1993) provide an excellent summary of the cognitive-behavioural treatment interventions that are commonly used for impulsive children and adolescents. These authors note that the focus of treatment should be to teach impulsive children new cognitive problem-solving skills given that impulsive teens and children have difficulty reliably generating successful solutions. Furthermore, given the impact of impulsivity on social functioning, and the importance of interpersonal relationships, Kendall and Braswell (1993) also note that instruction in cognitive problem-solving skills should be focused more on common social problems rather than on academic tasks. Popular cognitive-behavioural strategies for treating impulsivity with children and adolescents include self-instructional training and modelling. It is important to note, however, that the research support for the use of these cognitive-behavioural techniques to reduce impulsivity in children and adolescents is quite weak (Abikoff, 1985; Hinshaw, 2000). Indeed, if the impulsivity is extreme, then pharmacological treatments should also be considered, as recent research supports the use of medication, in conjunction with cognitive-behavioural strategies, to reduce ADHD symptomology (e.g. MTA Cooperative Group, 1999). Despite the lack of consistent support for cognitive-behavioural treatments for impulsivity, however, there is promise that the efficacy of cognitive-behavioural strategies can be enhanced with the addition of behavioural contingencies (e.g. self-reinforcement and contingency management) and social-skills training (Hinshaw, 2000).

Self-instructional training is one of the most popular and widely studied cognitive-behavioural interventions for impulsivity. Following the pioneering work by Michenbaum and Goodman (1971), impulsive children are taught to verbalise the various steps to solving a problem, and they are then assisted to make these verbalisations become covert and automatic. Within their social problem-solving approach, Kendall and Braswell (1993) suggest that impulsive adolescents should be taught to verbalise five steps to problem solving: problem definition ("what am I supposed to do?"); problem approach ("what are all the possibilities to solve this?"); focusing of attention ("I need to concentrate on only this problem now"); choosing an answer ("I think this is the one"); follow-up ("I did a great job" or "I'll try to concentrate harder next time and maybe I'll get it right"). After the therapist models a talking-aloud approach to problem solving, the adolescent then performs the tasks while talking aloud. Following practice with a number of tasks and a variety of self-instructional messages, the therapist then models task performance while whispering the self-instructions. This is followed by task performance by the therapist with only covert self-instruction with obvious pauses and other signs of reflection and thinking. Finally, the adolescent then practises performing a variety of tasks using only covert self-instruction. It is important to ensure that adolescents use language that is natural to them rather than simply mimicking the therapist. Adolescents who are eager to please adults typically employ the therapist's self-instructions with little modification, and it is doubtful they will generalise self-instructions beyond the therapy room. Indeed, it is often prudent to spend time assisting the adolescent to create a variety of self-statements related to each of the five steps for problem solving.

An intervention with significant overlap to self-instructional training is the use of modelling in teaching problem-solving skills. In essence, the therapist verbalises aloud as a variety of everyday problems are solved. In addition to the structured approach to problem-solving, one of the most important aspects of modelling is for the adolescent to observe how the therapist copes with difficulties and frustrations while performing the tasks (Kendall and Braswell, 1993). As such, it is essential for the therapist *not* to continually model perfect execution of tasks but, rather, to model how one copes with failure, errors and distractions.

Behavioural contingency-based interventions that are most commonly used to augment cognitive-behavioural procedures for reducing impulsivity include self-monitoring and self-evaluation (Ervin *et al.*, 1996). Self-monitoring requires the impulsive adolescent to observe and record specific behaviours when provided with external cues to do so. For example, an adolescent may be requested to note on a special recording form, at the sound of an audio signal, whether or not he or she is engaging in a specific behaviour. This form of monitoring does not involve prompting from adults or peers, and the goal is to encourage active self-awareness of targeted behaviours. Self-evaluation techniques are closely related to self-monitoring interventions; however, in addition to teaching the adolescent to be aware of target behaviours, self-evaluation treatment also requires that the adolescent learns to evaluate and reward successful task completion. A popular activity used to teach self-evaluation and self-reinforcement that can be used in group or individual therapy is the "Match Game" (Hinshaw, 2000). After teaching and role playing a new target skill, such as "cooperating with others", adolescents are asked to pay attention to how well they believe they are performing the specific task during an unrelated activity or game. When directed by the therapist (e.g. "It's time for the Match Game"), the adolescents rate their own performance of the targeted skill on a scale from one ("not at all good") to five ("great"). Therapists also rate each adolescent's skill performance, and the adolescent receives points according to therapists' ratings. Bonus points are awarded to the adolescents if their own ratings match the therapist's ratings. The span of self-evaluation periods can be increased gradually, and the frequency of this game during sessions can be reduced gradually to encourage less reliance on therapist ratings of performance. Hinshaw (2000) also notes that the more traditional behavioural interventions such as the use of carefully designed reinforcement and response-cost procedures lead to measurable short-term gains within the environments in which they are implemented (usually school or residential settings). Finally, it is essential to involve the important adults with whom the adolescent interacts if treatment gains are to be generalised. Parents, teachers and residential staff can assist to implement and monitor the impulsive adolescent's behavioural and cognitive-behavioural treatment programme, and there is promising research that simply providing behavioural training to teachers and parents can lead to significant reductions in ADHD symptomology for children (Hinshaw *et al.*, 1998). Kendall and Braswell (1993) outline a number of excellent strategies and exercises for providing training to parents and teachers.

## Prior victimisation

As in the case of poor social skills and low sexual knowledge, a common clinical assumption is that virtually all adolescents who commit a sexual offence are victims of childhood sexual abuse and, therefore, that sexual offending behaviours stem from early sexual victimisation. In a review of the literature related to this issue, Worling (1995c) found that sexual abuse histories varied from 19 per cent to 55 per cent across studies, and that researchers using pre-treatment data reported significantly lower rates (22%) than did researchers using post-treatment data (52%). This finding is consistent with the notion that adolescents are more likely to disclose their own personal victimisation once they have established a trusting relationship in treatment. At our community-based clinic in Toronto, it was found that 43 per cent of the male adolescents who offended sexually disclosed a childhood sexual victimisation history post assessment (Worling, 1995c).

Even though not all adolescents who offend sexually are victims of childhood sexual abuse, the 40 to 55 per cent victimisation rates that are observed by many researchers are at least four times higher than rates of childhood sexual victimisation observed in the general adolescent male population (Watkins and Bentovim, 1992). This is also the case with respect to the limited research with adolescent females who offend sexually where childhood sexual victimisation rates are closer to 75 per cent (Mathews *et al.*, 1997). While it is true that most child victims of sexual abuse do not become adolescents who commit sexual offences, there is a relationship between *some* forms of childhood sexual victimisation and later sexual offending for *some* adolescents.

In one recent investigation, it was found that adolescent sexual offenders who were abused sexually as children were more likely to repeat behaviours that they experienced as victims and to select victims such that there was a close match between their own personal victimisation and offending experiences (Veneziano *et al.*, 2000). For example, Veneziano *et al.* (2000) found that offending adolescents who were subjected to anal intercourse as younger children were fifteen times more likely to engage in this behaviour with their own victims. In another investigation, Burton (2000) found that the intrusiveness and complexity of the adolescents' sexual offence behaviours were significantly related to the intrusiveness and complexity of the adolescents' sexual victimisation history.

In addition to the social-learning aspects of the sexual victimisation history for some adolescents, there are additional sexual specific consequences of childhood sexual abuse that influence the adolescent's sexual thoughts, feelings, attitudes and behaviours. Some adolescent males who were abused by an older male struggle with questions regarding their own sexual orientation; particularly if their offender sexually aroused them during their own abuse (Watkins and Bentovim, 1992). For children who were abused by siblings and/or parents, a task in treatment is to alter the view that sexualised interactions within a family are "normal", and to help them see that love and affection can be expressed towards others without relying on sexual contact. In other cases, deviant sexual arousal may have been "shaped" by long-term abuse that has involved fear, violence and physiological arousal. Other sexual-specific symptoms include flashbacks, intrusive memories and sexual distress (e.g. becoming upset at the mere mention of sexual topics).

There is considerable variability with respect to the sequelae of childhood sexual abuse, and not all children are impacted equally. However, some of the more common nonsexual symptoms include depression, anxiety, social withdrawal, impulsivity, antisocial activities, increased anger and self-injurious behaviours (Kendall-Tackett *et al.*, 1993). Note that many of these are issues that are typically addressed in sexual-offence-specific treatment. These often impact negatively on the adolescent's social relationships, academic performance, family relationships and self-esteem.

There are some practitioners who believe that adolescents who sexually offend should not discuss their own victimisation as this will reinforce the view that these individuals are victims and, thus, not responsible for the sexual offences that they perpetrated. These clinicians forge ahead and provide sexual offence specific and relapse prevention treatment in the absence of addressing the adolescents' personal victimisation. Conversely, others argue that one should engage abused adolescents in offence specific treatment only after the adolescents have healed sufficiently from their personal victimisation. As an alternative to these polarised views, I would argue that it is important to address issues resulting from the adolescent's personal victimisation *concurrently* with sexual offence specific treatment. Regardless of victimisation history, the adolescent's risk to the community is of paramount importance; therefore, it is necessary to engage the adolescent in sexual offence specific treatment tasks from the outset. Similarly, the impact of childhood victimisation cannot be ignored until sexual offence specific treatment is completed. Take, for example, adolescents who are survivors of childhood sexual abuse and whose dissociation and anxiety are triggered by any sexual conversation. How would these adolescents be able to work on sexual offence specific tasks and talk about masturbatory practices, for example? Balancing the competing interests with respect to the adolescent's need to address community risk and personal victimisation requires that clinicians divide treatment time between offending and victimisation issues, and that they are familiar with techniques used to address difficulties associated with childhood victimisation.

Although much is written about the need to address childhood sexual victimisation for adolescents who have offended sexually, it is also important to address other forms of maltreatment. Some researchers have noted, for example, that many offending adolescents are also victims of physical abuse; particularly in the case of sibling incest (Worling, 1995b). Adolescents who have experienced physical abuse may have learned to use physical violence in their interpersonal relationships as a result of modelling their parents' behaviour (Worling, 1995a), and treatment will be necessary to ameliorate the impact of these experiences on the adolescents' attitudes and behaviours. Children who are victims of physical or emotional abuse or neglect also have difficulties in many other aspects of their lives such as peer unpopularity, poor affective regulation and expression, heightened anxiety, attentional difficulties and problems with independent functioning (Erickson *et al.*, 1989).

There is considerable empirical support for cognitive-behavioural treatment that is tailored specifically to the symptoms of post-traumatic distress for children and adolescents who have been sexually abused (Saywitz *et al.*, 2000). Although most of the research has focused on treating trauma resulting from sexual abuse, the success of cognitive-behavioural treatment has also been demonstrated with respect to childhood physical abuse (Cohen *et al.*, 2000). Deblinger and Heflin (1996) offer a detailed treatment manual for working with sexually abused children and their parents. Although many of the examples in the book are written for children up to age thirteen, the authors note that many of the strategies can be used with older adolescents with only slight modifications. The most significant modification required for working with adolescents is in the area of sexual education, as adolescents will require much more detailed information regarding issues such as sexual decision making, dating and consent. Furthermore, although many of the examples are written specifically for sexual victimisation, many of the techniques and exercises can easily be adapted for physical or emotional abuse as well.

The approach outlined by Deblinger and Heflin (1996) is based on three central components: coping skills training, gradual exposure and education. In coping skills training, abused adolescents learn and practise techniques that they can use to cope more effectively with the affective distress related to their traumatic experiences. Specific treatment elements include relaxation training, the identification and expression of feelings, and cognitive coping skills training that assists abused adolescents to refute inaccurate, abuse-related thoughts. A common abuse-related distortion in the case of physical abuse, for example, is that the adolescent is a "bad" person and, therefore, that they deserved the abusive discipline that they received.

After learning and practising new emotional coping skills, the second phase of treatment involves gradual exposure: an intervention that is based on a combination of systematic desensitisation and prolonged exposure.

Adolescents are initially exposed to low anxiety-provoking stimuli related to their abusive experience, such as a discussion of sexual abuse in the media or a discussion of a memory of their "least threatening" victimisation experience. As the adolescents are able to discuss such abuse-related stimuli without significant distress, they are asked to discuss progressively more anxiety-provoking victimisation experiences. The goal is for the adolescent to be able to think and speak about their abuse without maladaptive anxiety or avoidance behaviours such as traumatic flashbacks, dissociation or problematic stimuli-avoidance behaviours.

The third component of this approach is to provide the abused adolescents with education regarding healthy alternatives. In the case of sexual abuse, this would involve teaching adolescents about healthy sexuality (see Human Sexuality Education, above). In the case of physical abuse, the goal would be to provide the adolescent with educational information regarding alternatives to physical discipline. The rationale with this component is that, through their abusive experiences, the adolescents have likely incorporated a number of inaccurate thoughts and attitudes that would interfere in future interpersonal relationships.

A critical component of empirically supported treatment for abused children is the inclusion of parents in the treatment. Deblinger and Heflin (1996) outline specific steps and exercises for parents that parallel the adolescent's treatment. As such, treatment for parents includes aspects of coping skills training, gradual exposure and education. Although one aspect of this work is to assist parents to generalise their child's treatment gains by becoming familiar with the treatment tasks that are being used with their child, there is also often a need for parents to address their own personal issues connected with their son's or daughter's victimisation. For example, parents can often benefit from coping-skills training to deal with troubling thoughts such as "how could I have been such a fool to not know that the offender was abusing my child", or "my child will be damaged for the rest of their life because of the abuse". Parents of abused adolescents often must cope with feelings of anger toward their child's perpetrator, anger towards their child, and anger towards themselves, and coping skills training involves teaching parents relaxation techniques, enhancing parents' affective communication, and assisting them to refute dysfunctional thoughts.

Many parents also demonstrate significant anxiety when they must discuss their child's sexual victimisation; therefore, gradual exposure is an important feature of treatment for the parents. In addition to reducing the parent's own anxiety, gradual exposure for the parent will make it easier for the adolescents to discuss their own sexual victimisation. Of course, for those parents who are survivors of sexual abuse, it may be necessary to make a referral to the appropriate treatment resource to address these issues in more detail, as discussions of their child's sexual victimisation (or offending) may trigger significant emotional distress related to their personal victimisation. As in the case of coping skills training, gradual exposure exercises can be useful for parents of adolescents who offend sexually regardless of whether or not their children are also victims of abuse. Many parents become so distressed when discussing their child's sexual offences that it interferes with treatment.

The educational component of working with parents outlined by Deblinger and Heflin (1996) and others has two goals. First, parents are encouraged to participate in the sexual education exercises both to enhance their personal knowledge of human sexuality and to learn how to teach and discuss human sexuality issues with their children. Second, parents are taught management strategies for coping with their child's problematic behaviours such as non-compliance, nightmares and school avoidance.

Another excellent treatment resource for addressing sexual, physical and emotional victimisation issues for teenagers is the manual and accompanying client activity workbook by Karp *et al.* (1998). The treatment activities in this programme are grouped into four primary categories: building the therapeutic relationship; processing (cognitive and affective) the abusive experience(s); repairing the adolescent's sense of self; and helping the teen to become more oriented towards the future. Cunningham and MacFarlane (1996) also offer a number of excellent exercises for sexually abused children and young adolescents that can assist sexually abused clients to develop cognitive and behavioural coping strategies.

## Conclusion

In follow-up studies of adolescents who have offended sexually, the sexual assault recidivism rates following offence specific treatment are typically below 15 per cent after a period of approximately four years (Worling and Curwen, 2000). On the other hand, rates of nonsexual reoffending are often over 35 per cent for this same time period. Comprehensive and holistic treatment that addresses prosocial attitudes and behaviours, deficits in sexual knowledge, anger and impulse control and prior childhood victimisation, in addition to sexual offence specific goals, is likely to reduce the risk of both sexual and nonsexual recidivism. In Lipsey's (1995) review of effective treatment programmes for antisocial adolescents, it was stressed that positive outcome is related to multi-modal (e.g. individual and family and group) and behavioural programmes that teach adolescents new prosocial skills in a concrete fashion. The cognitive-behavioural and educational approaches discussed in this chapter are certainly consistent with this notion.

Many of the components of the cognitive-behavioural treatment outlined in this chapter are similar to those that are used in both offence specific treatment and relapse prevention (both discussed elsewhere in this volume) in that the aim of treatment is to teach adolescents to understand and manipulate the connections between thought, affect and behaviour. As such, many of the affective-coping and thought-correction skills discussed in the present chapter can be applied to treatment that addresses deviant sexual attitudes and arousal. Furthermore, several specific skills such as progressive muscle relaxation (Cautela and Groden, 1978), for example, can be used by adolescents in other aspects of their treatment such as covert sensitisation and relapse prevention.

## References

Abikoff, H. (1985). Efficacy of cognitive training interventions in hyperactive children: A critical review. *Clinical Psychology Review, 5*, 479–512.

Beck, R., and Fernandez, E. (1998). Cognitive behavioural therapy in the treatment of anger: A meta-analysis. *Cognitive Therapy and Research, 22*, 63–74.

Burton, D. L. (2000). Were adolescent sexual offenders children with sexual behaviour problems? *Sexual Abuse: A Journal of Research and Treatment, 12*, 37–48.

Cautela, J. R., and Groden, J. (1978). *Relaxation: A Comprehensive Manual for Adults, Children, and Children with Special Needs*. Champaign, IL: Research Press.

Cohen, J. A., Berliner, L., and Mannarino, A. P. (2000). Treating traumatized children: A research review and synthesis. *Trauma, Violence, and Abuse, 1*, 29–46.

Cunningham, C., and MacFarlane, K. (1996). *When Children Abuse: Group Treatment Strategies for Children with Impulse Control Problems*. Brandon, VT: Safer Society Press.

Deblinger, E., and Heflin, A. H. (1996). *Treating Sexually Abused Children and their Nonoffending Parents: A Cognitive Behavioral Perspective*. Thousand Oaks, CA: Sage.

Dodge, K. A., Price, J. M., Bachorowski, J., and Newman, J. P. (1990). Hostile attributional biases in severely aggressive adolescents. *Journal of Abnormal Psychology, 99*, 385–392.

Erickson, M. F., Egeland, B., and Pianta, R. (1989). The effects of maltreatment on the development of young children. In D. Cicchetti and V. Carlson (eds), *Child Maltreatment: Theory and Research on the Causes and Consequences of Child Abuse and Neglect*. Cambridge: Cambridge University Press, pp. 647–684.

Ervin, R. A., Bankert, C. L., and DuPaul, G. J. (1996). Treatment of attention-deficit/hyperactivity disorder. In M. A. Reinecke, F. M. Dattilio and A. Freeman (eds), *Cognitive Therapy with Children and Adolescents: A Casebook for Clinical Practice*. New York: Guilford Press, pp. 38–61.

Goldstein, A. P., and McGinnis, E. (1997). *Skillstreaming the Adolescent*, rev. edn: *New Strategies and Perspectives for Teaching Prosocial Skills*. Champaign, IL: Research Press.

Goldstein, A. P., Glick, B., and Gibbs, J. C. (1998). *Aggression Replacement Training*, rev. edn: *A Comprehensive Intervention for Aggressive Youth*. Champaign, IL: Research Press.

Graves, R., Openshaw, D. K., and Adams, G. R. (1992). Adolescent sex offenders and social skills training. *International Journal of Offender Therapy and Comparative Criminology, 36*, 139–153.

Hanson, R. K. (2000). *Risk Assessment*. Beaverton, OR: Association for the Treatment of Sexual Abusers.

Hanson, R. K., and Harris, A. J. R. (2000). *The Sex Offender Need Assessment Rating*

*(SONAR): A Method for Measuring Change in Risk Levels* (User Report 2000–1). Ottawa: Department of the Solicitor General of Canada.

Hazel, J. S., Schumaker, J. B., Sherman, J. A., and Sheldon, J. (1996). *ASSET: A Social Skills Program for Adolescents*, rev. edn. Champaign, IL: Research Press.

Hinshaw, S. P. (2000). Attention-deficit/hyperactivity disorder: The search for viable treatments. In P. C. Kendall (ed.), *Child and Adolescent Therapy: Cognitive-Behavioral Procedures*, 2nd. edn. New York: Guilford Press, pp. 88–128.

Hinshaw, S. P., Klein, R. G., and Abikoff, H. (1998). Childhood attention-deficit hyperactivity disorder: Nonpharmacalogic and combination approaches. In P. E. Nathan and J. M. Gorman (eds), *A Guide to Treatments that Work*. New York: Oxford University Press, pp. 27–41.

Howell, A. J., Reddon, J. R., and Enns, R. A. (1997). Immediate antecedents to adolescents' offences. *Journal of Clinical Psychology, 53*, 355–360.

Kaplan, M. S., Becker, J. V., and Tenke, C. E. (1991). Assessment of sexual knowledge and attitudes in an adolescent sex offender population. *Journal of Sex Education and Therapy, 17*, 217–225.

Karp, C. L., Butler, T. L., and Bergstrom, S. C. (1998). *Treatment Strategies for Abused Adolescents: From Victim to Survivor*. Newbury Park, CA: Sage.

Kendall, P. C., and Braswell, L. (1993). *Cognitive-Behavioral Therapy for Impulsive Children*, 2nd edn. New York: Guilford Press.

Kendall-Tackett, K. A., Williams, L. M., and Finkelhor, D. (1993). Impact of sexual abuse on children: A review and synthesis of recent empirical studies. *Psychological Bulletin, 113*, 164–180.

Kieren, D. K. (1988). *Growing Through Knowing: Issues in Sexuality*, 3 vols. Toronto: GLC.

Krepakevich, J., and Thompson, B. (producers), and Wynnyk, T. (director) (1997). *Unsuitable Actions*, film. Montreal, Quebec: National Film Board of Canada.

Lipsey, M. W. (1995). What do we learn from 400 research studies on the effectiveness of treatment with juvenile delinquents? In J. McGuire (ed.), *What Works: Reducing Reoffending, Guidelines from Research and Practice*. London: John Wiley and Sons, pp. 63–77.

Lipsey, M. W., and Derzon, J. H. (1998). Predictors of violent or serious delinquency in adolescence and early adulthood: A synthesis of longitudinal research. In R. Loeber and D. P. Farrington (eds), *Serious and Violent Juvenile Offenders: Risk Factors and Successful Interventions*. London: Sage, pp. 86–105.

Loeber, R. (1990). Development and risk factors of juvenile antisocial behaviour and delinquency. *Clinical Psychology Review, 10*, 1041.

Mathews, R., Hunter, J. A., and Vuz, J. (1997). Juvenile female sexual offenders: Clinical characteristics and treatment issues. *Sexual Abuse: A Journal of Research and Treatment, 9*, 187–199.

Michenbaum, D., and Goodman, J. (1971). Training impulsive children to talk to themselves: A means of developing self-control. *Journal of Abnormal Psychology, 77*, 115–126.

MTA Cooperative Group (1999). Fourteen-month randomized clinical trial of treatment strategies for attention-deficit hyperactivity disorder. *Archives of General Psychiatry, 56*, 1073–1086.

Nelson, W. M., III, and Finch, A. J., Jr (1996). *Keeping Your Cool: The Anger Management Workbook (Parts 1 and 2)*. Ardmore, PA: Workbook Publishing.

Novaco, R. W. (1975). *Anger Control: The Development and Evaluation of an Experimental Treatment*. Lexington, MA: D. C. Heath.

Rehm, L. P., and Sharp, R. N. (1996). Strategies for childhood depression. In M. A. Reinecke, F. M. Dattilio and A. Freeman (eds), *Cognitive Therapy with Children and Adolescents: A Casebook for Clinical Practice*. New York: Guilford Press, pp. 103–123.

Saywitz, K. J., Mannarino, A. P., Berliner, L., and Cohen, J. A. (2000). Treatment for sexually abused children and adolescents. *American Psychologist, 55*, 1040–1049.

Smith, W. R., Monastersky, C., and Deisher, R. M. (1987). MMPI-based personality types among juvenile sexual offenders. *Journal of Clinical Psychology, 43*, 422–430.

Spielberger, C. D. (1999). *State–Trait Anger Expression Inventory*, vol. 2: *Professional Manual*. Odessa, FL: Psychological Assessment Resources.

Stark, K. D., Sander, J. B., Yancy, M. G., Bronik, M. D., and Hoke, J. A. (2000). Treatment of depression in childhood and adolescence: Cognitive-behavioral procedures for the individual and family. In P. C. Kendall (ed.), *Child and Adolescent Therapy: Cognitive-Behavioral Procedures*, 2nd edn. New York, Guilford Press, pp. 173–234.

Steen, C., and Monnette, B. (1989). *Treating Adolescent Sex Offenders in the Community*. Springfield, IL: Charles C. Thomas.

Torrance, J. (producer) and O'Donoghue, A. (director) (1996). *Love Taps*, film. Montreal, Quebec: National Film Board of Canada.

Veneziano, C., Veneziano, L., and LeGrand, S. (2000). The relationship between adolescent sex offender behaviours and victim characteristics with prior victimization. *Journal of Interpersonal Violence, 15*, 363–374.

Watkins, B., and Bentovim, A. (1992). The sexual abuse of male children and adolescents: A review of current research. *Journal of Child Psychology and Psychiatry, 33*, 197–248.

Way, I. F., and Balthazor, T. J. (1990). *A Manual for Structured Group Treatment with Adolescent Sexual Offenders*. Notre Dame, IN: Jalice.

Worling, J. R. (1995a). Adolescent sex offenders against females: Differences based on the age of their victims. *International Journal of Offender Therapy and Comparative Criminology, 39*, 276–293.

Worling, J. R. (1995b). Adolescent sibling-incest offenders: Differences in family and individual functioning when compared to nonsibling sex offenders. *Child Abuse and Neglect, 19*, 633–643.

Worling, J. R. (1995c). Sexual abuse histories of adolescent male sex offenders: Differences based on the age and gender of their victims. *Journal of Abnormal Psychology, 104*, 610–613.

Worling, J. R. (2001). Personality-based typology of adolescent male sexual offenders: Differences in recidivism rates, victim-selection characteristics, and personal victimization histories. *Sexual Abuse: A Journal of Research and Treatment, 13(3)*, 149–166.

Worling, J. R., and Curwen, T. (2000). Adolescent sexual offender recidivism: Success of specialized treatment and implications for risk prediction. *Child Abuse and Neglect, 24*, 965–982.

Worling, J. R., and Curwen, T. (2001). Estimate of Risk of Adolescent Sexual Offence Recidivism (Version 2.0: The "ERASOR"). In M. C. Calder, *Juveniles and Children who Sexually Abuse: Frameworks for Assessment*. Lyme Regis: Russell House, pp. 372–397.

Chapter 11

# Relapse prevention with juvenile sexual abusers

## A holistic and integrated approach

*John Hunter and Robert E. Longo*

Although a mainstay of most juvenile and adult sexual offender treatment programmes today, relapse prevention originated nearly two decades ago as a treatment for substance abuse (Brownell *et al.*, 1986; Marlatt and George, 1984). The model, as conceived by Marlatt and colleagues, reflected an attempt to explain the acquisition and reoccurrence of addictive behaviours. While Marlatt's original model has been criticised for its lack of theoretical consistency, it is generally based on the tenants of social learning theory and an understanding of the influence of attributions on motivational processes (Hudson and Ward, 1996).

The Marlatt relapse prevention model assumes that maladaptive addictive behaviour results from a chain or sequence of interactive biological, psychological and social factors. Central to the model is the belief that "relapse" (a return to previous levels of addiction) is preceded by a "lapse" wherein the addicted individual cognitively and behaviourally rehearses the maladaptive behaviour. The model places an emphasis on understanding the antecedent chain of events that lead to lapses and eventual relapses, so that cycle re-enactment can be anticipated and interrupted. Critical to successful prevention of relapse is the identification and avoidance (when possible) of dangerous, event precipitant circumstances (i.e. "high risk" factors) and the acquisition of effective coping skills for maintaining self-control. Since its inception, relapse prevention has been applied to a number of psychosocial problems that lend themselves to an addiction model. These include the treatment of not only sexual offenders, but also a range of other unrelated conditions including, for example, obsessive-compulsive disorder (Hiss *et al.*, 1994).

### Relapse prevention with sexual offenders

The relapse prevention model was applied to the treatment of adult sex offenders beginning in the early 1980s with the seminal work of Pithers and colleagues (Pithers *et al.*, 1983). Pithers argued that sexual offending, like alcohol and drug addiction, reflects purposeful and planned behaviour and follows a series of synergistic events. Pithers' early work reflected an emphasis on delineating the antecedents of offending behaviour, including the manner in which negative affect (e.g. anger) can trigger sexual fantasies, and the role of cognitive distortions in reducing inhibitions to offence planning. Adaptations were made in the original Marlatt model, including redefining a "lapse" as engagement in a voluntarily induced risk behaviour (e.g. fantasising about deviant sexual behaviour) and "relapse" as any new sexual offence, not just a return to a previous level of offending (Pithers, 1990; Ward and Hudson, 1996).

Relapse prevention as a treatment model for adult sexual offending was soon introduced in a number of institutional settings for the treatment of adult sex offenders across the United States of America and abroad, including the Sex Offender Treatment Evaluation Project in California (Marques, 1988), the Vermont Program (Pithers and Cumming, 1989), and New Zealand's Kia Marama Programme (Hudson *et al.*, 1995). By 1994, a survey of providers suggested that relapse prevention, or some version thereof, was being used in nearly 90 per cent of the sexual offender treatment programmes in North America (Freeman-Longo *et al.*, 1995).

Relapse prevention models have evolved since their initial application to the treatment of adult sex offenders. Early models were viewed as in need of refinement based on a number of considerations. In their in-depth and comprehensive critique of relapse prevention models to date, Ward and Hudson (1996) pointed out that both Marlatt's original model, and Pithers' adapted model, were flawed in several respects. Chief amongst their criticisms were that the models did not reflect a parsimonious and current understanding of social cognition theory and overemphasised skill deficits and covert processes as mediators of high-risk situations. Ward and Hudson further criticised Pithers for creating conceptual conflicts in moving the lapse and relapse points back in the offence chain (i.e. incompatibility of the "problem of immediate gratification" and "abstinence violation effect").

Subsequent to this early work, a number of refinements have been introduced in an attempt to strengthen the basic model and improve its range of applicability. Pithers and Gray (1996) suggested that compliance with relapse prevention plans is improved by victim empathy work, the use of "reminder cards", and ongoing community supervision by the courts. They also pointed out that use of relapse prevention with juveniles requires modifications in both the formatting and presentation of materials. Amongst their recommended adaptations were the use of games and simpler language with children with sexual behaviour problems, and the concurrent conducting of relapse prevention groups for children and their parents.

Hudson *et al.* (1999) argue that relapse prevention models must account for diversity in pathways leading to sexual re-offending. Their analyses suggest that three major pathways exist in identified sexual offenders: (1) an appetitive, positive pathway; (2) a negative affect pathway with covert planning and restraint planning; and (3) a pathway that reflects a negative restraining process but with explicit planning. Laws (1996) contends that relapse prevention should be confined to disorders of impulse control and is best viewed as an intervention designed to reduce the frequency and intensity of offending in chronically predisposed individuals (i.e."harm reduction") rather than eliminate it. Laws (1999) also suggests model improvements, including revisions in the cognitive-behavioural chain and recognition of "cognitive deconstructionism" (impaired self-awareness and cognitive processing brought on by a conscious desire to indulge in the behaviour).

### *Relapse prevention effectiveness*

Empirical support for the effectiveness of relapse prevention in the treatment of addictive disorders is still somewhat tenuous. Irvin *et al.* (1999) conducted a meta-analysis of the effectiveness of relapse prevention in the treatment of alcohol, smoking and other substance use. Twenty-two published, and four unpublished, outcome studies involving over 9,500 participants were examined. A small (r = .14) but reliable treatment effect for reducing substance use was produced. A much larger effect (r = .48) was demonstrated for the effectiveness of relapse prevention in improving psychosocial functioning. Examination of moderator variables suggested that the intervention is more effective in the treatment of alcohol and polysubstance abuse than smoking. On a cautionary note, effect sizes diminished with biochemically validated self-report, comparison to alternative active interventions, and length of follow-up.

Even less evidence exists for the effectiveness of relapse prevention in the treatment of sexual offenders. As noted by Laws, the "greatest weakness of the RP model is that it has escaped empirical evaluation" (Laws, 1999, p. 285). Hanson (1996) notes that empirical support for the effectiveness of relapse prevention in the treatment of sex offenders is modest at best and that perhaps its greatest contribution to the field has been in focusing therapist attention on issues that explain the long-term risk of recidivism. Certainly, considerably more research is needed before it can be ascertained how relapse prevention can be most effectively applied to the treatment of juvenile sex offenders.

## The treatment of juvenile sexual offenders

Although the number of programmes for youthful offenders grew rapidly during the first half of the last decade, juveniles have been the focus of sexual offender treatment for at least twenty years (Freeman-Longo *et al.*, 1995). While the field is not new, conceptualisation of what constitutes effective treatment for this population is still evolving. Historically, juvenile sexual offender treatment has been heavily influenced by a "trickle down" of clinical approaches used with adult sexual offenders. Often this has occurred with little regard for developmental and contextual issues that need to be taken into consideration in treating adolescents or evidence that the areas of therapeutic focus (e.g. deviant sexual arousal) are relevant for the juvenile sexual offender population (Freeman-Longo, in press; Hunter, 1999). Most often treatment techniques and modalities used in treating adult sexual offenders have been directly applied to juvenile sexual abusers, or modified only slightly to make materials more easily understood, without taking into consideration learning styles and multiple intelligences (Gardner, 1983). High levels of confrontation are still common in many programmes with little regard for the potential impact these approaches may have on youth with histories of abuse and neglect.

The majority of juvenile sexual offender treatment programmes have generally adhered to a traditional adult sex offender model. Standard interventions include the teaching of relapse prevention and the sexual abuse cycle, empathy training, anger management, social and interpersonal skills training, cognitive restructuring, assertiveness training, journaling, and sex education (Becker and Hunter, 1997; Burton *et al.*, 2000; Freeman-Longo *et al.*, 1995; Hunter, 1999). Questions about the appropriateness and effectiveness of these approaches in the treatment of juveniles makes imperative the full development and testing of juvenile-specific intervention programmes.

In the following sections we present an approach to the teaching of relapse prevention to juveniles. This approach reflects the blending of traditional aspects of relapse prevention into a holistic, humanistic and developmentally consistent model for working with youthful sex offenders. New research is reviewed as it relates to refinement of relapse prevention strategies based on juvenile sex offender typology distinctions. In the described model, relapse prevention is but one component of a comprehensive treatment programme. Other areas of therapeutic focus are described and attention is given to the sequencing of treatment interventions.

## Teaching relapse prevention to juveniles

The teaching of relapse prevention, and the cycle of sexual abuse, can be readily blended into a holistic juvenile sexual offender treatment model (Freeman-Longo, 2001). When properly taught, the model is relatively easy to understand and serves as an umbrella for integrating a variety of traditional sexual abuser treatment interventions, ranging from anger management and empathy development to social skills and cognitive restructuring (Freeman-Longo and Pithers, 1992). Relapse prevention can help youth examine their acting-out cycle more closely, including identifying "high risk factors", "cues" (warning signs), and "lapses" that signal sexual offending.

Steen was one of the first professionals working with adolescent sexual abusers to help simplify the academic language of relapse prevention so that it would be more readily comprehended by youth (Steen and Monnette,

1989). We have used Steen's language, combined with additional changes, so that the relapse prevention model is more easily understood by youth. Key constructs in our model are described below.

### *Cognitive distortions*

The relapse process (the process that leads to re-engagement in offending behaviour) is facilitated by cognitive distortions. When a client's thinking becomes distorted and unhealthy, he is more likely to engage in thoughts, feelings and behaviours or put himself in situations that perpetuate the sexual abuse cycle. The cycle may look as follows:

> unpleasant affect → deviant fantasy → passive planning → *cognitive distortion* → disinhibition → deviant act (relapse of reoffence)
>
> (Gray and Pithers, 1993)

Cognitive distortions are essentially a mechanism for defending offending behaviour. They may take the form of minimisation of the impact of the behaviour on the victim, blaming the victim for occurrence of the behaviour, or rationalisation of the behaviour. Examples include: "young children can make decisions about having sex"; "if a child stared at my penis as I showed it to him/her, it meant they liked looking at it"; "girls who wear short dresses and tight clothes are asking for it"; and "children don't remember things that happen to them when they are young" (Hunter *et al.*, 1991). When the juvenile is capable of identifying and correcting these cognitive distortions, he may be able to return to abstinence and avoid engaging in the problem behaviour.

### *Risk factors*

Risk factors are thoughts, feelings, behaviours and situations that can initiate and perpetuate the relapse process and the sexual abuse cycle. Gray and Pithers (1993) have suggested that there are three types of risk factors youthful sexual abusers experience: 1) *predisposing* risk factors, 2) *precipitating* risk factors, and 3) *perpetuating* risk factors. "Predisposing" risk factors develop during a person's formative years and may include a history of various types of abuse, low self-esteem and poor social skills. "Precipitating" risk factors are those that an individual is most likely to experience as he gets closer to actually offending. They include emotional mismanagement, cognitive distortions and deviant sexual fantasies. "Perpetuating" risk factors are those ongoing risk factors that youth are likely to experience on a day-to-day basis and include anger, lack of supervision by caregivers, poor peer relations and family problems.

We have found that youthful clients are often confused and overwhelmed in

*Table 11.1* Risk factors common to juvenile sexual offenders

| *Predisposing* | *Precipitating* | *Perpetuating* |
|---|---|---|
| • Alcoholism in the family<br>• Physical abuse<br>• Sexual abuse<br>• Emotional abuse<br>• Substance abuse in the family<br>• Exposure to violent death of human or animal<br>• Neglect<br>• Family chaos<br>• Educational deficits<br>• Unhealthy thinking<br>• Learning deficit<br>• Family dysfunction<br>• Parental marital discord<br>• Maternal absence/neglect<br>• Parental divorce | • Gives up easily<br>• Feelings of inferiority<br>• Irresponsible<br>• Lack of confidence<br>• Intra/interpersonal problems<br>• Depression<br>• Anger<br>• Abusive fantasies<br>• Boredom<br>• Cognitive distortions ("thinking errors")<br>• Isolation/(withdrawal from others)<br>• Low self-esteem<br>• Peer pressure<br>• Depression<br>• Lack of empathy | • Emotional problems<br>• Stuffed feelings/emotions<br>• Over-controlled emotions<br>• Social skills deficit<br>• Feelings of inadequacy<br>• Rejection<br>• Drug/alcohol abuse<br>• Denial of problems<br>• Low self-esteem<br>• Living in a high risk neighbourhood |

learning about risk factors. Simplifying language and giving them a list of examples of risk factors can be helpful (Freeman-Longo, 2001). Table 11.1 describes risk factors common to juvenile sexual offenders.

### *Cues*

One of the most useful components of relapse prevention is teaching clients to identify cues that can warn them they are getting into trouble or experiencing problems. There are many kinds of cues, including: (1) emotional cues; (2) cognitive cues; (3) interpersonal cues; (4) self-statements; (5) physical cues; and (6) behavioural cues. Cues may also be risk factors. For example, feeling rejected can be a cue that one may soon begin to feel angry. Feelings of rejection can also be a risk factor separate from anger (e.g. lead to withdrawal and isolation). Table 11.2 lists examples of cues under each of the categories listed above.

### *Coping responses and maladaptive coping responses*

The relapse prevention model teaches that when youth first experience risk factors they should immediately use a coping response to counter it (e.g. if a young person begins to feel angry then he is to take deep breaths, count to ten, and use healthy thoughts to counter identified cognitive distortions associated with anger). However, clinical experience suggests that many youth

*Table 11.2* Cues for identifying risk factors

| *Emotional cues* | *Self-statements* | *Cognitive cues* |
|---|---|---|
| • Feeling all alone<br>• Worrying<br>• Fear of expressing feelings<br>• Feeling angry<br>• Feeling jealous<br>• Feeling depressed<br>• Faking happiness<br>• Stuffing feelings | • "Nothing is going right"<br>• "I should have done . . ."<br>• "I can't . . ."<br>• "There I go again . . ."<br>• "I always (or never) . . ."<br>• "No one cares about me" | • Dwelling on the past<br>• Suicidal thoughts<br>• Thinking about drugs<br>• Comparing myself to people to whom I feel inferior |
| *Physical cues* | *Interpersonal cues* | *Behavioural cues* |
| • Queasy stomach<br>• Sleeping excessively<br>• Feeling no energy<br>• Poor hygiene<br>• Not sleeping well<br>• Disregard for personal appearance<br>• Physically hurting myself | • Needing to win<br>• Getting others to feel sorry for me<br>• Bragging<br>• Making up stories<br>• Judging other people | • Staying by myself<br>• Nervous energy<br>• Skipping school<br>• Taking off work<br>• Horse play<br>• Risky behaviours (i.e. reckless driving)<br>• Being passive<br>• Putting things off<br>• Isolation |

will use "maladaptive coping responses". These are coping responses that may, in fact, be risk factors or create more problems for the client (e.g. drinking alcohol or using drugs to allay anger). Youth must be taught to recognise maladaptive coping responses and replace them with healthy ones. Healthy coping skills include relaxation exercises and positive imagery for anxiety, assertive behaviour for anger management and covert sensitisation exercises for impulse control.

### *"Giving-up" (abstinence violation effect)*

Giving up on changes that may prevent further sexual offending is referred to as the "abstinence violation effect" in the earlier literature (Pithers *et al.*, 1983). According to traditional relapse prevention models, giving up occurs after a client experiences a lapse (a more serious risk factor) and includes the following components: (1) self-deprecation; (2) an expectation of failure; (3) a need for immediate gratification; (4) erroneous attributions; and (5) an increased probability of relapse. Our clinical experience has been that the relapse process is more fluid than described in the earlier literature and that youth can experience "giving up" both before and after experiencing one or more lapses. As youths progress toward having a "lapse" (more serious risk factors), they often describe the feelings and desires of "giving up" before they actually engage in the lapse behaviour. This can be characterised as their giving up on using coping responses and interventions, and feelings of helplessness. It is at the time they are about to engage in the lapse behaviour that they begin to focus on the immediate gratification of engaging in the behaviour (e.g. the associated sexual arousal that comes with using pornography).

### *Lapses and high risk factors*

"Lapses" are more serious risk factors that threaten the client's ability to remain offence free. They usually occur further down a chain of events that may lead the client to sexual offending. Lapses increase the likelihood that the youth will offend. They include deviant sexual and violent fantasising, purchasing pornography, substance abuse and spending time alone with young children. Although lapses are temporally close to offending behaviour, youth must be taught that offending is not inevitable if a lapse occurs. To help prevent youth from seeing themselves as failures and giving up, we encourage them to think of lapses as mistakes that can be corrected through the use of well-practised coping skills.

### *The sexual abuse cycle*

In most relapse prevention programmes for juvenile and adult sexual offenders, the relapse process is taught in conjunction with an explanation of the sexual abuse cycle. The basic concept is that sexually abusive behaviour reflects a chain of thoughts, feelings and events that can become cyclical and habitual over time. Specifically, cycles may become stronger and more ingrained with repetition through an operant conditioning process. While traditional relapse prevention models for sexual offenders suggest that abuse cycles, and the relapse process, begin with negative affect, we have found it more useful to teach youth that these cycles can be triggered by the occurrence of any of their individual components.

We suggest that youth are taught that risk factors can be thoughts, feelings, behaviours and situations that threaten their sense of self-control. Cognitive distortions or unhealthy thinking can contribute to mismanaged emotions and behavioural problems and give justification to the anger that leads to sexual aggression. Anger, insecurity, rejection and feelings of low self-esteem and boredom are common in juvenile sexual offenders. Youthful sexual abusers are generally unskilled at recognising their own emotions and may also have difficulty recognising and understanding the feelings of others. They tend to think of feelings as "right or wrong" and subsequently seek to hide feelings they believe will lead to social ridicule or to being negatively judged by peers. Relapse prevention is a cognitive-behavioural model that emphasises the need for behavioural change. Behavioural management is essential to client success in treatment. Some of the core areas for behavioural change include: anger management, arousal control, social skills development, development and use of interventions and coping responses, assertiveness training and interpersonal skills development. Youths must be taught that behaviour is contextual and that their thoughts and feelings give direction to their behaviour. When teaching youths to identify problematic behaviours and behavioural risk factors, they must be encouraged to identify cues that are observable so that others can identify when they are experiencing problems and challenge them to change when coping responses and interventions are not forthcoming. Examples of observable behaviours that are risk factors and may also serve as cues for risk factors include: looking depressed; not talking to others; avoiding eye contact; distorting information; pacing the floor, chewing fingernails; becoming secretive; isolating and avoiding others; becoming sarcastic and argumentative; intimidating others; and, increasing use of profanity. In the language of relapse prevention, situations or triggers are events that stimulate sexual thoughts, feelings and/or behaviours. For example, if the juvenile offender sees a group of children playing at a playground, he may begin to fantasise about engaging one of the children and having sex with him/her. Or, if a youth has an argument with his parents or teacher, he may become angry and smoke marijuana after school. This, in turn, may impair judgement and impulse control and give rise to the expression of maladaptive sexual urges. Thus, situations are external events that can set off or "trigger" the youth's relapse process or sexual abuse cycle.

### *The four phases of the sexual abuse cycle*

Freeman-Longo (2001) has identified four sequential phases of the sexual abuse cycle: (1) the "pretends-to-be-normal" phase; (2) the "build-up" phase; (3) the "abuse or acting-out" phase; and (4) the "justification" phase (see Figure 11.1). One phase follows the other until the cycle is complete. Sometimes youths will experience "sub-cycles" that go back-and-forth between the "pretends-to-be-normal" phase and the "build-up" phase. If the sub-cycles are not interrupted, the youth will eventually progress through the entire cycle and sexually offend.

#### *The pretends-to-be-normal phase*

In the sexual abuse cycle, there are various problem areas that serve as early warning signals that the youth is at risk of re-enacting his cycle and relapsing. These warning signs indicate there is something wrong with how the youth is thinking, feeling or acting in response to life problems and situations. These often occur in the absence of any acknowledgement by the youth that trouble is looming, and he may, in fact, pretend everything is normal. In order for the youth to prevent re-enacting his cycle, he must identify the problem area

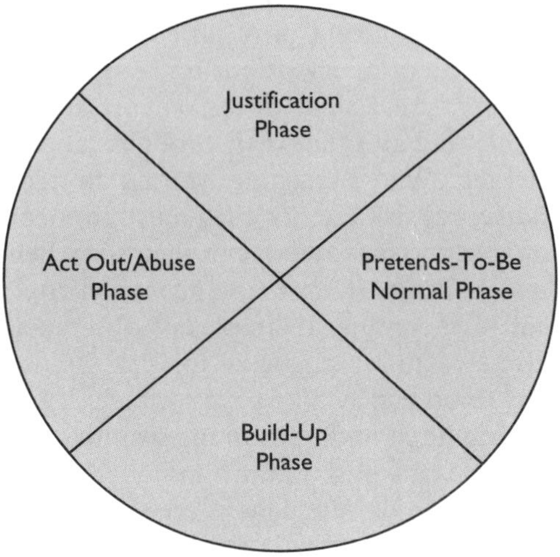


*Figure 11.1* The four phases of a sexual abuse cycle.

(or areas) being experienced and take positive steps to attenuate the risk. Problems in one or more of the following areas can serve as triggers to the "build-up" phase and sexual acting out: self-esteem; anger; family; peers, friends; social; school; employment; financial; drugs and alcohol; leisure time activities; marital/dating; health and physical appearance.

### *The build-up phase*

When problems are not addressed in the "pretends-to-be-normal" phase it leads to a "building-up" of the potential for relapsing. The build-up phase consists of several behavioural chains that are risk factors for sexual acting-out. These thoughts, feelings and behaviours usually build one upon another until the client enters into the pre-assault phase. When a youth enters the build-up phase it is important for him to understand his risk factors and to intervene as soon as he recognises the potential for lapsing.

Uninterrupted, lapsing follows the initial building-up of risk factors. Lapsing represents thoughts, feelings, behaviours and situations that place the youth at high risk for sexual re-offending. For example, the youth may place himself in a position of being alone with young children. In this situation, he may begin to "groom" the victim (i.e. "prepare" him) to be sexually abused. Maladaptive cognitions may be entertained that amplify the potential for acting-out, including the belief that it is hopeless to try to control the sexual urges or projection of blame for the potential behaviour onto others. At this point, the youth may feel justified in sexual acting-out.

### *The acting-out phase*

The "acting-out" phase represents engagement in the sexually abusive behaviour. It can serve several functions: (1) a temporary discharge of pent-up emotion, such as anger; (2) a means of gaining control and a sense of power over distressing environmental circumstances; and (3) a means by which to relieve tension and obtain sexual gratification.

### *The justification phase*

Once the youth has sexually re-offended, he may experience shame, guilt, fear and despair. A number of defence mechanisms may come into play, including minimisation and projection of blame. As the youth attempts to justify his acting-out behaviour, he may begin to feel sorry for himself and engage in a downward spiral of self-pity and self-absorption. During this phase, a number of youth have been observed to make short-lived promises to not offend again or attempt to convince themselves that their problem will simply go away with time. These maladaptive cognitions may only lead to re-entering the "pretends-to-be-normal" phase and, thus, cycle re-enactment.

## *Integrating models and modalities of treatment with adolescents*

We endorse the concept that treatment programmes for juveniles should be holistic and attentive to the overall developmental needs of the youth. This includes attention to their healthy psychosocial development and their familial, physical health and spiritual needs (Freeman-Longo, in press). Viewed in this context relapse prevention represents an important component of a comprehensive treatment programme for juvenile sex offenders, rather than the programme in its entirety. Because the relapse model has the potential for serving as a framework for integrating various aspects of sexual offender treatment, it is usually taught in the latter phases of the programme.

The formal teaching of the relapse model, and the formulation of a relapse prevention plan, is typically preceded by more fundamental work. This includes helping youth understand the importance of treatment and making a commitment to positive life changes. Attempts are made to infuse youth with a sense of optimism and confidence that they possess the capacity to make positive life changes if they remain fully motivated and are therapeutically diligent. Healthy masculinity is taught, including a respect for diversity and a commitment to the cessation of violence and the oppression of others on the basis of race, gender and sexual orientation. This work takes place in conjunction with examining the personal, interpersonal, familial and legal consequences of continued sexual and non-sexual offending.

We believe that juvenile sexual offender programmes must place a strong emphasis on building positive self-esteem and developing social competencies, not just identifying and correcting aberrant patterns of behaviour. While therapeutic attention is given to identifying and correcting distorted thought patterns that may support the continuance of offending behaviour, and helping youth explore cognitive-behavioural antecedents for their sexual acting-out, the acquisition of prerequisite skills for forming and maintaining healthy interpersonal relationships is equally stressed. This includes teaching basic and advanced social skills, healthy sexuality and anger management. It also involves teaching methods for improving impulse control and judgement and empathy training.

The relapse prevention model can be easily taught when preceded by therapeutic attention to the above. Following this work, youth have a fundamental understanding of the importance of behavioural control and a heightened motivation for change. They possess a basic understanding of the triggers of sexual re-offending and what for them constitutes high-risk factors. They also possess the necessary skills to interrupt maladaptive behaviour and maintain behavioural control. Most importantly, they have the underlying value system and prerequisite skills necessary to form healthy interpersonal relationships. For youth, this is critical as treatment adherence affords them more than an opportunity to contain "deviancy" – it represents a pathway to building a healthier and more fulfilling and rewarding life.

To be maximally effective, the youth's relapse prevention plan should be comprehensive and not only reflect an understanding of his sexual abuse cycle, but what the youth, his family and other important caretakers or mentors must do to help him achieve his positive life goals. It is best viewed as a collaborative endeavour representing the input of the youth, the treatment staff, the family and the referral and oversight agencies. For adjudicated youth, the latter should certainly include the probation/parole officer. The probation/parole officer can incorporate the terms of the relapse prevention plan into the terms of probation or parole and help ensure that all relevant parties are providing the youth with the support he needs to maintain his therapeutic gains.

## New typology research

Clinical observation and research suggest that juvenile sexual offenders are a heterogeneous population representing a variety of developmental pathways leading to offending behaviour and various patterns of offending. Some youth appear to be at high risk for re-offending and in need of institutionalisation, while many others appear to be at lower risk and highly amenable to community-based interventions. As such, it does not appear to be clinically, legally or fiscally prudent to formulate a "one size fits all" approach to their management. In an attempt to support an objective means by which to classify youth, and thus permit the development of more refined programming,

Hunter and colleagues have embarked upon research to develop a juvenile sexual offender typology. This research is reviewed here for its general relevance to the treatment of juvenile sexual offenders, and to relapse prevention planning in particular.

In a preliminary study, Hunter *et al.* (2000) analysed the criminal records of 126 juvenile sexual offenders in an attempt to compare the *modus operandi* of youths who sexually targeted peers or adults, to those who offended against children five or more years younger than themselves. Similar to the findings of Richardson *et al.* (1997), youths who offended against peers or adults were found to be more likely than those who targeted younger children, to commit a non-sexual crime in conjunction with their sexual offence and to demonstrate higher levels of aggression and violence in the course of their sexual offending. Peer/adult offenders were also found to be more likely to target females, and strangers or acquaintances.

In a follow-up study, Hunter *et al.* (2003) analysed survey data and archival clinical records on 200 residentially placed adolescent male sexual offenders. This was done to assess an explanatory model that linked aetiological influences, personality traits and offence characteristics. Factors were selected for study under each of these three major categories of interest based on both theoretical considerations and previous research findings. Aetiological influences that were examined included exposure to violence against women and male modelled antisocial behaviour, as well as childhood abuse experiences (physical and sexual). Personality constructs that were examined included: hostile masculinity (Malamuth, 1996, 1998; Malamuth and Malamuth, 1999), egotistical/antagonistic masculinity (Rowe *et al.*, 1997), general delinquency (Becker and Hunter, 1997; Figueredo *et al.*, 2000), and psychosocial deficits (Figueredo *et al.*, 2000; Hunter and Figueredo, 2000). The latter factor included measures of self-efficacy, anxiety and depression, social problems, and self-esteem. Three offence variables were also examined: (1) whether the offences were against same-age peers or adults; (2) the degree to which the offences were physically dangerous, involving escalated levels of aggression, use of weapons, and associated nonsexual offences; and (3) the degree to which the offences were perpetrated against victims who were strangers.

Structural equation modelling was used to assess the "goodness of fit" of the model in explaining the relationship between these variables. The obtained results suggested that the final model met all standard psychometric criteria for adequately explaining the theorised relationships (for details see Hunter *et al.*, 2003). Key findings are summarised as follows. Developmental exposure to violence toward women was found to predict deficits in psychosocial functioning in juvenile sex offenders. Exposure to male-modelled anti-social behaviour (e.g. drug and alcohol abuse, stealing) was found to be associated with more pronounced non-sexual delinquent attitudes and behaviour, and egotism/antagonism personality traits. A history of child abuse predicted deficits in psychosocial functioning and choosing a younger, prepubescent female victim. Juvenile offenders against pubescent females were found to be more violent in the commission of their sexual crimes, more likely to use a weapon, more likely to commit a non-sexual offence in conjunction with the sexual assault, and less likely to be related to the victim.

The above research is continuing under sponsorship from the Office of Juvenile Justice and Delinquency Prevention. It is planned to collect new survey, archival, and prospective (treatment outcome) data on an additional 325 juvenile male sexual offenders from both community-based and residential treatment programmes. The scope of explanatory constructs is being expanded to include psychopathy, sexual deviance, familial environment and peer affiliation. Measurement of the psychosocial deficits factors is being broadened to include reports of social competency deficits by third parties (e.g. therapist observations).

### *Clinical implications*

While additional research is needed before definite conclusions can be drawn, the research to date supports the contention that juvenile sexual offenders are indeed a heterogeneous clinical population. These youth may not only differ in the types of offences they commit, but also both in the early developmental experiences that have helped shape their offending behaviour and in their motivations for offending. Offenders against younger children appear to be more driven by deficits in social competency and self-esteem than is true for those who target peers and adults. The youth who offend against younger children show evidence of suffering from anxiety and depression, social ineptitude and loneliness. As such, their sexual offending may be more compensatory than reflective of underlying paraphilic interests. Younger children may be victimised more on the basis of frustration and availability rather than as a result of deviant sexual arousal. This hypothesis is bolstered by other research on juvenile sexual offenders showing that phallometric indices of deviant sexual interest in juveniles are less directly related to offence patterns than is the case for adult sex offenders. This suggests greater fluidity in the sexual interests of juveniles (Hunter and Becker, 1994).

Juveniles who target peers and adults demonstrate different offending patterns from those who target younger victims, and they also appear to have different motives for their behaviour. In general, these youth appear more criminal, violent and predatory. Violent behaviour may not only stem from the demands of the sexual assault (i.e. adults are more likely to resist than children), but also from personality traits. Hunter *et al.* (2000) found that the aggression of peer/adult offenders was often gratuitous in nature. The injuries sustained by their victims appeared in many cases to be in excess of what was required to gain control over the victim. They also appeared more likely than offenders against children to react to victim resistance with escalated aggression. It is hypothesised that upon further study these youth will show evidence of greater levels of psychopathy and a higher level of delinquent peer affiliation. Some support for the latter was found in Hunter *et al.* (2000) in that these youth were more likely than offenders against children to commit the sexual offence along with a co-offender.

While the above research is still in a preliminary phase, it suggests there may be significant differences in the sexual assault cycles of juveniles who target children and those who target peers and adults. In particular, the offending of the former may be more directly related to perceived and actual social rejection and frustrations. Highly relevant to the teaching of relapse prevention to these youth would be the identification of perceived negative self-attributions and the manner in which these cognitions give rise to feelings of depression, anxiety and hopelessness. These youth may also benefit from examining underlying cognitive distortions that exaggerate the magnitude of personal shortcomings or reduce their ability to attenuate skill deficits. Furthermore, therapeutic attention helping them to understand the reciprocal nature of cognitions and affect and the mutual, synergistic influence of both on behaviour would be of particular relevance. With some of this group this may include explaining avoidance conditioning paradigms and the role of anxiety in triggering dangerous lapses, such as spending time alone with children or deviant sexual fantasising. With this group of juveniles, a major thrust of relapse prevention programming will be the teaching of positive coping and social relationship skills.

Peer/adult offenders, on the other hand, appear more influenced by delinquent attitudes and values and negative peer-group affiliations. These youth may not suffer from low self-esteem and social anxiety. Instead, cognitive distortions may centre on beliefs that they are too clever to get caught, or that legal consequences if incurred would be minimal and easily endured. With this group of juvenile sexual offenders, cognitive distortions regarding women and the nature of male–female relationships are likely to be present. These youth may be much more likely to misinterpret social cues regarding women's attraction to sexually aggressive males or feel justified in engaging in sexual aggression based on negative sexual stereotypes. For peer/adult offenders relapse prevention strategies would include the confrontation and correction of distorted cognitions and beliefs, the teaching of healthy masculinity and pro-social values, and careful analysis of environmental factors that contribute to the maintenance of delinquent and sexually aggressive behaviour. The latter should include altering negative peer affiliations, building-in positive socialisation experiences and strengthening the external monitoring of the youth in the community. This may include enhanced parental monitoring, intensified probation and parole supervision, periodic polygraph assessment and, in more extreme cases, use of electronic monitoring devices.

## Conclusions

We believe that the teaching of relapse prevention to juvenile sexual offenders is a valuable endeavour. However, its fruitful employment depends on model and language adaptations, broadened clinical programming and an understanding of juvenile sexual offender sub-types. As reviewed, relapse prevention originates from an addictions model. Its application to sexual offending implies the belief that sexual acting-out is habitual and self-perpetuating. This premise, as applied to most juveniles, is questionable. At present, there is no solid scientific evidence that the majority of juvenile sexual offenders are destined to continue offending into their adult years or that deviant sexual arousal plays a prominent role in the offending of most of these youth. At issue is the wisdom of instilling in juvenile sexual offenders (and their families and the criminal justice system) the belief that their problem is chronic and can at best be managed, but not "cured". This potentially contributes to "self-fulfilling prophecy" and clinical programming and criminal justice policy that excludes youth from normalising socialisation experiences.

We suggest that youth be taught to understand patterns of sexual offending, including risk and protective factors, while still infusing them with a sense of hopefulness and optimism about their ability to lead healthy and productive lives. The success of the latter depends on programmes placing at least equal emphasis on accentuating and strengthening pro-social skills, competencies and values in these youth, as on teaching them to recognise and manage maladaptive cognitions, impulses and urges. It is also likely to require shifting the focus of interventions from the individual to systemic issues in the broader social environment that contributes to the maintenance of delinquent and aggressive behaviour (Huey *et al.*, 2000). Our hope is that needed refinements will be made in juvenile sexual offender treatment models and that competing models will be objectively evaluated through clinical trials. It will not be until then that the field will have a true understanding of what constitutes the most effective approach to the treatment of various types of juvenile sexual offenders.

## References


Becker, J. V., and Hunter, J. A. (1997). Understanding and treating child and adolescent sexual offenders. *Advances in Clinical Child Psychology, 19*, 177–197.

Brownell, K. D., Marlatt, G. A., Lichtenstein, E., and Wilson, G. T. (1986). Understanding and preventing relapse. *American Psychologist, 41(7)*, 765–782.

Burton, D., Smith-Darden, J., Levins, J., Fiske, J., and Freeman-Longo, R. E. (2000). *1996 Nationwide Survey of Treatment Programs and Models: Serving Abuse Reactive Children and Adolescent and Adult Sexual Offenders*. Brandon, VT: Safer Society Press.

Figueredo, A. J., Sales, B. D., Russell, K. P., Becker, J. V., and Kaplan, M. (2000). A

Brunswikian evolutionary-developmental theory of adolescent sex offending. *Behavioral Sciences and the Law, 18(2–3)*, 309–329.

Freeman-Longo, R. E. (2001). *Paths to Wellness*. Holyoke, MA: NEARI Press.

Freeman-Longo, R. E. (in Press). *A Holistic Approach to Treating Juvenile Sexual Abusers*.

Freeman-Longo, R. E., and Pithers, W. D. (1992). *A Structured Approach to Preventing Relapse: A Guide for Sex Offenders*. Brandon, VT: Safer Society Press.

Freeman-Longo, R. E., Bird, S., Stevenson, W. F., and Fiske, J. A. (1995). *1994 Nationwide Survey of Treatment Programs and Models: Serving Abuse Reactive Children and Adolescent and Adult Sexual Offenders*. Brandon, VT: Safer Society Press.

Gardner, H. (1983). *Frames of Mind: The Theory of Multiple Intelligences*. New York: Basic Books.

Gray, A. S., and Pithers, W. D. (1993). Relapse prevention with sexually aggressive adolescents and children: Expanding treatment and supervision. In H. E. Barbaree, W. L. Marshall and S. M. Hudson (eds), *The Juvenile Sex Offender*. New York: Guilford Press.

Hanson, R. K. (1996). Evaluating the contribution of relapse prevention theory to the treatment of sexual offenders. *Sexual Abuse: Journal of Research and Treatment, 8(3)*, 201–208.

Hiss, H., Foa, E. B., and Kozak, M. J. (1994). Relapse prevention program for treatment of obsessive-compulsive disorder. *Journal of Consulting and Clinical Psychology, 62(4)*, 801–808.

Hudson, S. M., and Ward, T. (1996). Relapse prevention: Future directions. *Sexual Abuse: Journal of Research and Treatment, 8(3)*, 249–256.

Hudson, S. M., Marshall, W. L., Ward, T., Johnston, P. W., and Jones, R. (1995). Kia Marama: A cognitive-behavioural program for incarcerated child molesters. *Behaviour Change, 12(2)*, 69–80.

Hudson, S. M., Ward, T., and McCormack, J. C. (1999). Offense pathways in sexual offenders. *Journal of Interpersonal Violence, 14(8)*, 779–798.

Huey, S. J., Jr, Henggeler, S. W., Brondino, M. J., and Pickrel, S. G. (2000). Mechanisms of change in multisystemic therapy: Reducing delinquent behavior through therapist adherence and improved family and peer functioning. *Journal of Consulting and Clinical Psychology, 68(3)*, 451–467.

Hunter, J. A. (1999). Adolescent sex offenders. In V. B. Van Hasselt and M. Hersen (eds), *Handbook of Psychological Approaches with Violent Offenders*. New York: Plenum.

Hunter, J. A. and Becker, J. V. (1994). The role of deviant sexual arousal in juvenile sexual offending: Etiology, evaluation, and treatment. *Criminal Justice and Behavior, 21(1)*, 132–149.

Hunter, J. A., and Figueredo, A. J. (2000). The influence of personality and history of sexual victimization in the prediction of offense characteristics of juvenile sex offenders. *Behavior Modification, 24(2)*, 241–263.

Hunter, J. A., Becker, J. V., Kaplan, M., and Goodwin, D. W. (1991). Reliability and discriminative utility of the Adolescent Cognitions Scale for juvenile sexual offenders. *Annals of Sex Research, 4(3–4)*, 281–286.

Hunter, J. A., Hazelwood, R. R., and Slesinger, D. (2000). Juvenile-perpetrated sex crimes: Patterns of offending and predictors of violence. *Journal of Family Violence, 15(1)*, 81–93.

Hunter, J. A., Figueredo, A. J., Malamuth, N. M., and Becker (2003). Juvenile sexual offenders: towards the development of a typology. *Sexual Abuse: A Journal of Research and Therapy, 15(1)*, 27–48.

Irvin, J. E., Bowers, C. A., Dunn, M. E., and Wang, M. C. (1999). Efficacy of relapse prevention: A meta-analytic review. *Journal of Consulting and Clinical Psychology, 67(4)*, 563–570.

Laws, D. R. (1996). Relapse prevention or harm reduction? *Sexual Abuse: Journal of Research and Treatment, 8(3)*, 243–247.

Laws, D. R. (1999). Relapse prevention: The state of the art. *Journal of Interpersonal Violence, 14(3)*, 285–302.

Malamuth, N. M. (1996). Sexually explicit media, gender differences, and evolutionary theory. *Journal of Communication, 46(3)*, 8–31.

Malamuth, N. M. (1998). An evolutionary-based model integrating research on the characteristics of sexually coercive men. In J. G. Adair and D. Belanger *et al.* (eds), *Advances in Psychological Science, Vol. 1: Social, Personal and Cultural Aspects.* Hove: Taylor & Francis.

Malamuth, N. M., and Malamuth, E. Z. (1999). Integrating multiple levels of scientific analysis and the confluence model of sexual coercers. *Jurimetrics, 39*, 157–179.

Marlatt, G. A., and George, W. H. (1984). Relapse prevention: Introduction and overview of the model. *British Journal of Addiction, 79(3)*, 261–273.

Marques, J. K. (1988). The sex offender treatment and evaluation project: California's new outcome study. *Annals of the New York Academy of Sciences, 52(8)*, 235–243.

Pithers, W. D. (1990). Relapse prevention with sexual aggressors: A method for maintaining therapeutic gain and enhancing external supervision. In W. L. Marshall and D. R. Laws (eds), *Handbook of Sexual Assault: Issues, Theories, and Treatment of the Offender*. New York: Plenum.

Pithers, W. D., and Cumming, G. F. (1989). Can relapses be prevented? Initial outcome data from the Vermont treatment program for sexual aggressors. In D. R. Laws (ed.), *Relapse Prevention with Sex Offenders*. New York: Guilford Press.

Pithers, W. D., and Gray, A. S. (1996). Utility of relapse prevention in treatment of sexual abusers. *Sexual Abuse: Journal of Research and Treatment, 8(3)*, 223–230.

Pithers, W. D., Marques, J. K., Gibat, C. C., and Marlatt, G. A. (1983). Relapse prevention with sexual aggressiveness: A self-control model of treatment and maintenance of change. In J. G. Greer and I. R. Stuart (eds), *The Sexual Aggressor: Current Perspectives on Treatment*. New York: Van Nostrand Reinhold.

Richardson, G., Kelly, T. P., and Graham, F. (1997). Group differences in abuser and abuse characteristics in a British sample of sexually abusive adolescents. *Sexual Abuse: Journal of Research and Treatment, 9(3)*, 239–257.

Rowe, D. C., Vazsonyi, A. T., and Figueredo, A. J. (1997). Mating effort in adolescence: Conditional or alternative strategy? *Journal of Personality and Individual Differences, 23(1)*, 105–115.

Steen, C., and Monnette, B. (1989). *Treating Adolescent Sex Offenders in the Community*. Springfield, IL: Charles C. Thomas.

Ward, T., and Hudson, S. M. (1996). Relapse prevention: A critical analysis. *Sexual Abuse: Journal of Research and Treatment, 8(3)*, 177–200.

Chapter 12

# Family intervention with young people with sexually abusive behaviour

*Jerry Thomas*

## Introduction

Whether traditional, non-traditional or even composed in part by institutions and their staff, it would be hard to overestimate the importance of family, or its absence, in the lives of young people. In all the years that I have worked with youth and their families, I have never heard anyone say that they did not want a family. Almost without exception their families were very important to them, even when they were severely dysfunctional. The children, regardless of whether they were the abused, non-abused or abusive siblings, wanted to be with their family, or any family, just without the abuse or neglect. In fact, often it is the abused sibling who most mourns the loss of the abusive sibling. And, regardless of what they may have done, most parents want all their children with them.

Family focused treatment recognises that the family is one of the most important influences on the shaping of any child's beliefs and behaviours. Therefore, whether overtly or covertly, knowingly or unwittingly, it is very possible that the family has in some way contributed to the shaping or supporting of sexually abusive behaviours. If this is true, then the family can learn to identify, interrupt and replace those patterns of behaviour with patterns of behaviour that support non-offending behaviour. Family focused treatment is also important because of the strong support system required by abuse specific treatment, particularly in the relapse prevention model. For youth the most influential and practical support system is the family. Further, the participation and support of family members contributes significantly towards many youth's own degree of involvement in treatment, achievement of treatment goals, and maintenance of a non-offending lifestyle.

Another community protection concern served by family focused treatment is the likelihood that these youth will establish families of their own some day. It is not at all unusual for the parents of sexually abusive youth to come from abusive backgrounds and to have recreated the dynamics of abuse in their own family environment. If there is no interruption of abusive dynamics, then the cycle of abuse is likely to continue generation by generation. In addition to the treatment and relapse prevention benefits, a family focused abuse specific approach also serves the community by interrupting the intergenerational transmission of abusive family culture.

Finally, in addition to the direct benefits to offender treatment, relapse prevention, healthy support systems and community protection, there are also benefits to the programme itself. As a result of the emphasis upon a comprehensive, collaborative approach which stresses teamwork and communication, a family focused offence specific approach improves programme efficiency and safety. To a certain extent, the reason why improved teamwork, effectiveness and communication make a programme more efficient (cost-effective) and safer are self-evident. For a fuller treatment of these and the other benefits of a family based abuse specific approach, please see Thomas (1991).

As a last note, it is equally important to keep a family perspective when the existing family is rejecting or otherwise unavailable to the youth in treatment. The attachment problems which result from these circumstances not only prevent healthy development, but are also a major deterrent to treatment success. Keeping a family perspective means that you will seek to reverse this damage by focusing treatment on attachment issues, and any other problems that have resulted from the absence or alienation of family in a youth's life. Logically, the devastating effects that the absence of family have upon a youth's life, health and development must be repaired as part and parcel of treatment, just as treatment must address and repair any abuse or dysfunction in participating families. Youth with little or no family experience are likely to have even less realistic understanding of what a family or being part of a family means than youth from dysfunctional families. Without this understanding, they will go through life lost, abandoned and unattached.

The following chapter will outline the information that treatment providers need in order to develop a family focus for any contingency or circumstance, which serves both youths whose families are present and available, and those whose families are absent or nonexistent. In all cases, the ultimate goal of all family focused treatment is the prevention of abusive behaviour, the healing of the wounds that it has already caused and the development of a healthy family lifestyle.

## Who is family in the twenty-first century?

If we are to provide an effective approach to family treatment then we must be ready to give up our traditional views of family. In fact, we must be ready to accept definitions of family which are not only non-traditional, but which challenge our preconceptions of what family means. The definition of family used here is both simpler and more complex than the traditional one. Simple in that it describes family as the group that takes care of you, is there for you through thick and thin, which helps mould your beliefs and values, provides for your physical, emotional and spiritual development, and which loves you unconditionally. Complex, in that it views family as a collection of interpersonal relationships and resources which may be as unique as the circumstances of each individual child.

An inclusive definition of family can involve not only biological and adoptive parents, but foster and group home parents, caseworkers, older siblings, grandparents, neighbours, big brothers or sisters, teachers, and/or any caregiver which has been a constant in the child's life. It may include the sort of non-relatives children commonly call "aunt" or "uncle" in the American South, who can be anyone from a parent's best friend, to your fourth cousin twice removed. It may even include treatment or agency staff. However, the most important consideration when defining family is to identify the people who have been the greatest constants and supports in any particular child's life. The defining quality of family for any of us is the characteristic of the interactions over time. From this perspective a functional family is not a group of parents and offspring, but a social system which collectively provides for the emotional, physical and mental needs of a specific child.

## Defining abuse specific family treatment

There is not a great deal of professional literature or formal research on the use of a family focused approach with sexually aggressive youth. There is, however, a large body of research confirming that the family is critical in the development of beliefs and behaviour, and that family involvement is an important factor in the treatment success for other populations of youth. There is also a great deal of shared clinical experience that corroborates the efficacy of involving family in the treatment of sexually abusive youth.

It was not until very recently that our understanding of the treatment needs of sexually abusive youth changed from an adult model to one that was developmentally and contextually appropriate for a population under twenty-one. When we began to see this population as young people with specific characteristics and needs, we then began to appreciate the role of family as part of the treatment process.

Just as we must be non-traditional in our concept of family, we must also be non-traditional in the kind of family intervention that we provide. In order for the approach to be abuse specific there has to be a melding of three very different approaches to family work – those of mental health, juvenile justice and social work. This means that clients are sometimes involuntary, confidentiality is limited, treatment is often mandated, and the therapist may be directive and take a value stance. The focus is not just on the identified problem youth, but also on that youth within a particular family and community system. This means that an abuse specific approach requires multidisciplinary collaboration, and the coordination of the efforts and services of several different agencies and disciplines, the treatment team and the family.

For this reason this approach cannot work unless it is flexible, eclectic and individualised. Static methodology is based on generalisations, not idiosyncrasies, and is designed to serve homogenous populations not individuals. The more diverse a population, the less likely it is that a standardised methodology will provide effective treatment. There are few populations as diverse as sexually aggressive youth.

## Special issues for the family therapist

### *The need for competency and courage*

To provide family treatment for a family which includes a sexually abusive youth and may also include a sibling victim is a formidable undertaking. It means accepting the fact that the work will be difficult and emotionally draining, that the therapist will be working with complex relationships over long periods of time, and that he may not even have the reinforcement of being liked or having grateful clients. It means that it is necessary for the therapist to have a wide variety of knowledge about numerous subjects related to child sexual abuse, multidisciplinary teamwork and family treatment. It also means that he will provide more than individual family therapy. Sometimes the helping professional will be a teacher, a systems coordinator, a resource person, or a case manager – to name just a few of the likely roles. Unfortunately, it is rare for any of this to be taught in either undergraduate or graduate schools. However, there is professional literature, training and supervision available that provides helpful information (Burnham *et al.*, 1999; Burton *et al.*, 1997; Kaplan, 1986; Pithers *et al.*, 1998; and Warsh *et al.*, 1994).

Even though the work is difficult and time-consuming, the hardest part for many therapists is a willingness to enter into the family turbulence and chaos. Doing so can be intellectually challenging, emotionally draining and terribly frustrating. It often brings up personal and professional issues that may be very painful to face (Erooga, 1994). In spite of this, or perhaps because of this, involving families in treatment provides a number of rewards for treatment providers, not the least of which is their own professional growth and development. Inevitably it teaches many important things about families, life, pain, perseverance and resilience, and about our ability to meet challenges and adapt to complex situations.

### *Overcoming professional resistance*

Despite the growth of knowledge and understanding in the field, despite our recognition that children are not miniature adults, many professionals still resist involving family in the treatment of sexually abusive youth and there is a practically institutionalised jargon of reasons that have developed to support this. In addition to: "We don't have the funding", and "They won't come in", there is, "The families are physically distant", "The family is too dysfunctional/will undermine treatment", and, "We struggle just to meet the treatment needs of the youth themselves, much less taking on their families too!" Although these objections are all reality based, they are also precisely the reason why we must be non-traditional in our approach and think flexibly and creatively about working with the families of sexually abusive youth.

It is not possible to attempt this work alone. However, overcoming the possible resistance of your colleagues or agency may be necessary as this approach requires intensive and comprehensive staff effort in collaboration internally, and with outside systems and the young person's family. Agencies that prefer a "tight ship", where control is strongly vested in the programme and none given to the clients or families, will actively resist this approach. This may put treatment providers and administrators in the position of being family treatment advocates within their institutions or even at the local, state or national level to obtain the changes necessary. Yet the potential benefits, more effective treatment, a stronger relapse prevention plan, an abuse free support system, and safer, more efficient treatment programmes, are well worth the effort.

Overcoming professional resistance requires a strong belief in the importance of a family perspective and the ability to inspire change in others. It calls for a strong belief that most families have the capacity to change if they are given adequate support and resources, that most families really care about their children, want the best for them, and in the current circumstances are doing the best that they can. This approach rests on a belief that most families have the capacity, the strength and the resources to make changes that will promote the growth and development and emotional well-being of all family members. It is true that people may choose not to change, and that helping professionals may not have adequate support and resources to offer them. Yet even in these situations failure may be mitigated by initiating a therapeutic process that may result in some degree of positive change.

### *Working with a co-therapist*

For many reasons it is preferable that co-therapist teams conduct family therapy when working with this population. It is difficult for one person to be able to guide the process and note all of the nuances occurring simultaneously. It is also difficult for one person to handle all of the preparation, documentation, and emotional stress alone. Co-therapists share the work load of each case, provide each other with moral and psychological support, allow for more creative, team-based therapeutic approaches and bring at least two minds and perspectives to bear on the case and on therapy sessions.

Mixed gender co-therapy teams are especially desirable. They provide opportunities for the therapeutic modelling of healthy male–female relationships based on mutual respect and cooperation. When one member of the team clearly has more seniority or experience than the other, this modelling of collaborative teamwork is even further emphasised. Families may also ask about the sexual relationship of mixed gender co-therapy teams. Many are completely unfamiliar with the concept of nonsexual intimacy between a man and a woman. These questions open the door to a variety of extremely valuable discussions of inter-gender sexual and asexual relationships and should be welcomed and approached openly.

Some organisations are legitimately unable to afford to pay more than a single family therapist, but this does not necessarily mean that co-therapy cannot be attempted. Instead, these organisations should simply approach this situation as another opportunity to be creative and use their problem-solving skills. For example, in my own community qualified therapists from other fields, interns, practicum students, etc., are happy to serve as co-therapists *pro bono* because of the tremendous training and experience it provides.

## Establishing a collaborative professional relationship with parents

Parents are shocked by the disclosure that one of their children has been sexually abusive and feel embarrassed, ashamed, scared and responsible. Feelings of shame and humiliation are compounded when the victimised child is a sibling. Most parents tend to feel guilty and humiliated over even the simplest public problems with their children. For example, imagine a child who gets a failing grade in school and the teacher requests a family conference. Many parents in this situation automatically feel guilty, like a failure, and are embarrassed or humiliated. And if the teacher treats the parents as if they are at fault and makes disparaging remarks about their parenting skills, then they are likely to feel even worse. In comparison we can only respect the courage that parents have to exhibit in order to respond to the needs of all their children when child sexual abuse is disclosed. If one or more of the children have been removed from the home, and if treatment has been mandated, then it would not be unusual for parents to also feel helpless and out of control. No one likes their family autonomy taken away from them.

Because the familial and societal impact of sexual offending is so negative and overwhelming, it is important for the treatment provider to present a trustworthy, caring and helpful demeanour. Credibility must be established, not by coercion or threats, but through effort, listening, showing respect, and actively seeking the family's involvement. In doing so you are also therapeutically modelling empathy, which is often an important treatment issue for many families.

It should not be assumed that the family will want to be involved in treatment. It is not at all unusual or even unreasonable for the treatment provider to have to actively pursue parents and encourage them to become active participants. This is essential since many families will actually make their decisions on whether to participate based on their interaction with the treatment programme representative or through their experiences with the representatives of other systems.

It is up to professionals to overcome all the barriers to collaboration and form a working relationship with the family of a young person who has engaged in abusive behaviour. The process of engagement is really nothing more than the professional extending herself to another person or persons and winning their confidence, trust and cooperation. Having someone simply tell parents that they need to participate – or, alternatively, telling them the programme or courts require participation – is rarely ever enough. Feelings of helplessness, hopelessness and inadequacy may lead families to take the line of least resistance – leave the youth for the treatment programme to fix and return only to retrieve him or her when that is done. As a treatment provider we should be able to empathise, given how tempting the line of least resistance is for us as well.

The same strategies that are used to engage birth families should also be used to engage foster families, group home parents or caseworkers in the treatment programme. Here are some suggestions that will be helpful for successful engagement:

*(1) Use your "self".* Ask yourself this – are you able to form relationships? The most powerful therapeutic tool that the therapist or treatment provider has is one that they always have with them. That is the self, and that self's ability to form relationships. We commonly use this ability when we begin friendships, apply for a job, want to make a good impression, and so on. Since we often teach relationship skills to the youth in our programmes, we obviously know what it takes to do this. These are the four qualities that are particularly helpful in forming relationships – empathy, warmth, humour and genuineness. Empathy means being understanding, sensitive, caring, patient, genuine and compassionate, and having a willingness to listen. It is a cornerstone of offence specific treatment. Warmth means to be nurturing, sharing and accepting. Humour is a survival skill as well as a disposition, and means that we are generally able to find something to laugh about even in difficult situations – many times ourselves and sometimes just the common everyday things of life that touch all of us. And, last, to be genuine means to be open, human, natural, responsive, congruent – using the whole self rather than just the expert self. These are four powerful qualities that are not costly, time-consuming, or difficult to understand that will be very powerful in forming a positive, collaborative relationship with families (Baldwin, 2000).

*(2) Give parents many areas of choice.* The more areas of choice you can give parents the better. Choices give a feeling of control, and feeling out of control is a common source of hostility and suspicion. For example, allow

parents to choose what day and time they can come for family therapy. This may seem like a small matter, but for a parent whose job is tenuous, or who has small children with no caretaker this is a very large concern. Another way to give back some control is by enlisting parents' help with treatment tasks, even if it is only a small thing like providing their child with materials needed for the treatment programme.

*(3) Be open-minded and non-judgemental.* Let parents know that you are impartial, and that you do not pre-judge them. Begin with the presumption of competence and good intention of one individual toward another. Families need reassurance that sexual abuse can happen in any family, yours included. Reassurances such as this will go a long way toward reducing the family's anxiety and gaining their confidence. This does not mean being naive, but being fair and reasonable. This is often exactly how we would like to have families and youth to behave and feel toward us. Modelling these behaviours is one of the most effective ways to teach them.

*(4) Value the power of listening.* Listen without inappropriate statements of support such as "I know what you are going through." Ask families for their side of the story, how they learned of the behaviour, how they feel about it, and about everything that has happened since the disclosure. Assure parents that they can ask you anything, and if they do not respond, tell them what other parents have asked previously. See if that is helpful to them. Let them ventilate all they want. Nothing can feel better than being allowed to ventilate by someone who simply listens non-judgementally. This is valuable as much for the way it adds to feelings of control and confirms that they are a legitimate part of the process, as it is for the information itself. Also be willing to listen to constructive feedback about either the programme or yourself from family members. We cannot always be right or get things correct. Willingness to accept responsibility for mistakes goes a long way toward establishing your credibility and your humanness.

*(5) Use the family's strengths.* We generally spend an inordinate amount of time identifying familial problems and deficits. Yet it is the strengths we identify that help us solve problems and deficits. Ask the family what they think is needed to help their family, and what suggestions they would make. Besides being engaging and empowering this is an important assessment-gathering tool and a very good way to enhance your knowledge for treatment planning.

*(6) Be multilateral.* When working with very complex families there is always the danger of becoming over-identified with a family member, or of treating one family member more harshly than another. This can quickly bring about an alignment of family members against the therapist, and create

divisions within the family. You can avoid this by the use of a family therapy technique called multi-laterability. This just means that the therapist attempts to act responsibly toward everyone, meet every family member's needs, and respect their rights. Multi-laterability both demonstrates the therapist's trustworthiness to every family member, and encourages collaboration. You will know that you have been successful at practising multi-laterability if every member of the family has been mad at you at least one time during the treatment process. This often happens when individual family members try unsuccessfully to get you to align with them or give them special attention. If the therapist is prepared for this, then these manipulations can be avoided and the therapist can continue to present a fair front to all.

*(7) Do your job.* I often wonder what percentage of families that treatment providers call resistant and hostile would not present in this way if the therapist were doing a better job of engaging them in the first place. How many families that drop out of treatment prematurely would stay if the therapist were simply more patient and understanding? Admittedly, some families can be hostile, oppositional, destructive and extremely unhealthy. Yet it is our job to overcome that. As well, lest we become arrogant, there are also some treatment providers who can be thoughtless, controlling, overbearing and ill-equipped for the job. It is not the parent's job, however, to overcome this kind of attitude, but our own.

*(8) Impart hope.* There is abundant medical research to show that both negative and positive emotions can produce powerful changes in the body's chemistry, and intensify illness or promote health and healing. Millennia ago Hippocrates insisted that medical students give full weight to the emotions, both as a contributing cause of disease and as a factor in recovery. Throughout history and to the present time, physicians have emphasised the importance of the patient's will to live when fighting critical illness (Cousins, 1989). In periods of intense exasperation, rage or frustration it is not unusual for people to become victims of their own emotions, their despair and defeatism hampering their health and ability to adapt to new situations, and to cope even with normal daily activities. Depression, inertia, hopelessness, despair, anxiety, psychosomatic illness and other complaints are all common in the families of sexually aggressive youth. The following questions should be addressed concerning hope in the context of the family based treatment of child sexual abuse. Should we offer hope unless it is real? What is real hope? Is real hope the same for all of us – for any of us? Is our hope for families the same as what they hope for themselves? And what is the purpose of treatment if there is no hope? It is vital to answer these questions before beginning the treatment process or in order to do an adequate job of engagement, assessment, treatment-planning or developing outcome goals (Cousins, 1989).

## Influencing the course of treatment

The following are some of the common but easily correctable mistakes treatment providers make that can negatively influence the course of family treatment.

*(1) Do not rush to therapy.* It is a serious mistake to rush right into a therapeutic agenda because it seems essential to get in a certain number of sessions within a set amount of time mandated by some static guideline. Failing to develop a relationship with the family, assess dynamics and develop a treatment plan before beginning the treatment agenda produces pervasive problems that will plague the entire course of treatment. It is not possible to be successful if the first few steps are skipped due to a hurry to get going. It is not even good common sense to attempt a clarification session when a family is hostile and resistant, or when you do not know all of the family members and their unique perspectives. Planning, patience and persistence will eventually pay off.

*(2) Do not ignore cultural issues.* A second mistake is being unaware of or insensitive to cultural and subcultural differences, particularly their subtleties. In addition to the obvious differences that may exist between therapists and client families, there can be a thousand small variances of lifestyle and meanings. The therapist's official position and perceived power over the lives of client families may make them especially sensitive to those differences. Some families will enter treatment openly and aggressively convinced that the therapist will not and cannot appreciate their particular values and ways of life. Others may not be outwardly hostile, yet inwardly may be just as certain of an unwillingness to understand them, their beliefs and lifestyle, in their own terms.

In the very beginning differences between therapists and clients should be openly acknowledged and a willingness to learn about and understand the family's cultural and ethnic background should be expressed. In addition to providing valuable information, this will help personalise and demystify the therapist's role and position for the family. Understanding cultural differences is simply an additional tool and aid to communication and understanding rather than an obstacle. The more divergent a particular family's subculture is from the majority culture, the more obvious the therapist's efforts to meet client families on their own terms will be, and this in itself will establish a more positive working relationship. As the therapist's understanding of other cultures increases, it usually emerges that there are resources in those cultures (community elders or religious authorities, for example) that may be able to contribute significantly to treatment success.

Being sensitive is only the first step. Competency is the next. Programmes offering offence specific services must also have the requisite competency to adapt abuse specific methods, language and techniques to any culture represented within their treatment population. Different cultures define gender roles differently, have various perspectives on masturbation, use different language to discuss sexual issues, and/or do not use direct language at all (for example they may address such issues through the use of metaphor). Being ignorant of these issues will not only result in repeatedly finding your foot in your mouth, but will result in interventions based on erroneous assumptions, and the setting up of poor treatment goals.

*(3) Avoid labelling.* Avoid at all costs the tendency of some treatment professionals to label and therefore effectively dehumanise the families of sexually aggressive kids. I sometimes hear treatment providers talking in a very negative way about family systems, categorising families either upon their initial attitude of hostility or denial, their history of previous abuse and neglect, or, alternatively, their presentation as the perfect family. A treatment provider who applies simplistic and dehumanising labels to families will not only alienate them, but also fail to accurately assess their characteristics and needs. Either mistake greatly increases the odds of treatment failure, and all but guarantees an inability to engage families in the treatment process. It is a much more easily understood mistake on the part of parents toward treatment providers than of professionals toward parents.

*(4) Do not act in a controlling or authoritarian manner.* In therapy the goal is collaboration not the exercise of authority or control. Learning to conduct a collaborative effort is essential in working with sexually aggressive youth because of the many systems that impact on the identification, investigation, assessment, placement and treatment of this population. Our cooperative efforts must reach out into the community and join together with law enforcement, juvenile justice, the court, peripheral mental health professionals, child protective services, the abused child's therapist and, sometimes, attorneys. Doing this reduces the effort for any one person or system and improves the effectiveness of all the systems involved in a case, just as learning the art of collaboration with the family enhances the success of the treatment process. Working in a collaborative effort means a change in perspective from being controlling to being in control as we collaborate.

Collaboration with the family requires the therapist to present as a guide, a helper, and as part of a team which includes the family, and avoids presentation as an authority figure. This not only is a philosophical base for family therapy, but encourages rapport. Since many families do not attend services voluntarily but have been mandated into treatment, this issue should be addressed immediately. For example, a therapist might say:

I know you don't want to be here and that the court has ordered you to come. I would have preferred that you had come in voluntarily. I am here only to help your child stop his/her abusive behaviour and to help you in any way that I can. We are a team here. My part in that team is to be your guide and coach. Are you willing to work with me to do that?

If the answer to the last question is no, then the therapist should simply ask the family why this is the case, and what can be done to overcome their objections. If the family's objections cannot be overcome at first, then the therapist should be prepared to be patient and show by her actions that she can be trusted.

*(5) Do not forget to mention sex.* One very harmful and even ludicrous mistake some therapists make is thinking that they can do this work without talking about sex. Despite the nature of our work, there are professionals who are so uncomfortable with the subject of sexuality that they will work with a family for a year and artfully avoid ever using the word "sex". Although sex of any kind can be very difficult to talk about, it is ironic that dysfunctional/unhealthy sexuality is often easier for professionals to deal with than normal sexuality. As clinicians, we can distance ourselves from "it" as a professional subject which we have been trained to deal with objectively. Normative human sexuality, however, is more personal and subjective, and a surprising number of treatment providers have difficulty discussing it with families. Both deviant and normative sexuality will be a critical part of the treatment process. If the therapist is not comfortable talking about sex and sexuality then certainly no one will be. Staff training, role-plays and desensitisation exercises are just some of the methods that can be very helpful in dealing with this problem.

*(6) Do not try to be superman or superwoman.* Some of us are so determined to work with every family no matter what that we become unrealistic. There are some families that we will not be able to work with because they are so chaotic, multi-problematic, sabotaging, criminal, mentally ill and set in denial and refusal to support change that working with them is simply impossible. However, it is important not to rush to the conclusion that this is the case. Assess, evaluate, utilise the treatment team and supervision, and listen to the client and family.

*(7) Be sure not to forget to have a life.* As the saying goes: "If you've made treatment into a religion, then you've become a missionary, and missionaries get eaten by cannibals."

## Putting together a family focused programme

The modality options available for the development of a family focused programme are not so much limited by the resources of time, energy and financial support as they are by a lack of imagination, creativity, determination and positive energy. If you utilise the latter you may be able to overcome the former. There are actually many options that might be considered when making a decision about family focused programming, and each agency needs to use or develop what is pertinent to their client population, level of care, and context. The only essential modalities are family engagement, assessment, treatment planning, and the provision of family therapy. The rest can be added as or when needed, or not at all. The necessary work can be done in different modalities or combined into one. The development of different modalities in order to cover the essential material, however, can have the advantage of utilising a number of staff people instead of just one, and this will make the work go more quickly.

The following descriptions of modalities are just some suggestions to consider. Some will be described briefly and some in more detail. For more complete details on assessment, individual family therapy and multi family therapy see Thomas (1991).

### *1 Family assessment and evaluation*

The clearest and most comprehensive definition of assessment and evaluation was made by Maddock and Larson (1995).

> Assessment is the process of gathering information and applying expert knowledge in order to judge the status of a client's problem and to understand the context within which the problem is occurring. Evaluation is the application of some criteria and forming of judgements. Data gathering is the obtaining of information about the client. Observation is looking at patterns of language, non-verbal behaviour and behaviour as a whole. A pattern is a process of behaviour that is observed over a period of time.

Families influence growth and development in all aspects of a child's life. This influence can also unwittingly support, allow or foster the development of offending behaviour. In addition, you cannot truly understand the individual adolescent or his/her needs for community reintegration except in the context of his/her family, community and life context. However, it is important not to jump to the conclusion that the promotion of family therapy in the treatment of child sexual abuse is based upon a belief that the family is causal in the development of offending behaviour. As Becker and Kaplan (1993) have pointed out, there are many different and diverse paths both singly and in combination that effect the development of sexually aggressive behaviour.

Therefore, it is important to assess and evaluate how the behaviour was shaped or allowed to occur, so that you can identify what skills need to be developed in order to enable the family to provide an environment that is low-risk. Although there are instruments that clinicians can use to assess family dynamics, it is my belief that the family as individuals and as a unit is the most important source of data that you have, and that the clinical interview is the hallmark of assessment. Prior to the clinical assessment it is important that you gather data from all previous sources of information, such as every professional and agency with any prior involvement, clinical interviews at the time of admission and throughout treatment, and observation. Clinical observation will be an important source of data. Note how family members act in the first encounters – are they open, defensive, or deviant? Are the children over-compliant, or completely out of control? The interpretation of your observations gives meaning to the data and gives rise to assumptions about the motives and capabilities of others. There can be numerous interpretations of the same data, however, and all must be considered until they are dismissed or validated.

Since family circumstances are as diverse as the youth themselves it is not a good idea to try to use a generic assessment or treatment plan. It is better to assess and evaluate the unique family circumstances of each and every youth in order to individualise our data. The unique family circumstances will not only include any deficits or problems, but will also include an identification of the family's strengths and assets. Knowing assets and strengths will help in planning how to strengthen or rebuild the family structure. The strengths within the system will support the family's involvement in treatment, the ability to overcome problems, and the development of a non-offending environment. For example, it is important to assess family strengths such as problem solving skills, stress management and communication skills, the availability of external support systems, and the emotional resilience of family members. Six different areas of strength within the family system should be considered: (a) the strengths of the individual adolescent, (b) the strengths of individuals in the family, (c) the family unit strengths, (d) the resources available to them as a family, (e) their cultural strengths, and (f) the resources available to them in the community.

An abuse specific assessment should consider each of the following issues within the family: family enmeshment, isolation, external and internal stresses, intergenerational sexual or physical abuse, communication styles, conflicting relationship styles, emotional deprivation, abuse of power and sexualised environments – all of which can impact on the development of sexually abusive behaviour. In addition it should allow a consideration of family members' perception of the sexual abuse, how they have reacted to the disclosure, and the reaction of the extended family. It is important to assess family values concerning sex and sexuality. This should include an exploration of the following issues. How sex education is taught and the sexual environment within the home; the level of comfort with the subject and specifics of sexuality; and the degree that language, environment, television, music and clothing are sexualised.

Remember that assessment is not a static, time-limited procedure, but an ongoing process, which continues throughout treatment. It begins immediately with the first contact with the parents and continues as new information is revealed. This will always occur as the family begins to trust the therapist, and as their developing understanding and skills alter their perception of themselves, each other and events. With continual assessment it is sometimes difficult to tell when the assessment ends and treatment begins. Keep in mind that the family members' individual and collective perceptions of facts, regardless of their objective accuracy, are as important to the structure and operation of family dynamics as the facts themselves.

It is also important to note that the process of assessment is more than just a preamble to treatment. It is an opportunity to connect with each family member on a human level, to connect with the family as a whole, to gain the family's trust, to observe family dynamics, to check out collateral information. It is also an opportunity for the therapist to establish herself as a competent expert in the field and to convince the family to join her in a collaborative effort to help their children. Finally, the meeting with the parents to review the information obtained as a result of the assessment and evaluation is a good opportunity for the parents to generate questions and identify problem areas for inclusion in the treatment plan; to discuss previous treatment interventions or placements, what helped create direction and focus, and which plans they felt were directionless; to label themes and redirect the family for solutions to the treatment planning.

### 2 *Family treatment plan*

The treatment plan, developed from the assessment data, is a treatment roadmap, complete with signposts indicating how much further to the final destination. With a treatment plan, no one has to wonder what the treatment is trying to accomplish because it is documented and detailed. The plan is a guide that structures the focus of treatment toward the ultimate goal, the prevention of abusive behaviour. It is completed by: identifying and interrupting the family patterns that may have allowed or supported abusive behaviour; replacing those with patterns that support non-abusive and pro-social behaviour; interrupting the cycle of intergenerational abuse; healing the wounds caused by family membership or non-membership; teaching self-management skills to the sexually abusive youth; outlining the standards of care for victim clarification and family reunification; and learning what it means to be a part of a healthy family.

Some treatment providers are intimidated by the necessity of developing individualised treatment plans. Jongsma *et al.* (1996) recommend that the process of developing treatment plans involves the following logical series of steps. First, select the problem. The problem selected should be clear from the data collected in the assessment. Second, define the problem. This simply means that you define how this problem is evidenced in the family. Third, develop a goal or goals. These are usually global, long-term goals for the resolution of the targeted problem. Fourth, construct objectives. Objectives are stated in terms of measurable behaviour and broken into steps. They are the steps toward achieving the short-term goals or the series of steps towards accomplishing the long-term goal. Place the objectives in the order that you think is primary for their achievement. Fifth, create suitable interventions. Appropriate interventions are the actions of the clinician designed to help the family reach their objectives. If any particular intervention is not helpful to the client in achieving their objectives then new interventions and descriptions of the modalities in which these interventions are to occur should be added. Sixth, state who is responsible for the intervention. This is particularly important when the therapist is part of a team. Seventh, state a proposed target date for completion. A target date for the accomplishment of each objective should be stated. If after review on this target date the objective has not been reached the target date can be expanded. Finally, make a statement of accountability for following up the plan. State the date of the review of the treatment plan, by whom it is to be reviewed, and with whom the information will be shared. A fictional example of a treatment plan for the Smith family is given in Figure 12.1.

As is evident from the above, a treatment plan is simply an outline of goals, the objectives necessary to meet those goals, the interventions that will be utilised to meet those objectives, and the modalities, staff members and time frame for completion of those interventions. Because the plan is meant to be used by the family as well as staff, it must be written in concrete, child and family friendly terms. One suggestion that may be appropriate is to write the treatment plan with the family present so that they can be part of a discussion that clarifies details of the plan.

It is important to keep breaking the problem down into understandable and clear elements. For example, sexual offending and family dysfunction in general may be what brings youth and their families into treatment, but to simply label either as a problem area is too broad. Sexual offending can be broken down into numerous problem areas such as deviant arousal, denial, minimisation and projection of blame, and cognitive distortions, and so on. Similarly, family dysfunction is not a single discrete phenomenon. It is important to break it down into the various dynamics that make up the dysfunction, such as impaired communication style, inability to share feelings on a verbal level, emotional detachment, inadequate supervision. In doing so objectives can be tailored more specifically to the described problem area.

Since issues can change during treatment, the plan should be seen as a dynamic document that can and must be updated to reflect any major change

**Team treatment plan for the Smith family**

**Problem:** Mr and Mrs Smith have tended to minimise Ted's sexual abuse of his sister (Mary) as play. They feel that Mary shares much of the blame for what has happened.

**Goal:** To help the Smith family acknowledge Ted's responsibility for his sexually abusive behaviour without minimisation or projection of blame.

**Interventions:** Family therapy sessions; multi-family therapy

**Objective 1:** The Smiths will begin multi-family therapy so that they can benefit from learning about the experiences of other families in similar situations.

**Objective 2:** The Smiths will watch *One Can Hurt for a Lifetime* or a similar film which will help break through denial. They will process this experience with their therapist after the film.

**Objective 3:** When appropriate Ted will give a full and accurate account during a family session of his sexually abusive behaviour.

**Staff member responsible for implementing the Smiths' plan:** Jane Kahn, family therapist.

**Time frame:** Review date: 10 June, 2004.

*Figure 12.1* A fictional example of a family treatment plan for the Smiths.

of problem, goal, objective or intervention. By describing the goals and objectives in detail the family can see at every review what has been done, what work is in progress or ongoing, and what objectives remain unaddressed. Again, be sure and get family input on this treatment plan and their approval of it before you begin. This involvement of the family in planning shows respect for their opinions, gives them ownership in the plan, and is empowering to family members at a point in the process when they feel most helpless and out of control.

### 3 *Family contact*

When families are asked what they need most from a treatment provider, the reply often given is availability and contact. Availability means that when there is a family concern or crisis the person in the programme closest to the family is available to speak with them. Contact can mean many different things – personal phone contact by the therapist or another programme representative, weekly structured conference calls with family members, individual family therapy sessions, multi-family sessions, family retreats, family visits, or even communication by writing, video or audio tapes.

### 4 Individual family therapy

Individual family therapy is the cornerstone of family involvement. In some cases where distance is a factor (for example, if the youth is in out-of-home placement in another city), families may be asked to see a family therapist in their community who coordinates her work with the rest of the intervention system. Some programmes also use an exchange of videotapes, telephone conferencing and longer intensive sessions scheduled either once a month or during retreats. If natural or adoptive parents are not available, the therapist should encourage group home parents, foster parents, caseworkers or others designated as a support system to work with the programme.

### 5 Multi-family therapy

Bringing families together who have common concerns, problems and issues is logical and reasonable. This is particularly true when there are limited resources, staff, time and financial support. It is economical, efficient, non-threatening and non-intrusive, yet engaging and therapeutically effective. It provides an environment in which children and their families can emotionally support one another and other families while they work together exploring, confronting and changing problematic behaviours within the family. It reduces the isolation of parents and families while providing a supportive link to others who are facing similar problems dealing with the emotional and behavioural impact of sibling abuse. It is a forum where family and relationship problems can be addressed and enables them to gain insight through observation and identification with other families. Greater detail about multifamily groups is available in Ryan and Lane (1997).

### 6 Family psycho-educational groups

One of the responsibilities of the family treatment provider is to teach the family what they need know in order to provide a safe environment for all of their children. Families must be educated about child sexual abuse because they are part of a general public that generally does not understand the issues, dynamics, behaviours and emotions of child sexual abuse or sexually abusive youth. Without this understanding families are not able to intervene with their children in a constructive way. Understanding the subject empowers parents to respond in a constructive fashion to identify, address, and even prevent abuse, and helps them adequately supervise sexually abusive youth. In addition to this understanding of the dynamics of child sexual abuse, we can teach parents how to negotiate the legal, law enforcement, child protection services, education and child care systems, an overwhelming task even for the most sophisticated of us.

There are several different ways to teach the necessary material. It can be taught individually by the family therapist or treatment provider or in a family group. Groups are the most efficient use of the treatment provider's time and energy. Besides psycho-educational parent groups and psycho-education as a part of family therapy, there are other modalities that will be helpful in transferring the needed information. One of these is the development of a family resources and education packet. Although this is meant to be an adjunct to the psycho-educational group, in some circumstances it may be the only available resource. Although it is usually best to share this with them after some level of a relationship has formed, this packet should be provided soon after admission. It is also important to take the time to process the information with them so that they do not refuse to look at it. Be sure to personalise the packages of information for each family, recognising their particular culture as well as reading skills. Figure 12.2 provides an example of the contents of a typical parent pack that I have used. The following

**Suggestions for developing a programme specific parents pack**

Typically, the contents of a programme specific parents pack would include:

- A cover letter personally addressed to parents that is simultaneously an introduction to the programme and conveys an acknowledgement of the importance of their family in the life of the young person who has engaged in sexually abusive behaviour.
- An outline of the philosophy of the programme.
- Information on the identity of each staff member working on the programme.
- A clear description of the various treatment interventions and modalities utilised in the programme.
- A description of client/family rights, and any grievance procedures.
- A clear description of any service policies that affect families.
- Guidelines on the service's view of family responsibilities.
- Suitable information gleaned from the available literature (see Figure 12.3 for suggestions on sources of information).
- Any other information that might be useful for the parents or other family members.

*Figure 12.2* Suggestions for material to include in a parents pack.

*Children Who Molest: A Guide for Parents of Young Sex Offenders* by Eliana Gil (1987), Launch Press, PO Box 31491, Walnut Creek, DC 94598.

*Facing the Future, A Guide for Parents of Young People who Have Sexually Abused* (2001), by Simon Hackett, Russell House, Lyme Regis, England.

*Understanding Children's Sexual Behaviours: What's Normal and What's Not?* by Toni Cavanagh Johnson, 1101 Fremont Avenue, Suite 101 South Pasadena, CA 91030.

*Helping Children with Sexual Behavior Problems - A Guidebook for Parents and Substitute Caregivers,* by Toni Cavanaugh Johnson, 1101 Fremont Avenue, Suite 101 South Pasadena, CA 91030.

*Because There is a Way to Prevent Child Sexual Abuse: Facts About Abuse and Those who Might Commit It.* Edited by Joan Tabachnich, The Safer Society Press, PO Box 340, Brandon, Vermont 05733-0340 802-247-3132.

*Siblings At War: How to Reduce the Combat in your Home,* by Toni Cavanagh Johnson, 1101 Fremont Avenue, Suite 101 South Pasadena, CA 91030.

*Pathways Guide for Parents of Youth Beginning Treatment* (1990), by J. Kahn, The Safer Society Press, PO Box 340, Brandon, Vermont 05733-0340 802-247-3132.

*From Trauma to Understanding: A Guide for Parents of Children with Sexual Behavior Problems* (1993), Cunningham, Pithers, Gray, and Lane, The Safer Society Press, PO Box 340, Brandon, Vermont 05733-0340 802-247-3132.

*Childhood Sexuality: A Guide for Parents* (1998) Gail Ryan and Joanne Blum, Kempe Center, 1825 Marion Street Denver, C0 80218.

*The Feeling Good Again Guide for Parents and Therapists* (1998), by Burt Wasserman, The Safer Society Press, PO Box 340, Brandon, Vermont 05733-0340 802-247-3132.

*The Brother/Sister Hurt: Recognizing the Effects of Sibling Abuse* (1996), by Vernon Wiehe, The Safer Society Press, PO Box 340, Brandon, Vermont 05733-0340 802-247-3132.

*Figure 12.3* Resources for compiling information for a parents pack.

suggestions are not meant to be followed verbatim, but to provide some ideas about possible contents.

The literature on young people who engage in sexually abusive behaviour includes a number of brochures, pamphlets, and books that provide useful information to include in a parents pack. Figure 12.3 provides details of some possible sources of information. Certainly including all of them in a family package at one time would be overwhelming. It is best to pick what most suits your needs, utilising community resources where available, audios and videos when appropriate, and to regularly update the information included. Although any of the following are useful, they are most helpful when processed with the therapist afterwards providing an opportunity for parents to ask questions and talk about their feelings.

### 7 *Therapeutic family visitation*

When youth are in out of home care while they are in treatment, therapeutic visitations will be the heart of any family reunification plans. These provide opportunities for family members not only to maintain family ties, but to learn and practise new behaviours and styles of communicating. They also provide therapists with valuable measures of the family's progress toward reunification

Family visitation begins with brief planned visits in the facility, and progresses along a continuum until, in ideal cases, the visits culminate with three- to four-day unsupervised visits in the home. Home visits begin with short supervised daytime visits, progress to unsupervised overnight visits, and ultimately to unsupervised three- to four-day visits until everyone is assured that reintegration is going to be possible and safe. This continuum of increasingly open and potentially stressful formats helps families gradually gain competence in applying new skills in real life situations while still being supported and guided.

The family therapist provides homework assignments for visits, and these provide the children and families with opportunities to learn, practise, and demonstrate new behaviour and patterns of interaction. There should also be some kind of form that outlines the purpose of the visit, the therapeutic task to be accomplished, and any feedback on either the success of the visit or the problem areas encountered. Following visitations, the family therapist or other designated staff person evaluates and documents the visit to identify progress or problem areas. Decisions about visitation are made by the treatment team, which establishes the criteria that must be met for each level of visitation in collaboration with the parents and any other agencies that must be advised.

### 8 *Family retreats*

Family retreats are simply occasions in which the parents, non-abused or non-abusive siblings, the abused sibling and abusive youth come together in order to have an intensified, time-limited family experience with other families. It can be one or two days in length, depending on your clientele and your environment. Retreats may be held in the programme building, or at a community facility. They are very useful when parents are at a great distance, or work and childcare make it difficult for parents to participate on a consistent basis.

Beginning day one of the retreat with some kind of therapeutic recreation allows families to have an opportunity to relax and be prepared to face the more stressful events of the day. In addition, learning to enjoy being together is a basic treatment goal for youth and their families, and it is hard to overestimate the therapeutic value of these experiences. Simply having a good time together as a family can go a long way toward healing and removing the distance and barriers created by a previous history of arguments, boredom, misunderstanding and alienation. The rest of the first day can be devoted to a combination of psycho-educational group, parent support group, sibling groups and multi-family therapy. Meals are conducted family style, and if there is a need for an individual family session then this takes place as well.

Many programmes find that one day is enough, others like to have a second day that is not as work-oriented. If day two falls on a Sunday, then some sort of values clarification class, religious service or a short class on moral and ethical behaviour may be appropriate, depending on the situation. For example a short contemplative service can feature music by the youth and/or be conducted by the youth. After a family mealtime together, sports activities such as basketball, volleyball, fishing or board games may be organised. Some programmes that are experientially based have the family join in a challenge course experience, hiking, or river rafting.

Budgeting retreats is a concern for many programmes. Some have this cost written into their *per diem* as part of the programme. Some programmes have found creative ways of overcoming their cost limitations. These include providing overnight lodging for families, such as constructing a multi-purpose building that includes apartments, having motel chains donate rooms, and the utilisation of community resources such as churches or a Ronald McDonald house. Meals are sometimes donated, and cookouts or picnics can be planned and executed by the families.

### 9 Discharge

Discharge is based on the completion of treatment, which simply means that the family has met the goals that have been outlined on the treatment plan. It is possible for the family work to be completed before the treatment programme has been successfully completed by the youth. It can be very confusing for families if their perception of treatment completion is the completion of workbooks, modules or some programmatic steps. Completion must be dependent upon measurable outcomes such as decrease in sexual behaviour, increase in management of impulsive behaviour, or ability to manage anger in an appropriate way. The time to prepare parents for the discharge criteria is during the treatment planning phase.

### 10 Aftercare services

Even when families have successfully completed treatment it is still necessary to continue to provide support after the youth is discharged from a programme. Treatment providers often make the mistake of thinking that aftercare is an additional and optional component. On the contrary, it is a critical part of the programme. The initial period after discharge is a very fragile time for the reunited family. The treatment provider needs to tailor aftercare services to the needs of the family, the capabilities of the agency and their accessibility to the client and his/her family. This may include individual family therapy, multi-family therapy, home visits, and regular telephone checks. The involvement of families who have completed treatment can also be very valuable to other families in multi-family groups.

Discharge from the programme does not end the programme's involvement with a family, particularly when the family has reunified. Aftercare services may be essential in order for the family to stay together. This is particularly true if the child is in out of home placement for any length of time, since he will come home changed to a family which has itself changed, and therefore the dynamics of living together may be very different. In addition, if a child is in residential treatment he may have lived within a structure that makes freedom a scary prospect. The parents themselves are scared because they may not really believe that they can yet cope with what they may see as an overwhelming task and responsibility. The number of services and length of aftercare is very individualised. If the youth is in out of home placement and the family does not live in the immediate vicinity, then the treatment provider is responsible for making appropriate referral to the home community.

## Family focus when the family is absent or unavailable

When a youth's family is absent, nonexistent or unavailable, a family focus is still important. Because a family is not available to be involved in the treatment process with the youth does not mean that the youth does not need to deal with the issues of being a part – or not a part – of that family. There are also youth with families who are available who suffer from some of the same problems as those without families – the effects of loss, separation, lack of attachment or abuse and neglect, for example. These youth will also benefit from the treatment interventions recommended here. There are three important issues common to youth who have no family: (1) loss, abandonment and separation problems; (2) attachment problems; and, (3) a lack of any concept of the meaning of family.

*Loss, separation and abandonment.* There are some losses that can be called very significant losses and these typically fall into one of three categories: loss of health, loss of loved ones, or loss of self-esteem. A good percentage of young people with sexually abusive behaviour have suffered all three of these types of losses. Loss of health from being abused and neglected, loss of parents and/or siblings due to court action, rejection or placement, and loss of self-esteem due to guilt, inadequacy and inability to control what is happening. By the time youth who have been physically or sexually abused, neglected or emotionally maltreated get into the treatment system, they have already developed a very confusing worldview of parent–child relationships and family life in general. It will not be easy to alter that worldview or for them to give up the coping skills that they have developed to deal with a world which can include neglect and abandonment, deceit and trickery, intolerance and verbal, physical and/or sexual abuse.

*Lack of attachment.* In order for children to grow and develop normally they require a healthy emotional attachment to an adult. This healthy attachment provides the foundation for relationships, the development of conscience, the ability to think logically and manage impulses, the development of positive self-esteem, an awareness of their own and others' feelings, and the ability to get along with others. Children subjected to mistreatment form unhealthy attachments, becoming more comfortable with failure and misery than success and happiness, and as a result often set themselves up for failure. Youth who suffer attachment disorders may need special help in developing their consciences, controlling their impulses, having better self-esteem, getting along with others, being more self-assured, thinking more logically and minimising developmental delays. Achieving this task will take patience and perseverance.

*Abnormal concept of the meaning of family.* Growing up in a family that has been abusive and rejecting, influences a young person's concept of family, reflecting that experience. Expectations of "real" families may become based on dysfunctional family experiences, nor derived from the unrealistic portrayals of family life in popular media and culture. Children who have not had normative family experience need the chance to learn that neither the dysfunctional nor idealistic models of family are healthy or realistic. They need the opportunity to learn both that healthy families have problems too, and the ways that healthy families cope with these problems in the real world.

### *Special therapeutic interventions when the family is absent or unavailable*

In order to help a young person deal with loss the therapist needs to be frank, open and sensitive about loss and separation issues and listen non-judgementally. Youth will need help in understanding that their feelings of abandonment, anger and grief are normal, and, then, in finding appropriate ways to express these feelings. They will need support and guidance as they go through the grieving process identified by Kubler-Ross (1969) (shock, denial, anger, resolution). Even though this sounds easy, youth are often very resistant to fully completing this process. It is helpful to begin by a focus on feelings rather than behaviours or thoughts. Young people may need permission to feel scared, anxious, worried, and angry and to know that they have a right to those feelings. Without acknowledging those feelings and having them validated, it is impossible to work through or resolve them or learn ways to express those feelings so that they do not hurt themselves or others.

Building attachments takes time, and meeting a person's interpersonal needs takes more time. During this time it is necessary to set realistic expectations of youth and families because this may be a lengthy process. There are some additional things that the therapist can do to help build attachment with children and to teach their parents, group home parents, foster parents, extended family group, about attachment related issues. These include helping them develop their family history. Life books have been used for years for children in foster services to tell their family stories and their personal history while outlining their emotional lifelines. Usually this simply involves a scrapbook that children put together about their lives, which includes birth parents, extended family, foster family, group home parents. Factual information, memories of happy times and memories of unhappy times are all recorded. Since lives are unique then so are the scrapbooks; some may be computer generated art, some may be drawings and stories, some may be photographs, or even a copy of a birth certificate. Life books give youth a sense of belonging, of having a history that says that they matter. Providing reliable information on placement plans, providing appropriate reassurance and support during intervention, and acting as a role model for the healthy processing and expression of emotion, are all useful attachment-related interventions. Be prepared to continually answer questions about the unknown (even if not directly asked by the young person), especially questions such as "How long will I be here?" "Where will I go next?" "Who is making decisions about me?" "What do I do if I get sick or hungry?" and "Will I be safe here?" The therapist and other members of the intervention network should also provide appropriate reassurance to the young person as needed. Appropriately repeated reassurance conveys a message to the young person that he will be protected and that he is worthwhile and valued.

It may in part be helpful to teach a young person about family just as you would teach them about aspects of other subjects such as geography, for example. Topics covered could include how most of us learn about family life through our personal experience; what we need to know in order to be part of a functional family; what makes us a good family member; and, what being in a family really means.

## Conclusion

This chapter does not contain all the information that you need to know in order to work with the families of sexually aggressive youth. In fact, I do not know if any one source could provide all of that information. However, it hopefully provides a useful starting-point. Most of us with expertise in the family treatment of juvenile sexual aggression rely upon the limited available literature, and on each other for insight and support in this relatively new and ever growing field. We also learn a great deal from our clients themselves.

## References and Bibliography

Baldwin, M. (2000). *The Use of Self in Therapy*. New York: Haworth Press.

Barbaree, H., Marshall, W., and Hudson, S. (eds) (1993). *The Juvenile Sex Offender*. New York: Guilford Press.

Becker, J., and Kaplan, M. (1993). Cognitive behavioral treatment of the juvenile sex offender. In H. Barbaree, W. Marshall and S. Hudson (eds), *The Juvenile Sex Offender*. New York: Guilford Press.

Bera, W., Hindman, J., Hutchens, L., McGuire, D., and Yokley, J. (1990). *The Use of Victim–Offender Communication in the Treatment of Sexual Abuse: Three Intervention Models*. Brandon, VT: Safer Society Press.

Blanchard, G. (1995). *The Difficult Connection: The Therapeutic Relationship in Sex Offender Treatment*. Brandon, VT: Safer Society Press.

Burnham, J., Moss, J., Debrelle, J., and Jamieson, R. (1999) Working with families of young sexual abusers: Assessment and intervention issues. In M. Erooga and H. Masson (eds), *Children and Young People who Sexually Abuse Others*. London: Routledge.

Burton, D. L., Nesmith, A., and Badten, L. (1997). Clinicians' views on sexually aggressive children and their families: A theoretical exploration. *Child Abuse and Neglect, 21(20)*, 57–70.

Carlo, P. (1991). Why a parental involvement program leads to a family reunification: A dialogue with childcare workers. *Residential Treatment for Children and Youth, 9(2)*, 37–48.

Cousins, N. (1989). *Head First: The Biology of Hope*. New York: Dutton.

Edmunds, S. (ed.) (1994). *Impact: Working with sexual abusers*. Brandon, VT: Safer Society Press.

Erooga, M. (1994). Where the professional meets the personal. In T. Morrison, M. Erooga and R. Beckett (eds), *Sexual Offending against Children: Assessment and Treatment of Male Abusers*. London: Routledge.

Garner, H. (1988). *Helping Others Through Teamwork: A Handbook for Professionals*. New York: Child Welfare League of America.

Gil, E. (1987). *Children Who Molest: A Guide for Parents of Young Sex Offenders*. California: Launch Press.

Greene, J., and Holden, M. (1990). A strategic-systemic family therapy model: Rethinking residential treatment. *Residential Treatment for Children and Youth, 7(3)*, 51–55.

Haaven, J., Little, R., and Petre-Miller, D. (1990). *Treating Intellectually Disabled Sex Offenders: A Model Residential Program*. Brandon, VT: Safer Society Press.

Hilman, D., and Solek-Tefft, J. (1988). *Spiders and Flies: Help for Parents and Teachers of Sexually Abused Children*. Lexington, MA: Lexington Books.

Isaacs, M., and Benjamin, M. (1991). *Toward a Culturally Competent System of Care*. Washington, DC: National Technical Assistance Center for Children's Mental Health.

Jongsma, A., Peterson, M., and McInnis, W. (1996). *The Adolescent Psychotherapy Treatment Planner*. New York: Wiley and Sons.

Kaplan, L. (1986). *Working with Multiproblem Families*. Lexington, MA: Lexington Books.

Kubler-Ross, E. (1969). *On Death and Dying*. New York: Macmillan.

Landry, S., and Peters, R. (1992). Toward an understanding of a developmental paradigm for aggressive conduct problems. In R. Peters, R. McMahon and V. Quinsey (eds), *Aggression and Violence Throughout the Life Span*. Thousand Oaks, CA: Sage.

Laws, D. R., and Marshall, W. L. (1990). A conditioning theory of the etiology and maintenance of deviant sexual preference and behavior. In W. L. Marshall, D. R. Laws and H. E. Barbaree (eds), *Handbook of Sexual Assault: Issues, Theories and Treatment of the Offender*. New York: Plenum Press.

Lewis, A. D. (1999). *Cultural Diversity in Sexual Abuser Treatment*. Brandon, VT: Safer Society Press.

Long, P., and Jackson, J. (1994). Childhood sexual abuse: An examination of family functioning. *Journal of Interpersonal Violence, 9(2)*, 270–277.

Maddock, J., and Larson, N. (1995). *Incestuous Families: An Ecological Approach to Understanding and Treatment*. New York: Norton.

Mayer, A. (1983). *Incest: A Treatment Manual for Therapy with Victims, Spouses and Offenders*. Holmes Beach, FL: Learning Publications.

Morrison, T. (1994). Learning together to manage sexual abuse: Rhetoric or reality? *Journal of Sexual Aggression, 1(1)*, 29–44.

Morrison, T., Erooga, M., and Beckett, R. (eds) (1994). *Sexual Offending against Children: Assessment and Treatment of Male Abusers*. New York: Routledge.

National Adolescent Perpetrator Network (1988). Preliminary report from the national task force on juvenile sexual offending. *The Juvenile and Family Court Journal, 39(2)*.

O'Brien, M., and Bera, W. (1986). Adolescent sexual offenders: A descriptive typology. *Preventing sexual abuse, 1(3)*, 1.

Peters, R. D., McMahon, R. J., and Quinsey, V. (1992). *Aggression and Violence Throughout the Life Span*. Newbury Park, CA: Sage.

Pithers, W., Gray, A., Cunningham, C., and Lane, S. (1993). *From Trauma to Understanding: A Guide for Parents of Children with Sexual Behavior Problems*. Syracuse, NY: Safer Society Press.

Pithers, W., Gray, A., Busconi, A., and Houchens, P. (1998). Caregivers of children with sexual behavior problems: Psychological and familial functioning. *Child Abuse and Neglect, 22(2)* 129–141.

Ryan, G. (1991). Theories of etiology. In G. Ryan and S. Lane (eds), *Juvenile Sexual Offending: Causes, Consequences and Correction*. Lexington, MA, Lexington Books.

Ryan, G. (1998). The relevance of early life experience to the behavior of sexually abusive youth. *Irish Journal of Psychology, 19(1)*, 32–48.

Ryan, G., and Lane, S. (eds) (1991). *Juvenile Sexual Offending: Causes, Consequences and Correction*. Lexington, MA, Lexington Books.

Ryan, G., and Lane, S. (eds) (1997). *Juvenile Sexual Offending: Causes, Consequences and Correction*, 2nd edn. San Francisco, CA: Jossey-Bass.

Ryan, G., Blum, J., Law, S., Christopher, D., Weber, F., Sundine, D., Astler, L., Teske, J., and Dale, J. (1988). *Understanding and Responding to the Sexual Behavior of*

*Children: Trainers Manual*. Denver, CO: Kempe National Center, University of Colorado Health Sciences Center.

Ryan, G., *et al.* (1999). *Web of Meaning: A Developmental-Contextual Approach in Sexual Abuse Treatment*. Brandon, VT: Safer Society Press.

Steele, B. F. (1987). Abuse and neglect in the earliest years: Groundwork for vulnerability. *Zero to Three, 7(4)*, 14–15.

Steele, B. F., and Ryan, G. (1997). Deviancy: Development gone wrong. In G. Ryan and S. Lane (eds), *Juvenile Sexual Offending: Causes, Consequences and Correction*, 2nd edn. San Francisco, CA: Jossey-Bass.

Thomas, J. (1991). The adolescent sex offender's family in treatment. In G. Ryan and S. Lane (eds), *Juvenile Sexual Offending: Causes, Consequences and Correction*. San Francisco, CA: Jossey-Bass.

Thomas, J., and Viar, W. (1994). *The Familial Roots of Sexual Aggression*. Unpublished keynote presentation for the 1994 National Organisation for the Treatment of Abusers (NOTA) Conference, UK.

Thomas, J., and Viar, W. (1995). *Modelling in Therapeutic Environments*. Residential Treatment Staff Manual and Training Packet. Memphis, TN: J. Thomas Consulting Services.

Trepper, T., and Barret, M. (1988). *Treating Incest: A Multiple Systems Perspective*. Binghamton, NY: Haworth Press.

Van Derber, M. (1992). *One Can Hurt a Lifetime*. Washington, DC: One Voice Foundation.

Ward, T., and Hudson, S. (1998). The construction and development of theory in the sexual offending area: A metatheoretical framework. *Sexual Abuse: A Journal of Research and Treatment, 10(1)*, 47–63.

Warsh, R., Pine, B., and Maluccio, A. (1994). *Teaching Family Reunification: A Sourcebook*. Washington, DC: Child Welfare League of America.

Wiehe, V. (1996). *The Brother/Sister Hurt: Recognizing the Effects of Sibling Abuse*. Brandon, VT: Safer Society Press.

# Part IV

# Special client groups

Chapter 13

# Adolescents with intellectual disabilities who sexually harm

## Intervention design and implementation

*David O'Callaghan*

### Introduction

Although it appears that individuals with intellectual disabilities do not offend at any greater frequency than the general population (Lindsay, 2002) sexual offending appears disproportionately represented among this group when we consider indices reflecting the characteristics of sexual offender populations (Day, 1993; Thomas and Singh, 1995). British community-based programmes for adult sexual offenders have reported around 10 per cent of clients have an intellectual disability (Allam *et al.*, 1997; Doyle and Gooch, 1995) and surveys of intellectually disabled victims of sexual abuse have consistently identified other service users as the most frequent perpetrators (Beail and Warden, 1995; Brown *et al.*, 1995; Thompson, 1997). There is little by way of follow-up studies with this group, but Klimecki *et al.* (1994) in investigating re-offence rates among offenders with an intellectual disability found a recidivism rate of almost 31 per cent (30.8%) for sexual offences, with the vast majority of re-offences (84%) occurring within the first twelve months.

To date the specific needs of young people with intellectual disabilities have received limited attention in the literature devoted to adolescents who sexually harm. This is more notable given the apparent over-representation of this group within surveys of young sexual abusers. Beckett (1999), Dolan (1996), Epps (1991), Hawkes *et al.* (1996), Monk and New (1996) and Vizard (2000) are examples of UK studies of adolescent sexual offenders that identify between one-third and one-half of their samples as intellectually disabled or having significant educational problems. Farmer and Pollock (1998) studied young victims and perpetrators of sexual abuse within the UK care system and found that being identified as intellectually disabled was one of the features which was more prevalent within the abuser group. This apparent over-representation of young people with intellectual disabilities may be due to a number of factors including imprecise use of the term intellectual disability, difficulties in the assessment of learning ability, and the impact of adverse life experiences, such as trauma and neglect, on many young people's psycho-social and educational development. Less able young people may also be more likely to have their behaviour identified by agencies due to the higher levels of scrutiny and observation they experience. However, based on the available data, both anecdotal evidence and our clinical experience suggest that there is a particular gap in services for this group of young people.

Available evidence suggests that the developmental adversities associated with the onset of problematic sexual behaviours in youth generally (such as trauma, disruption of attachment bonds, and family dysfunction) are also features of the life histories of intellectually disabled sexual offenders (Day, 1993; Lindsay, 2002; Thompson and Brown, 1998). However, particular issues that may adversely affect the development of positive sexual identities for intellectually disabled youth include a limited opportunity for social development, social isolation, limited sexual education, a lack of privacy, a lack of opportunity to experience normative and appropriate sexual interactions, specific difficulties in communication, and the impact of specific genetic and medical factors.

## Assessment

Clinical assessments of offenders with intellectual disabilities must take account of the following factors (Clare, 1993; Clare and Gudjonsson, 1993): General literacy difficulties and problems in the comprehension of complex language; specific deficits in speech and communication, such as limited vocabulary, or the need to use signs or symbols to facilitate communication; level of conceptual understanding; presence of memory deficits; and level of suggestibility. Commonly, assessment frameworks developed for adolescent sexual offenders are based on a format of clinical interviews supported by psychometric testing and information-gathering. Although there have been attempts to adapt or apply existing psychometric measures for use with intellectually disabled clients (Riding, 1999; Rose *et al.*, 2002) these appear to encounter the difficulties previously identified in attempts to employ measures originally designed for intellectually able clients with individuals who have an intellectual disability (Clare, 1993; Murphy, 1997). However, a positive example of an attempt to design resources specifically designed to meet the needs of this group is the QASCO, which is an attitudinal scale specifically for sexual offenders with intellectual disabilities developed by Lindsay *et al.* (1998).

O'Callaghan (2002b) outlines a model for the initial assessment of intellectually disabled young sexual abusers based upon a detailed developmental and behavioural review which covers each of the nine areas outlined below.

1 *Family of origin factors.* Including parents' level of intellectual functioning; development and functioning of siblings; family attitudes towards sexuality (particularly in respect of the child with a learning disability); and current family relationships and level of contact.

2 *Personal health history.* Including specific known genetic conditions such as fragile X, Down's syndrome, autistic spectrum disorders; other medical factors impacting on development, such as brain trauma; use of medication; and impact of other physical conditions if present.
3 *Developmental history.* Including point at which developmental delay was identified; and other behavioural problems that have been following a developmental trajectory.
4 *Care history.* Including bonding and attachment experiences; issues related to loss or separation, such as being subject to respite, substitute or hospital care; care concerns such as neglect, lack of stimulation, abuse, trauma, lack of supervision; response of parents to their child being identified as having a learning disability.
5 *Educational history.* Including attendance at mainstream or special schooling; point at which Statement of Special Educational Needs was drafted; academic and social experience of schooling to date; and behaviour within the school setting.
6 *Assessment of general cognitive functioning.* Including memory and retention of information skills; attention and concentration skills; problem solving abilities; language, communication, and literacy skills; capacity for conceptual thinking; and ability to transfer and generalise solutions.
7 *Social functioning.* Including access to social networks, activities and opportunities; relationships with peers; independence skills, such as mobility within the community, and use of public transport; level of supervision in the community; assertiveness skills.
8 *Psycho-sexual history.* Including known information on sexual maturity, for example when did the young person experience the onset of puberty, physical development, erectile response, use of masturbation; information known on the young person's past sexual experiences; known experiences of sexual victimisation.
9 *History of problematic sexual behaviour.* Including the range of behaviours demonstrated (exposure or contact offences); at whom has the behaviour been targeted to date (children or adults? was the direction of the behaviour gender-specific or not?); relationship to those victimised (was the person a family member, fellow student, fellow service user, neighbour, or stranger?); how has the young person gained access or made contact with those victimised?; what were the settings and circumstances of the behaviour?; was there evidence of planning or targeting specific and more vulnerable people such as less able peers or certain care staff?; what responses have adults and involved agencies made to problematic sexual behaviours to date (have they been ignored, attempts made to distract the young person from the behaviour, has the young person been subjected to sanction, restriction or removal, have the police been involved, and is the young person subject to legal sanction)?; have there been any previous attempts at therapeutic intervention?

Information from these nine areas may be integrated into a formulation and provide the basis for treatment plans for young people with intellectual disabilities who sexually abuse others.

## Treatment

In this section the literature on some of the most frequently used approaches to therapeutic intervention for people with an intellectual disability who have engaged in sexually abusive behaviour will be reviewed. These programmes may be classified as those which focus on the modification of deviant sexual arousal; applied behavioural analysis programmes which target both sexual and other behaviours; group work programmes; multi-component programmes; and programmes that explicitly address relapse prevention.

### *Modifying deviant sexual arousal*

Deviant sexual arousal is a central risk factor requiring modification for a proportion of intellectually disabled sexual offenders (Coleman and Haaven, 1998). Specific interventions to address this risk factor have been a component of a number of sexual offender treatment programmes (Crawford, 1984; Murphy *et al.*, 1983; O'Connor, 1996, 1997). However, few studies have been conducted on the effectiveness of these methods in modifying deviant arousal in adolescents (Fisher and McGregor, 1997) and there is even less information on the modification of deviant arousal in young people with intellectual disabilities. One of the earliest examples is provided by Kolvin (1967) in his account of the use of aversive imagery with an adolescent male. Withers and Gaskell (1998) outline the use of a "minimally aversive" technique to eliminate the inappropriate masturbation of an eleven-year-old boy with mild intellectual disabilities. Lund (1992) notes an unsuccessful attempt to apply slide assisted covert sensitisation to reinforce the consequences of continued sexually offending behaviour with one client.

Murphy (1997) in reviewing the potential application of such techniques with intellectually disabled clients notes the need to ensure clarity of task and the importance of establishing a high level of motivation and honesty. O'Callaghan (1999) suggests four minimum criteria that should be met before such techniques are considered for use with adolescents, particularly those with intellectual disabilities. These are: (1) The young person experiences the arousal as problematic and is motivated to work on this area. (2) Experience would support a view of the young person as open and communicative about their sexual drives and interests. (3) The pattern of deviant sexual fantasy is reasonably distinct and consistent. (4) The young person is supervised and receives considerable support from carers.

### *Behavioural intervention*

Programmes developed within the Applied Behavioural Analysis (ABA) tradition have been widely used within the field of intellectual disability to modify a range of challenging behaviours and also to promote skills development (Emerson, 2001). The ABA model assumes that all behaviour, including challenging behaviour, has a function, which can be assessed through an analysis of the setting events and background factors that precede the behaviour and the consequences that follow from it. In the case of challenging behaviour, once its function is understood, the individual can be taught new behaviours that achieve the same function. Within the ABA field, treatment outcome studies typically involve controlled single case designs. A small handful of studies have been conducted in which the impact of ABA programmes on adolescent sexual offenders with intellectual disabilities has been assessed.

Wright, Herzog and Seymour (1992) describe an intervention with a young man with Down's syndrome in which it was concluded that unacceptable sexual behaviours occurred when (a) staff made demands on the young man, and (b) he wished to gain attention. Behavioural change was promoted by staff consistently ignoring negative attention-seeking behaviours and rewarding positive ones. Taylor (1996) presents an example of the application of ABA to therapeutic work with intellectually disabled sexual offenders based on the STAR approach (Setting conditions, Triggers, Actions, Results). The programme described combines direct contingency management with educative work on consequences, cognitive-behavioural counselling and role-play. O'Connor (1996; 1997) has described an attempt to merge ABA with the relapse prevention model.

### *Groupwork programmes*

Group programmes have emerged as the dominant treatment modality for adult sexual offenders in the UK (Allam and Browne, 1998). There are, as yet, only sporadic examples of groups run specifically for intellectually disabled offenders, many of which are described below.

Swanson and Garwick (1990) describe a treatment group for clients with a broad ability range (from moderate to borderline intellectual disability) addressing victim harm, non-abusive sexuality and social skills. Sexual recidivism over an unspecified time period was reported to be 40 per cent. The Social Sexual Group Treatment Programme outlined by Cox-Lindenbaum and Lindenbaum (1994) emphasised the role of social isolation and intimacy deficits in sexual offending and provided therapeutic input on feeling identification, anger management, social skills, cognitive restructuring and relapse prevention. Charman and Claire (1992) provide an account of an education group for male in-patients in a hospital setting that focused on laws, social boundaries and social rules of sexual behaviour. They found the group process was particularly effective in offering a safe environment for the discussion of sensitive issues including the men's sexual offences and their own victimisation. In contrast, the experience of Gardiner *et al.* (1996) in running a group for five men who had sexually offended within a community-based service for people with intellectual disabilities was that it proved difficult to establish a sense of group cohesion in which group members adopted a shared commitment to the process and an interest in each other's contribution.

Allam *et al.* (1997) reviewed the experience of the West Midlands Probation Service in developing an adapted group programme for male sexual offenders with intellectual disabilities. Interestingly, they found that less focus on the development of victim empathy and insight into offending behaviour was required, and that it was preferable to emphasise the promotion of impulse control, social skills, sexual knowledge, interpersonal relationships and relapse prevention skills.

Lindsay *et al.* (1998) provide a detailed evaluation of a community based cognitive group programme for men with intellectual disabilities who offended against children, in which the explicit focus was tackling attitudes, including responsibility for the offence, denial of intent and understanding harm inflicted on the person victimised. Over a follow-up period of four years, none of the participants re-offended. Evaluation of attitudinal change was assessed using specifically designed measures. Acceptance of responsibility for the offence and acknowledging harm to the victim were the attitudes most resistant to change. Lindsay stressed the need for a lengthy period of input and follow-up to ensure retention of key messages.

Riding (1999) provides a preliminary review of an in-patient group treatment programme that applied adapted versions of the psychometric measures used to evaluate the UK community and prison programmes (Beckett *et al.*, 1994). Riding found some evidence of attitudinal change but concluded that it will be necessary to extend the study to establish whether observed treatment gain is generalisable to community settings.

The British Prison Services Sex Offender Treatment Programme (SOTP) has recently been adapted for incarcerated sexual offenders who have a degree of intellectual disability. The emphasis of the adapted programme is on the self-management of risk to avoid the negative consequences of re-offending and makes use of vivid symbols, drawings and clearly expressed messages.

Rose *et al.* (2002) have developed a sixteen-session community-based programme. Although they found that the programme led to gains in basic sexual knowledge and awareness of social rules of sexual behaviour, it was difficult to interpret the impact of the group on other areas of personal functioning. This is because some of the evaluation measures were not designed for use with individuals with an intellectual disability. Encouragingly, a twelve-month follow-up of the five men who attended the group identified no serious incidents of concern or re-offences.

### *Multi-component interventions*

Multi-component programmes for young sexual offenders with intellectual disabilities typically involve educational, cognitive and skill development components (Murphy *et al.*, 1983; Griffiths *et al.*, 1985; Griffiths *et al.*, 1989). For example Hames (1987) described a programme undertaken with five sixteen- to seventeen-year-old males living in a residential treatment unit. All had victimised children and the programme utilised individual counselling with sexual education, and a social skills group. A follow-up of four clients over six months found that one young man had re-offended.

Haaven *et al.* (1990) provide an example of a model residential programme, which they described as a "modified therapeutic community". A core principal of Haaven's model is that all behaviour is seen as relevant to the individual's treatment goals. The total environment and activity of the unit is, therefore, geared to promoting the ethos of positive respect and the development of skills such as honesty, taking responsibility and supporting the growth of self-esteem. In their description of the programme Haaven *et al.*, identified a number of common techniques in sexual offender treatment practice that did not appear constructive for those with an intellectual disability, including masturbatory satiation, the use of fantasy logs and victim empathy training. They did employ certain behavioural techniques aimed at redirecting deviant sexual arousal, but these were considered a relatively minor part of the programme. For a majority of the men who attended the service anxiety and poor social and relationship skills were considered to be major inhibitors in the development of appropriate sexual relationships. Descriptions of therapeutic approaches are striking with the use of vivid art and drama techniques and an emphasis on the provision of accessible messages. Sexual behaviours were not isolated as a specific issue and all examples of the men being sharing, supportive, respectful to others and working on positive personal goals were considered important. In their more recent update on this programme Coleman and Haaven (1998) emphasise the importance of integrating motivational systems, for example, by providing smaller more discrete rewards for specific achievements, and developing rituals for acknowledging treatment and social or interpersonal gains. They comment that "a culture in which status is gained by participation in the programme needs to be nurtured and a sense of responsible self-identity encouraged" (1998, p. 281).

Lund (1992) also describes a residential programme for adult and adolescent males that merges a number of elements, such as attempts to promote behavioural change, cognitive restructuring, anger-management training, victim empathy training, problem solving and dealing with personal victimisation components. Delivery was via individual, group-work and token economy programmes. Graduated independence and unsupervised mobility in the community was based on the extended absence of problem behaviours.

Evaluation in terms of quality of life criteria and the provision of less restrictive environments was positive. However, Lund found that the total number of treatment components, and exposure to specific treatment components, did not systematically affect outcome.

### *Generalising self-management skills across community settings*

A major task for clinicians with this client group is to devise strategies to promote skill development, particularly self-management of risk, across a range of settings. O'Connor (1997) suggests that the principles of relapse prevention, with a heightened emphasis on designing a supportive social network, can be adapted for use with intellectually disabled clients. Dowrick and Ward (1997) describe the use of video techniques to promote self-management of risk in a young man with mild intellectual disabilities who demonstrated a high level of arousal to children. This involved his watching of prepared videos demonstrating appropriate responses to risky situations. They concluded that this intervention produced a more rapid, consistent and longstanding change in behaviour than previous attempts to teach this self-management strategy by more traditional counselling and educational techniques. Demetral (1994) found that sexual offenders with intellectual disabilities were more likely to apply coping strategies effectively if they have a supportive and reinforcing network. O'Connor (1996; 1997) provides an example of a programme in which attempts were made to measure treatment gain across therapeutic and community settings. The service model drew heavily from applied behaviour analysis, which emphasises the function of the behaviour for the person concerned and the influence of the setting in which it is displayed. O'Connor's programme additionally employed techniques more common to sexual offence specific treatment such as covert sensitisation. The achievement of target goals was assessed both by self-report and by direct observation in other settings. The critical importance of this external monitoring was demonstrated by the fact that most participants were able to retain the verbal component of the intervention, but behavioural change occurred for only some participants.

### *The G-MAP intervention programme for intellectually disabled youth who sexually harm*

This section describes how we have implemented some of the ideas described in the previous section on intervention at the G-MAP Programme in the UK. (G-MAP originally stood for the Greater Manchester Adolescent Programme, but now is a programme name in its own right.) Although the structure and themes are of our G-MAP programme for young people with intellectual disabilities are similar to the G-MAP mainstream ability group programme, the process is designed specifically to meet the learning needs of the participants. We view the programme not as an adapted version of the mainstream programme, but as a programme existing in its own right that has evolved from the experiences of delivering groups to intellectually disabled young men over a number of years.

The G-MAP service delivery model (O'Callaghan, 2002a) identifies six areas around which a holistic, individual and developmentally sensitive service should be organised. These are: (1) offence specific problems; (2) family issues; (3) the young person's sexuality; (4) influences on the young person's participation; (5) social functioning; and (6) non-sexual conduct problems. A comprehensive assessment process structured around these six domains is used to identify specific areas of need, existing or potential strengths, and issues of continuing uncertainty regarding the young person. An assessment based on these six areas can be used to develop and record an individualised, discrete and ongoing plan for appropriate intervention work. The overall intervention package will usually include both direct treatment components and other indirect interventions and supports. The intervention plan locates the various goals relevant to that young person on a single document. These goals should be specific, achievable, progressive, time limited and subject to regular evaluation and review. This approach to intervention planning is illustrated in Figure 13.1, using information provided in the case study for Alan (a pseudonym which is used to protect the identity of the client, all other identifying details have also been changed).

## *Case study: Alan*

Alan is sixteen years of age and currently placed in a small mixed-sex residential unit for young people with intellectual disabilities and challenging behaviour. He is the eldest of three siblings and was cared for by his mother until aged six at which point he and his sisters moved to the care of his grandmother and aunt. This was instigated by social services due to the general neglect of all the children and mother's current partner having a history of physically abusing children in a previous relationship. When his grandmother's health failed his aunt felt she could not care for Alan as he was becoming increasingly disruptive. Aged nine Alan moved to the first of many foster placements. This placement broke down when the foster carers found him sexually stimulating the family's pet dog. Over the next six years Alan had six placement changes and concerns regarding his sexual behaviour became increasingly dominant. In his last foster placement Alan took a six-year-old child with Down's syndrome into a shed during a game of hide and seek (organised by Alan amongst the younger children in the street) and coerced her into performing oral sex. There had been a series of other incidents with younger children. None led to prosecution. Alan has now begun college and attends a course for young people with special needs. He feels this will help him as he can "get himself a girlfriend". He appears to involve himself particularly with less able young women and there have been concerns about his inappropriate sexual behaviour in places such as the college cafeteria. Socially he is overbearing and risks being rejected by other students. Supervision has now been extended to the college setting. Staff report concerns about Alan's evident sexual interest in children when out in the community and he is often aggressive towards female staff in particular. His sisters have remained living with his aunt and he has contact with them which is supervised by his aunt. Staff have been concerned at how tactile he is with his youngest sister (aged eleven years) in particular.

### *The G-MAP challenge group*

G-MAP has been developing group-work programmes for intellectually disabled adolescents for some years. Our clinical experience and reports in the literature suggest that although group-based treatment programmes can be an effective format for work with intellectually disabled adolescents, the programme content and process need to be geared to the learning needs of the participants. The application of the following principles have enhanced the effectiveness of our practice with this client group:

- Reduce the number of messages per session or block of sessions and aim to produce these as simple verbal and/or visual statements.
- Ensure that each session's message is explicit (for example: "This session's topic is 'How can I spot a risky thought?' ").
- Regularly reinforce session messages.
- Check message retention by returning to the topic, or using spot checks, or by asking the young person to explain the message to others, or apply it to a suggested scenario.
- Use concrete examples that are meaningful to the young person and his everyday life using real places, people and situations.
- Identify desirable versus negative behaviours and promote clear labelling of behaviour by agreed language and self-talk.
- Aim to promote a model of healthy sexual expression rather than

| Area of input | Desired outcomes | Area of input | Desired outcomes |
|---|---|---|---|
| **1. Offence specific work**<br>• Pathway into abuse<br>• Distorted thinking<br>• Consequences<br>• Victim awareness<br>• Sexual thoughts/fantasies (nature; frequency; intensity)<br>• Influences on arousal pattern (e.g. mood states)<br>• Identification of risk (situational/internal)<br>• Self-management of risk | • Establish links between past & present: connections/exploring unexplored areas of life.<br>• Education process: boundaries; consent; consequences.<br>• Clarify arousal pattern.<br>• Behavioural methods & tools to decrease deviant arousal & thoughts.<br>• Monitoring: openness; honesty; internal risk awareness.<br>• Create open dialogue between Alan & care staff. | **4. Participation/motivation**<br>• Denial (acceptance; honesty; openness)<br>• Motivation<br>• Locus of control<br>• Anxiety<br>• Learning disability<br>• Communication skills<br>• Behavioural (ADHD)<br>• Trauma (PTSD)<br>• Mental health | • To be totally honest about arousal & sexual thoughts.<br>• Techniques to lessen anxiety (breathing techniques; positive feedback).<br>• Reduce anxiety linked with issues of sexual arousal & behaviour by proving potential for new directions.<br>• Therapists' style & materials sensitised to intellectual functioning/communication & retention skills.<br>• Aware of own abuse & family response (accommodation process).<br>• Mental health assessment. |
| **2. Family issues**<br>• Attachment issues<br>• Coping styles<br>• Safe care/protection<br>• Level of participation (e.g. information giving; supportive; fully participative) | • Family involvement in training process.<br>• Family involvement in planning & treatment goals.<br>• Frequent feedback & communication.<br>• Practical issues: contact & problems arising (family chaos and conflict; Alan's contact with sisters).<br>• Engaging family in supporting core messages. | **5. Social functioning**<br>• Self-esteem<br>• Assertiveness<br>• Intimacy/perspective taking<br>• Core social skills<br>• Problem solving skills<br>• Self-care skills<br>• Education/occupation<br>• Activities<br>• Networks/ friendships | • Positive attitude of staff: conflicting needs – empowering v. controlling.<br>• College course/social network/self-care skills/activities/holidays.<br>• Employment & role in self-image/self-esteem.<br>• Empowerment through behavioural techniques and application across settings.<br>• Working on compatibility with other clients in accommodation. |
| **3. Sexuality**<br>• Experience<br>• Knowledge<br>• Sexual scripts<br>• Orientation<br>• Masculinity<br>• Relationship skills<br>• Sexual abuse experiences | • Sex education programme.<br>• Understanding relationships with peers: roles; gender; steps towards intimacy.<br>• Understanding own abuse and impact on his life. | **6. Non-sexual conduct problems**<br>• Anger/violence<br>• Impulsivity<br>• Non-sexual criminality<br>• Substance misuse | • Behavioural programme based on positive reinforcement re: anger management. |

*Figure 13.1* G-MAP intervention planner – Alan.

exclusively focusing on the elimination or suppression of problematic sexual behaviours.

- Emphasise the importance of the identification of risk and the use of others to support self-management strategies.
- Emphasise consequences for individuals that are meaningful as opposed to promoting emphatic concern as the main motivation for change.
- Deliver the programme through a variety of participative, active and multi-sensory techniques to maximise interest and engagement, ensuring that you link emotion to learning.
- Mark and celebrate small gains.
- Develop a group culture where high status is achieved by participation which is reinforced for the young person through positive feedback.
- Link progress in all areas to self-management skills.
- Develop group rituals and icons for positive behaviour.
- Emphasise the negative consequences of sexually abusive behaviour for the group participant and not victim.
- Set realistic timescales for delivery of a specific component and allow flexibility so that you can stay with it until you have delivered it adequately.
- Allow a lot of behavioural rehearsal through role play.
- Design resources that allow participants to continue to learn from the intervention programme outside of the therapeutic setting (for example, provide take-home folders, exercises, posters and reminder cards).
- Brief carers on how to use these resources and ensure they are familiar with the key messages you are trying to deliver to the young person.

In designing the G-MAP group programme for young men with intellectual disabilities and problematic sexual behaviour, known as the Challenge Group, we developed a modular structure with the following eleven programme blocks: (1) Beginning the group. (2) Sexual development. (3) What is sexual abuse. (4) Four steps to abusive behaviour. (5) Old life/new life. (6) The consequences of sexual abuse. (7) Communication. (8) Relationships with others. (9) Staying safe/staying in control. (10) Being assertive/coping with anger. (11) Making choices.

The core messages of the group concern taking responsibility for sexual behaviour problems, being honest and being respectful of others. Concurrent individual work is a requirement of the group programme and is provided by members of the G-MAP clinical team. Throughout each topic block the link with individual therapy is focused around three questions. These are (a) How does this help me understand my sexual behaviour problem? (b) How can I get better at this or learn more about it? and (c) How will this help me better manage my sexual behaviour problem? The ethos of the group is supportive rather than confrontational and group members are encouraged to bring current issues for consideration and advice. Given the general social isolation, low self-esteem and experience of rejection and exclusion by peers common to these young men, the group is generally valued highly. Typical comments by participants include "it's safe here", "nobody picks on you" and "you can say what your problem is".

Group rules are very important; they provide boundaries that ensure participants feel safe, and encourage participation. In the Challenge Group the following rules are applied. (1) No name-calling. (2) Don't be rude to each other. (3) Let people finish what they are saying. (4) We all listen to each other. (5) No swearing. (6) No bullying. (7) Say what you want to say. (8) Try your best. (8) Say if you find it difficult. (9) Group things are confidential. (10) Try to be honest.

In the Challenge Group activities are dynamic and interactive with use of expressive mediums such as role-play, video, sculpting, games, drawing and collage. Group leaders join in many of the activities, particularly fun games aimed solely at warm-up and tension release. For any given programme module group leaders frequently provide the initial role-plays. Group members then vote on what they have seen in the role plays (for example they may be asked to judge whether the behaviours that were role played were OK, not OK, or if they fall into a "not sure" category). Although activities that involve physical movement are encouraged for their benefit in promoting client participation (for example "voting" is by running to labelled corners of the room), they do not involve touch between group members. Where text is used there is an emphasis on clear and simple language (such as, "what helps or does not help in managing anger").

Group members have portfolios with sections for each of the programme blocks. They save their work in this along with summaries of the key points from sessions. These are then reviewed and elaborated within individual sessions and made accessible to carers. At the outset of a topic block each participant commits to a relevant behavioural goal (for example, to improve their relationship with a particular individual). At the outset of each session group members provide feedback on how they have progressed with their goal. Each topic block lasts for six weeks and the concluding session is attended by the young person's carer. Group members take a lead in presenting what the group has learned from the topic block and group members' individual therapists participate in this group process. There are breaks during which the individual workers and group members work individually to consider specific issues such as what the young person has gained from the block and targets for the next block.

Topic blocks are designed as self-standing modules. New group members can enter at the outset of a programme block and progress through all modules from this point. The group is seen as only one intervention component that is part of a broader intervention plan. It may be used during the early stages of individual therapeutic intervention, or after a considerable amount of individual therapy has meant that a young person is now functioning at a level where they can gain from the group. There is very limited focus within the group on the group members' own offences, though all group members provide summaries of their offending behaviour.

While active participation in the group is likely to be a positive indicator, progress is defined by demonstrable change on a number of individual targets that are set and monitored outside of the group. The group provides the young person with experiences and messages that are aimed at being supportive of individual therapy and general goals. The group process allows these to be delivered by more dynamic methods than individual therapy, facilitates behavioural rehearsal (particularly of social and interpersonal skills) and aims to support and promote motivation. In the following section we will look at two specific skills developed in our group: developing a sense of a new life characterised by positive goals, and developing skills for the self-management of risk.

### *New Life/Old Life*

The organising concept for the development of positive personal goals in the group is that of New Life/Old Life (see Figure 13.2). Haaven and Coleman (1990) pioneered the concept of New Me/Old Me as a framework for engaging intellectually disabled sexual offenders to identify positive, concrete and achievable goals. This was linked to self-talk statements associated with Old Me behaviours and corresponding New Life self-statements. All therapeutic work within the community, in this programme, was linked to the concept of assisting the individual achieve his New Me. Recently there has been considerable interest in employing such "success orientated" paradigms into work with adult sexual offenders to heighten their motivation.

In adapting this concept for use with intellectually disabled adolescents we wished to use it in a dynamic manner that facilitated the following:

- Recognition that change is an ongoing process that allows incidents of Old Life behaviours not to lead to a sense of hopelessness but provide an

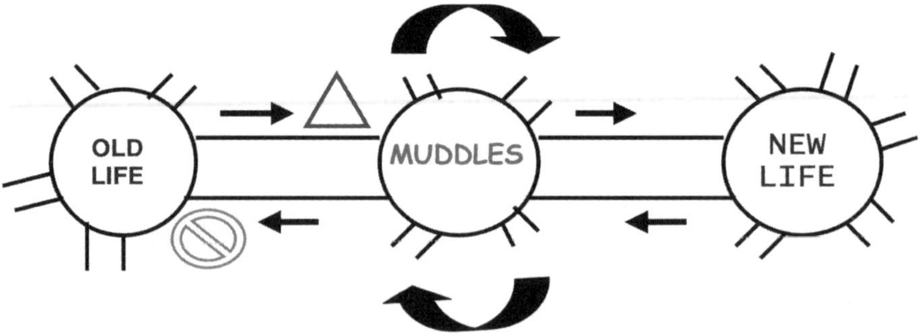


*Figure 13.2* My road map to a new life.

opportunity for participants to reaffirm their positive goals and learn from the occurrence of negative and risky behaviours.
- Through use of a New Life rather than a New Me concept, acknowledgement that others, such as family members and carers, have a significant role to play in shaping the quality of a young person's life and will need to contribute to the change process.
- Provision of a method for clearly labelling negative Old Life and positive New Life behaviours.
- Monitoring of progress by young people in the programme.
- Exploration of ideas and behaviours that young people struggle to label as reflecting either Old or New Life.

The resulting concept of a "Roadway to New Life" (see Figure 13.2) allows for the inclusion of a "Muddle Round-About" which is the area used by young people to explore issues that generate confusion such as response to sexual interests in peers, feelings regarding individuals who have abused them and difficulties with honesty. "Roadsigns" are present on either lane of the motorway and are colour coded so that red signifies Old Life attitudes and behaviours while blue indicates New Life. Typical Old Life signs signal "lying", "not listening" and "no respect". Signs representing New Life attitudes and behaviours typically reflect "honesty", "taking control" and "asking for help".

It is important that young people have a clear vision of their New Life. To facilitate this they are asked to produce posters, collages and paintings depicting Old and New Life. Typically the Old Life work young people produce depicts feelings of loss, pain and restriction expressed through images of sadness, abuse, bullying, rejection, rules and supervision. Police, prison and court also feature heavily, even when young people have not been subject to criminal processes given the fear of this as a consequence if they continue in Old Life behaviours. New Life imagery often involves improved relationships with family, acceptance by peers, freedom from restrictions and success in education, work or material possessions. It is important to develop a New Life concept that is meaningful and has gains rather than emphasising the loss of a desired inappropriate activity such as sexual contact with children. Carers need to be involved with the ongoing development of this concept and responsive to opportunities to develop positive and safe interests. For example, Michael (a pseudonym) is a seventeen-year-old with Asperger's syndrome who is attracted to very young boys and has assaulted a number of them in the community. Given his level of attraction his New Life plan necessarily requires components that involve limiting his contact with children. Michael ostensibly has commited to this but persistently begins to subvert his "child free" New Life plan and introduce opportunities for contact with children (for example, by moving from a plan of having a cat for company to breeding cats and selling the kittens door to door). At this stage Michael is not fully committed to a New Life plan which avoids offending opportunities and we have found detailed work on New Life plans are one effective way of evaluating motivation.

Through the course of the group, other modules will feed into the New Life plan and group members will identify specific targets such as New Life *relationships* ("I will not argue with my mum so much"), New Life *communication* ("I will talk to my key-worker when I feel upset") and New Life *assertions* ("I will say when I don't like something").

### *Promoting risk management*

A primary role of individual therapy and group-work is the reduction of problematic sexual behaviours through the development of self-management or relapse prevention (RP) skills. Risk of continuing sexual aggression may be conceptualised in three domains:

*Predisposing risks:* Such as traumatic sexualisation; attachment/intimacy/empathy problems; and difficulties with general social functioning.

*Precipitating risks:* Such as arousal; impulsivity; and opportunity.

*Perpetuating risks:* Such as lack of support or supervision; the absence of a model of healthy sexuality; and poor social and self-regulatory skills.

Overall progress may result from positive gains in all domains but self-management strategies are best if they focus on precipitating factors (for example, developing specific responses to high risk situations that are the immediate precursors to offending). Individuals with intellectual disabilities can develop self-management skills but require a framework that recognises and adapts to particular difficulties.

A useful approach towards promoting risk management skills is the introduction of the "Toolkit" (see Figure 13.3). This is introduced in the group programme. The toolkit is a series of self-management principles which young people are taught. They can use them to take responsibility for their problem behaviours. They can also use them to elicit help from others in managing risk. The toolkit comprises a series of six icons which the young men have available within their own portfolios and on wallet cards. Each icon represents one of the following:

1 *Danger* (identifying dangerous situations or thoughts).
2 *Stop* (any activity that is increasing risk or is wrong).
3 *Escape* (get out of risky situations).
4 *Talk* (go to someone and discuss your risky behaviour).
5 *Listen* (to what they say or to your own safe thoughts).
6 *Think* (about what is said).

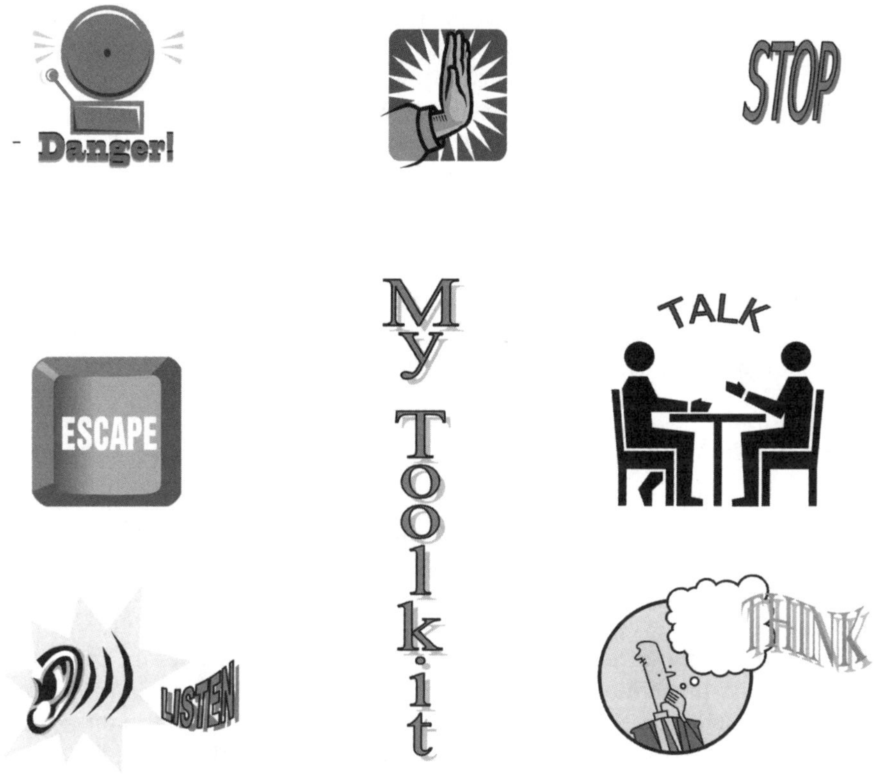


*Figure 13.3* The toolkit.

Our clinical experience supports an emphasis on designing clear behavioural targets, which can be measured by family, carers or other involved professionals in a variety of settings. Self-management of risk is premised on a number of factors including an appreciation of the process leading up to offending; the ability to consistently label risky thoughts and behaviours as such; strategies to intervene and escape from risky situations; and the motivation to do so.

Many young people are subject to high levels of supervision. There is often considerable anxiety about this being reduced and the individual being allowed any unsupervised access within the community or settings in which there may be potential victims such as school or college. Decisions for reducing supervision need to be based upon evidence of skills being transferred from therapeutic to community settings. Such evidence comes from observations made during behavioural rehearsal and observations of young people's capacity to use a variety of risk management strategies in their day-to-day lives. Therapists may accompany young people in community settings and review directly with them their ability to identify risky situations.

In addition, young people may be helped to design reminder cards which can act as cues for using risk reduction strategies. These are then produced in a laminated "credit card" format and can be carried everywhere and read in potentially risky situations. It is also useful to help young people produce individualised diary sheets or logs so that they can self-monitor aspects of risk management. Young people may also be encouraged to produce visual resources, such as posters, which convey messages about using self-management skills, and they may then place these in their rooms as reminders. Considerable weight is given to the role and observations of carers and key workers who have frequent contact with the young people. They are best placed to both reinforce and evaluate the extent to which young people have retained and applied self-management skills in community settings.

## Conclusions

This chapter has outlined the need for the promotion of specialised approaches to help young people with intellectual disabilities who develop sexually abusive behaviour problems to effectively address their difficulties. A comprehensive framework for assessment is required which, on the one hand, takes account of the competencies and constraints associated with this population and, on the other, covers a wide range of factors relevant to sexual abuse and its prevention. A variety of intervention programmes have been developed including those which focus on modification of deviant sexual arousal; those based on applied behavioural analysis; those which take a group skills training approach; multi-component programmes; and programmes that explicitly address relapse prevention. Lessons learned from all of these approaches and from the assessment literature have been incorporated into the G-MAP programme. A comprehensive assessment process is used in this programme to identify specific areas of need and potential strengths. An individualised plan is developed for each programme participant. Overall intervention packages usually include both direct treatment components and other indirect interventions and supports. The Challenge Group is typically a central part of most G-MAP intervention packages. This group incorporates a series of six-week modules on a range of themes including sexual development, sexual abuse, goal setting using an old life/new life framework, relationships with others, anger management and self-management risk reduction skills. The programme facilitates risk reduction by helping young people develop positive life goals and skills for recognising and coping with potentially abusive behaviour within a context of support and monitoring by key individuals in the young person's life such as family and carers. Further work is needed to develop user-friendly frameworks for practice, and to evaluate the effectiveness of intervention.

## References and Bibliography


Allam, J., and Browne, K. (1998). Evaluating community-based treatment programmes for men who sexually abuse children. *Child Abuse Review, 7*, 13–29.

Allam, J., Middleton, D., and Browne, K. (1997). Different clients, different needs? Practice issues in community based treatment for sex offenders. *Criminal Behaviour and Mental Health, 7*, 69–84.

Bancroft, J. (1989). *Human Sexuality and Its Problems.* London: Churchill Livingstone.

Barber, J. D. (1992). Relapse prevention and the need for brief social interventions. *Journal of Substance Abuse Treatment, 9*, 157–158.

Beail, N., and Warden, S. (1995). Sexual abuse of adults with a learning disability. *Journal of Intellectual Disability Research, 39(5)*, 382–387.

Beckett, R. (1999). *The Latest Research on Young Abusers.* Paper presented to Info-log Conference: Young Abusers: The Hidden Crime of Children who Sexually Abuse Children. Royal Overseas House, Park Place, London, 5 October 1999.

Beckett, R., Beech, A., Fisher, D., and Fordham, A. (1994). *Community-Based Treatment for Sex Offenders: An Evaluation of Seven Treatment Programmes.* London: Home Office.

Bentovim, A., and Williams, B. (1998). Children and adolescents: victims who become perpetrators. *Advances in Psychiatric Treatment, 4*, 101–107.

Brown, H. (1997). Introduction to special issue on sexuality. *Journal of Applied Research in Intellectual Disabilities, 10(2)*, 80–82.

Brown, H., and Barrett, S. (1994). Understanding and responding to difficult sexual behaviour. In A. Craft (ed.), *Practice Issues in Sexuality and Learning Disabilities.* London: Routledge.

Brown, H., Stein, J., and Turk, V. (1995). The sexual abuse of adults with learning disabilities: Report of a second two-year incidence survey. *Mental Handicap Research, 8(1)*, 3–24.

Cambridge, P. (1997). At whose risk? Priorities and conflicts for policy development in HIV and learning disability. *Journal of Applied Research in Intellectual Disabilities, 10(2)*, 83–104.

Cambridge, P., and McCarthy, M. (1997). Developing and implementing sexuality policy for a learning disability provider service. *Health and Social Care in the Community, 5(4)*, 227–236.

Carr, E. G., and Durand, V. M. (1985). Reducing behaviour problems through functional communication training. *Journal of Applied Behaviour Analysis, 18*, 111–126.

Carrell, S. (1993). *Group Exercises for Adolescents: A Manual for Therapists.* London: Sage.

Charman, T., and Clare, I. (1992). An education group for male sexual offenders with mild mental handicaps. *Mental Handicap, 20*, 74–80.

Clare, I. (1993). Issues in the assessment and treatment of the male sex offender with mild learning disabilities. *Journal of Sexual and Marital Therapy, 8(2)*, 167–180.

Clare, I., and Gudjonsson, G. H. (1993). Interrogative suggestibility, confabulation, and acquiescence in people with mild learning disabilities (mental handicap): Implications for reliability during police investigations. *British Journal of Clinical Psychology, 32*, 295–301.

Cooke, L. B., and Sinason, V. (1998). Abuse of people with learning disabilities and other vulnerable adults. *Advances in Psychiatric Treatment, 4*, 119–125.

Coleman, E., and Haaven, J. (1998). Adult intellectually disabled sexual offenders: Program considerations. In W. Marshall, Y. A. Fernandez, S. Hudson and T. Ward (eds), *Sourcebook of Treatment Programs for Sexual Offenders*. New York: Plenum.

Corbett, A. (1996). The role of attachment in working with people with learning disabilities who commit sexual offences. *NAPSAC Bulletin*, March, 14–17.

Corbett, A. (1996). *Trinity of Pain: Therapeutic Responses to People with Learning Disabilities who Commit Sexual Offences*. London: Respond.

Cormack, E. (1993). Group therapy with adults with learning disabilities who have sexually offended. *Groupwork, 6(2)*, 162–176.

Cox-Lindenbaum, D., and Lindenbaum, L. (1994). A modality for treating aggressive behaviours and sexual disorders in people with mental retardation. In N. Bouras (ed.), *Mental Health and Mental Retardation: Recent Advances and Practices*. Cambridge: Cambridge University Press.

Craissati, J., and McClurg, G. (1997). The challenge project: A treatment program evaluation for perpetrators of child sexual abuse. *Child Abuse and Neglect, 21(7)*, 637–648.

Crawford, D. (1984). Behaviour therapy. In M. Craft and A. Craft (eds), *Mentally Abnormal Offenders*. London: Bailliere Tindal.

Cullen, C. (1993). The treatment of people who offend. In K. Howells and H. Hollin (eds), *Clinical Approaches to the Mentally Disordered Offender*. London: Wiley.

Davidson, G. C., and Neal, J. M. (1990). *Abnormal Psychology*, 5th edn. New York: Wiley.

Day, K. (1993). Crime and mental retardation. In K. Howells and H. Hollin (eds), *Clinical Approaches to the Mentally Disordered Offender*. London: Wiley.

Day, K. (1994). Characteristics, management and treatment of mentally handicapped sex offenders. In *Mentally Handicapped Sex Offenders: A Symposium*. Supported by Schering Health Care. Merit.

Day, K. (1994). Male mentally handicapped sex offenders. *British Journal of Psychiatry, 165*, 630–639.

Demetral, G. D. (1994). Diagrammatic assessment of ecological integration of sex offenders with mental retardation in community residential facilitates. *Mental Retardation, 32*, 141–145.

Department of Health and the Home Office (1992). *Review of Health and Social Services for Mentally Disordered Offenders and Others Requiring Similar Services. Final Report Summary (The Reed Committee Report)*. London: HMSO.

Dolan, M., Holloway, J., Bailey, S., and Kroll, L. (1996). The psychosocial characteristics of juvenile sexual offenders. *Medicine, Science and the Law, 36(4)*, 342–352.

Dowrick, P. W., and Ward, K. M. (1997). Video feedforward in the support of a man with intellectual disability and inappropriate sexual behaviour. *Journal of Intellectual and Developmental Disability, 22(3)*, 147–160.

Doyle, P., and Gooch, T. (1995). The mentally handicapped as offenders. In *Mentally Handicapped Sex Offenders: A Symposium*. Supported by Schering Health Care. Merit.

Emerson, E. (2001). *Challenging Behaviour: Analysis and Intervention in People with Severe Learning Disabilities*. Cambridge: Cambridge University Press.

Epps, K. J. (1991). The residential treatment of adolescent sex offenders. In

M. McMurran and C. McDougall (eds), *Proceedings of the DCLP First Annual Conference. Issues in Criminological and Legal Psychology, 17(1)*, Leicester: British Psychological Society.

Epps, K. J. (1996). Sexually abusive behaviour in an adolescent boy with the 48, XXYY syndrome: A case study. *Criminal Behaviour and Mental Health, 6*, 137–146.

Fairburn, G., Rowley, D., and Bowen, M. (1995). *Sexuality, Learning Difficulties and Doing What's Right*. London: David Fulton.

Farmer, E., and Pollock, S. (1998). *Sexually Abused and Abusing Children in Substitute Care*. New York: Wiley.

Finkelhor, D. (ed.) (1984). *Child Sexual Abuse: New Theory and Research*. New York: Free Press.

Fisher, D., and McGregor, G. (1997). Behavioural treatment techniques. In M. Hoghughi, S. R. Bhate, and F. Graham (eds), *Working with Sexually Abusive Adolescents*. London: Sage.

Gardiner, M., Kelly, K., and Wilkinson, D. (1996). Groups for male sex offenders with learning disabilities. *NAPSAC Bulletin*, March, 3–6.

Griffiths, D., Hingsburger, D., and Christian, R. (1985). Treating developmentally handicapped sex offenders. *Psychiatric Aspects of Mental Retardation, 4(1)*, 49–52.

Griffiths, D., Quinsey, V., and Hingsburger, D. (1989). *Changing Inappropriate Sexual Behavior*. New York, Brookes.

Gross, G. (1985). *Activities of the Developmental Disabilities Adult Offender Project*. Olympia, WA: Washington State Developmental Disabilities Planning Council.

Haaven, J., and Coleman, E. (2000). Treatment of the developmentally disabled sex offender. In D. R. Laws, S. M. Hudson and T. Ward (eds), *Remaking Relapse Prevention with Sex Offenders: A Sourcebook*. Thousand Oaks, CA: Sage.

Haaven, J., Little, R., and Petre-Miller, D. (1990). *Treating Learning Disabled Sex Offenders: A Model Residential Programme*. Orwell, VT: Safer Society Press.

Hames, A. (1987). Sexual offences involving children: A suggested treatment for adolescents with mild mental handicap. *Mental Handicap, 15*, 19–21.

Hawkes, C., Jenkins, J., and Vizard, E. (1997). Roots of sexual violence in children and adolescents. In V. Varma (ed.), *Violence in Children and Adolescents*. London: Jessica Kingsley.

Hayes, S. (1991). Sex offenders. *Australia and New Zealand Journal of Developmental Disabilities, 172*, 221–227.

Hedderman, C., and Sugg, D. (1996). *Does Treating Sex Offending Reduce Reoffending?* Home Office Research and Statistics Directorate, No. 45. London: Home Office.

Herzog, D., and Money, J. (1993). Sexology and social work in the case of Klinefelters (47 XXY) syndrome. *Mental Retardation, 3(3)*, 161–162.

Hird, J. (1997). Working in context. In H. Hoghughi, S. R. Bhate and F. Graham (eds), *Working with Sexually Abusive Adolescents*. London: Routledge.

HM Inspectorate of Probation (1998). *Exercising Constant Vigilance: The Role of the Probation Service in Protecting the Public from Sex Offenders. Report of a Thematic Inspection*. London: Home Office.

Home Office (1990). *Circular 66/90: Provisions for Mentally Disordered Offenders*. London: Home Office.

Home Office (1995). *Statistics of Mentally Disordered Offenders: England and Wales 1994*. London: Home Office.

Humel, P., Ashcroft, W., Blessman, F., and Anders, O. (1993). Sexually aggressive acts of an adolescent with Klinefelter Syndrome. *Uprax-Kinderpsychologie-Kinderpsychiatrie, 42(4)*, 132–138.

Jones, A. M., and Bonnar, S. (1996). Group psychotherapy with learning disabled adults. *British Journal of Learning Disability, 24*, 65–69.

Klimecki, M., Jenkinson, J., and Wilson, L. (1994). A study of recidivism amongst offenders with an intellectual disability. *Australia and New Zealand Journal of Developmental Disabilities, 19*, 209–219.

Knopp, F. H. (1990). Introduction. In J. Haaven, R. Little and D. Petre-Miller (eds), *Treating Intellectually Disabled Sex Offenders*. Orwell, VT: Safer Society Press.

Kolvin, I. (1967). Aversive imagery treatment in adolescents. *Behaviour Research and Therapy, 5*, 245–248.

Lindsay, W. R. (2002). Integration of recent reviews on offenders with intellectual disabilities. *Journal of Applied Research in Intellectual Disabilities, 15*, 111–119.

Lindsay, W. R., Neilson, C. Q., Morrison, F., and Smith, A. H. (1998). The treatment of six men with a learning disability convicted of sex offences against children. *British Journal of Clinical Psychology, 37*, 83–98.

Lindsay, W. R., Smith, A. H. W., Law, J., Quinn, K., Anderson, A., Smith A., Overend, T., and Allan, R. (2002). A treatment service for sex offenders and abusers with intellectual disability: Characteristics of referrals and evaluation. *Journal of Applied Research in Intellectual Disabilities, 15*, 166 –174.

Lisak, D., and Ivan, C. (1995). Deficits in intimacy and empathy in sexually aggressive men. *Journal of Interpersonal Violence, 10(3)*, 296–308.

Lund, C. A. (1992). Long-term treatment of sexual problems in adolescent and adult developmentally disabled persons. *Annals of Sexual Research, 5*, 5–31.

McCarthy, M., and Thompson, D. (1997). A prevalence study of sexual abuse of adults with intellectual disabilities referred for sex education. *Journal of Applied Research in Intellectual Disability, 10(2)*, 105–124.

Malekoff, A. (1997). *Group Work with Adolescents: Principles and Practice*. New York: Guilford Press.

Mishna, F. (1996). In their own words: Therapeutic factors for adolescents who have learning disabilities. *International Journal of Group Psychotherapy, 46(2)*, 265–273.

Monk, E., and New, M. (1996). *Report of a Study of Sexually Abused Children and Adolescents, and of Young Perpetrators of Sexual Abuse who were Treated in Voluntary Agency Community Facilities*. London: Department of Health, HMSO.

Murphy, G. (1997). Treatment and risk management. In J. Churchill, H. Brown, A. Craft and C. Horrocks (eds), *There Are No Easy Answers*. Nottingham: ARC/NAPSAC.

Murphy, W. D., Coleman. E. M., and Haynes, M. R. (1983). Treatment and evaluation issues with the mentally retarded sex offender. In J. G. Greer and I. R. Stuart (eds), *The Sexual Aggressor: Current Perspectives in Treatment*. New York: Van Nostrand Reinholt.

Murrey, G. H., Briggs, D., and Davies, C. (1992). Psychopathically disordered, mentally ill and mentally handicapped sex offenders: A comparative study. *Medicine, Science and the Law, 32*, 331–336.

Noelly, D., Muccigrosso, L., and Zigman, E. (1996). Treatment successes with mentally retarded sex offenders. In E. Coleman, S. M. Dwyer and N. J. Palone (eds),

*Sex Offender Treatment: Biological Dysfunction, Intrapsychic Conflict, Interpersonal Violence*. New York: Haworth Press.

O'Callaghan, D. (1999). Young abusers with learning disabilities: Towards better understanding and positive intervention. In M. Calder (ed.), *Working with Young People who Sexually Abuse: New Pieces of the Jigsaw*. Lyme Regis: Russell House.

O'Callaghan, D. (2002a). Providing a research informed service for young people who sexually harm others. In M. Calder (ed.), *Young People who Sexually Abuse: Building an Evidence Base for Your Practice*. Brighton: Russell House.

O'Callaghan, D. (2002b) A framework for undertaking assessment of young people with intellectual disabilities who present problematic/harmful sexual behaviours. In *Working with Children and Young People who Display Sexually Harmful Behaviour: Assessment Manual*. The AIM Project

O'Callaghan, D., and Print, B. (1994). Adolescent sexual abusers: Research, assessment and treatment. In T. Morrison, M. Erooga and R. Beckett (eds), *Sexual Offending Against Children*. London: Routledge.

O'Connor, W. (1996). A problem solving intervention for sex offenders with an intellectual disability. *Journal of Intellectual and Developmental Disability, 21(3)*, 219–235.

O'Connor, W. (1997). Towards an environmental perspective on intervention for problem sexual behaviour in people with an intellectual disability. *Journal of Applied Research in Intellectual Disabilities, 10(2)*, 159–175.

Parkin, W., and Green, L. (1994). Sexuality and residential care: Research in progress. Paper presented at the British Sociological Association Annual Conference. *Sexualities in Context*. University of Central Lancashire, 28–31 March.

Perry, B. D. (1994). Neurobiological sequelae of childhood trauma: PTSD in children. In M. Murry (ed.), *Catcholamines in Post-Traumatic Stress Disorder: Emerging Concepts*. Washington, DC: American Psychiatric Press.

Pithers, W. D. (1990). Relapse prevention with sexual aggressors: Method of enhancing therapeutic gain and enhancing external supervision. In W. L Marshall, D. R. Laws and H. E. Barbaree (eds), *Handbook of Sexual Assault: Theories and Treatment of the Offender*. New York: Plenum.

Riding, T. M. (1999). An abuse of disability? Assessing treatment outcome in sexual offenders with learning disabilities. *Journal of Learning Disabilities for Nursing, Health and Social Care, 3(4)*, 188–193.

Rose, J., and O'Connor, C. R. (1998). Sexual offending and abuse perpetrated by men with learning disabilities: An integration of current research concerning assessment and treatment. *Journal of Learning Disabilities for Nursing, Health and Social Care, 2(1)*, 31–38.

Rose, J., Jenkins, R., O'Connor, C., Jones, C., and Felce, D. (2002). A group treatment for men with intellectual disabilities who sexually offend or abuse. *Journal of Applied Research in Intellectual Disabilities, 15*, 138–150.

Schilling, R. F., and Shinke, S. P. (1989). Mentally retarded sex offenders, fact, fiction and treatment. *Journal of Social Work and Human Sexuality, 7*, 33–48.

Segal, Z. V., and Stermac, L. E. (1990). The role of cognition in sexual assault. In W. L. Marshall, D. R Laws and H. E Barbaree (eds), *Handbook of Sexual Assault: Theories and Treatment of the Offender*. New York: Plenum.

Sigelman, C. K., Budd, E. D., Winer, J. L., Schoenrock, C. J., and Martin, W. (1982).

Evaluating alternative techniques of questioning mentally retarded persons. *American Journal of Mental Deficiency, 86(5)*, 511–518.

Sobsey, D. (1994). Sexual abuse of individuals with a learning disability. In A. Craft (ed.), *Practice Issues in Sexuality and Learning Disabilities*. London: Routledge.

Stanley, P. D., Dai, Y., and Nolan, R. F. (1997). Differences in depression and self-esteem reported by learning disabled and behaviour disordered middle school students. *Journal of Adolescence, 20*, 219–222.

Sulzer-Azaroff, B., and Mayer, G. R. (1991). *Behavior Analysis for Lasting Change*. Fort Worth: Holt, Rinehart and Winston.

Swanson, C. K., and Garwick, G. B. (1990). Treatment for low functioning sex offenders: group therapy and interagency co-ordination. *Mental Retardation, 28(3)*, 155–161.

Taylor, J. (1996). The sex offender with a learning disability: the role of psychological therapies and counselling. *Journal of the APLD, 12(4)*, 11–21.

Thomas, D. H., and Singh, T. H. (1995). Offenders referred to a learning disability service: A retrospective study from one county. *British Journal of Learning Disability, 23*, 24–27.

Thompson, D. (1997). Profiling the sexually abusive behaviour of men with intellectual disabilities. *Journal of Applied Research in Intellectual Disabilities, 10(2)*, 125–139.

Thompson, D., and Brown, H. (1997). Men with intellectual disabilities who abuse: A review of the literature. *Journal of Applied Research in Intellectual Disabilities, 10(2)*, 140–158.

Thompson, D., and Brown, H. (1998). *Response-ability: Working with Men with Learning Disabilities who have Difficult or Abusive Sexual Behaviours*. Brighton: Pavilion.

Thompson, D., Clare, I., and Brown, H. (1997). Not such an "ordinary" relationship: The role of women support staff in relation to men with learning disabilities who have difficult sexual behaviour. *Disability and Society, 12(4)*.

Verberne, G. (1990). Treatment of sexually deviant behaviours in mildly mentally retarded adults. In A. Dosen, A. Van Gennep and J. Zwanikkeen (eds), *Treatment of Mental Illness and Behavioural Disorders in the Mentally Retarded*. Leiden: Logon.

Vizard, E. (2000). *Characteristics of a British Sample of Sexually Abusive Children*. Keynote presentation to the BASPCAN National Congress, University of York, September.

Withers, P. S., and Gaskell, S. L. (1998). A cognitive-behavioural intervention to address inappropriate masturbation in a boy with mild learning disabilities. *British Journal of Learning Disabilities, 26(2)*, 58–61.

Wright, G., Herzog, D., and Seymour, J. (1992). Treatment of a constellation of inappropriate sexual and social behaviours in a 20-year-old man with Down's syndrome. *Sexuality and Disability, 10*, 57–61.

Chapter 14

# Bridging the gender gap

## Addressing juvenile females who commit sexual offences

*Nancy Halstenson Bumby and Kurt M. Bumby*

What are little boys made of, made of?
What are little boys made of?
Snips and snails and puppy dogs' tails.
And that's what little boys are made of.

What are little girls made of, made of?
What are little girls made of?
Sugar and spice, and all that's nice.
And that's what little girls are made of.
(*The Real Mother Goose*, 1916)

As reflected in the age-old and familiar poem, stereotypical assumptions about fundamental differences between the genders have been long-standing and widespread. There is, however, a significant body of existing and continually evolving empirical literature within the medical and social sciences that supports the existence of gender differences across a variety of domains. It is this research, coupled with the popular press, that has, to some extent, fuelled an increased awareness and popularity of the examination of gender differences over the past several decades.

Within criminal and juvenile justice systems, however, the recognition of gender differences has ironically led to a significant dismissal and minimisation of female offenders. This has been in part due to perceptions that crimes committed by females are less serious, violent and harmful (Chesney-Lind and Shelden, 1998; Maniglia, 1996; 1998). Moreover, it is impossible to ignore the statistics reflecting males as primarily responsible for the vast majority of crimes perpetrated by both adults and juveniles (FBI, 2001). Recent crime data, however, has revealed a significant increase in the number of female offenders coming to the attention of law enforcement and child welfare agencies (FBI, 2001; Poe-Yamagata and Butts, 1996). Consequently, it has become increasingly difficult to continue the historical tendency to overlook the need for gender-specific programming in the criminal justice field, and in juvenile justice systems in particular.

From 1991 to 2000, arrests for juvenile males under eighteen years of age decreased by 3 per cent, yet there was a 25 per cent increase in arrests of juvenile females under age eighteen (FBI, 2001). While juvenile males are more likely to come to the attention of law enforcement for crimes against persons, property offences, and violent crimes, girls who enter the juvenile justice system are typically charged with status offences such as truancy, running away, under-age drinking, curfew violations and incorrigibility (Chesney-Lind and Shelden, 1998; Poe-Yamagata and Butts, 1996). Interestingly, it is almost exclusively juvenile females, not males, who are presented to juvenile authorities for certain types of sexual behaviours such as early sexual activity and sexual promiscuity, behaviour which is often perceived as incorrigibility by parents or guardians (Chesney-Lind, 1995; Chesney-Lind and Shelden, 1998). Indeed, the sexual behaviours of girls tend to be more closely scrutinised and frowned upon by parents and others in authority roles. Conversely, the sexual experiences and practices of boys are not only monitored less, but also implicitly and explicitly condoned (Chesney-Lind, 1995). Given the differential responses that suggest an unbalanced scrutiny of girls' sexual behaviours, it is both ironic and troubling that for decades sexually offending behaviours perpetrated by juvenile females have either escaped detection or been largely ignored.

A variety of hypotheses have been postulated regarding the failure to recognise and attend to female sexual offenders. First, it has been argued that, to some degree, there has existed a professional bias that sexual offences committed by females are not possible or are less serious or harmful (Elliott, 1993; Jennings, 1994). In addition, stereotyped views of female sexuality may serve to inhibit professionals' tendency to report potential abuse (National Adolescent Perpetrator Network (NAPN), 1993). Under-reporting by victims is believed to be a significant issue as well. For example, male victims may be hesitant or ashamed to acknowledge having been victimised by a female, perhaps fearing a reaction of disbelief. Female victims, too, may be unlikely to disclose female-perpetrated sexual abuse, due to the magnified trauma, additional socio-cultural stereotypes, and desire to avoid stigmas attached to same-gender victimisation (Allen, 1991; Elliott, 1993; Jennings, 1994). Yet another suggested factor that may contribute to both the identification and under-reporting of sexual abuse committed by females is the "legitimate" contact that accompanies certain care-giving activities such as bathing. This may blur the ability to recognise or define the contact as inappropriate (Allen, 1991; Elliott, 1993; Margolin, 1991; NAPN, 1993). Finally, and perhaps most influential, has been the historic perception that sexual offending is a "male only crime", a belief that is continually reinforced by statistics indicating that females account for a small percentage of all sexual offences committed (Allen, 1991; Elliott, 1993).

Recently, however, professionals in the child welfare, mental health and juvenile justice systems have anecdotally reported increases in adolescent females who have come to their attention for sexual behaviour problems. Indeed, it is now more commonly accepted that juvenile females may be responsible for a larger percentage of sexual offences than initially believed (Mathews *et al.*, 1997). Ten-year arrest trends from 1991 to 2000 corroborate these professional experiences and reports, reflecting a striking 23 per cent (22.8%) increase in arrests for sexual offences (excluding forcible rape and prostitution) perpetrated by females under the age of eighteen. Conversely, the number of juvenile males arrested for sexual offences parallels the downward trend in the arrest rate for juvenile male-perpetrated crimes in general, with a decrease of 6 per cent (6.2%) between 1991 and 2000 (FBI, 2001).

These statistics represent only the data provided by participating law enforcement agencies rather than total law enforcement agencies, and therefore reflect an underestimate of the true arrest rate nationwide. Further, the low prevalence rates may also be more indicative of the societal response to offending by females, which will be discussed later in this chapter. Nonetheless, estimations of absolute numbers, while relatively small, do in fact reflect a significant number of victims and subsequent impact. As such, the importance of attending to this population is evident.

## Characteristics and offence patterns

Within the sexual offender field, it was initially assumed that juvenile sexual offenders were simply a reflection of adult male offenders. However, as is demonstrated in the more contemporary literature, and as recognised elsewhere in this volume, juvenile male sexual offenders differ from adult offenders in significant ways (see Becker, 1998; Righthand and Welch, 2001). A similar error in logic would be to assume that juvenile female sexual offenders mirror juvenile male offenders across all domains. Consequently, it is critical to identify the various gender differences with respect to sexual offending, recognising that these distinctions will have important implications for effective prevention, intervention and management efforts.

Research on juvenile females who commit sexual offences remains limited. Much like their adolescent male counterparts, females who perpetrate are believed to be a relatively heterogeneous group. Notwithstanding, the available literature suggests both common and distinguishing characteristics. In one of the first contributions to the literature on adolescent female sexual offenders, Fehrenbach and Monastersky (1988) provided descriptive information on a sample of twenty-eight females who received outpatient services at a juvenile sexual offender treatment programme. Upon review of their offence patterns, it was revealed that these young women engaged in a range of sexually abusive acts against young children who were known to them (i.e. relatives or acquaintances), with the offences generally occurring in a care-giving (i.e. babysitting) context. Victims of both genders were targeted, although a greater overall proportion of the victims was female. The authors noted that these female perpetrators tended to lack a history of conduct-related difficulties outside of the exhibited sexual behaviour problems. Finally, a history of sexual maltreatment during childhood was identified for many of the females.

Similar characteristics were revealed in an examination of twelve adolescent female perpetrators in an inpatient psychiatric setting (Bumby and Bumby, 1993; 1997). More specifically, the females victimised both males and females, and with the exception of one perpetrator who targeted a same-aged peer during a sleepover, the sexually abusive acts occurred against children during care-giving activities. All of the female offenders in the sample were either related to or otherwise acquainted with their victims. None perpetrated against a stranger. The majority of the females in the sample evidenced significant social maladjustment, psychological disturbance, academic performance deficits, substance abuse, delinquency, previous maltreatment or family dysfunction. Given the nature of the setting, however, these co-morbid behavioural health, conduct and family issues were not particularly surprising. More remarkable, however, was that each of the female perpetrators in the sample had themselves experienced sexual victimisation, often beginning at an early age, by multiple perpetrators, both within and outside of their families.

In a more comprehensive investigation, Hunter *et al.* (1993) studied ten female sexual offenders in a residential treatment programme for youth with emotional and behavioural disturbances. Similar to the females in the previous research (Bumby and Bumby, 1993; Fehrenbach and Monastersky, 1988), these offenders were found to have victimised young children of both genders. In contrast, male victims were found to be more prevalent within this sample. Most of the targeted victims were young relatives or children with whom the offenders were acquainted, although a substantial proportion of the females perpetrated against strangers as well, a striking differentiation from the findings of previous researchers. Further, while earlier investigations were less clear with respect to chronicity or persistence, Hunter *et al.* (1993) identified repetitive acts of perpetration including fondling, oral sex, and more intrusive behaviours such as penetration against multiple victims. The use of force was also reported by a significant proportion of the female offender sample. It was further revealed that the majority of the females fantasised about the offending behaviours, with such fantasies often preceding the offences. Taken together, these findings led the authors to suggest that the female offenders were not simply acting solely out of curiosity or experimentation.

Consistent with their residential placement, but nonetheless significant, the female offenders in the Hunter *et al.* (1993) study evidenced behavioural health concerns as well as extensive and long-standing histories of sexual and other maltreatment. Many of the girls reported having been sexually victimised by multiple offenders, both male and female, who were either related or otherwise known to them. These victimisation experiences tended to begin at an early age and were generally quite intrusive, with the presence of force commonly reported. Further, most of the girls reported experiencing both eroticism and psychological distress on at least one occasion during victimisation. Subsequently, Hunter *et al.* (1993) suggested an aetiological link between the early onset of extensive and long-standing sexual victimisation, the experiencing of pronounced but psychologically disturbing sexual arousal during one or more of the sexual victimisation experiences, and the development of sexually offending behaviours of adolescent females. Overall, based on the descriptive data, the female offenders appeared similar to male adolescent offenders in terms of the deliberateness and persistence of the offending behaviours, targeting of both male and female victims, the suspected development of deviant interests for some, and a strong association between prior victimisation and resultant offending.

To more systematically compare gender differences and adolescent sexual offenders, Mathews *et al.* (1997) examined data on sixty-seven female juvenile sexual offenders in community-based and residential treatment programmes and seventy juvenile male sexual offenders referred for community-based or residential treatment. The majority of both female and male offenders had a history of prior mental health treatment, nearly half had experienced suicidal ideation or attempts, and approximately one-third of both samples evidenced runaway behaviours. Both groups experienced childhood maltreatment, although a substantially greater percentage of the female offenders had been subjected to such abuse. More specifically, while less than half of the males had been physically abused, approximately 60 per cent of the females were previously subjected to physical maltreatment. Gender differences were most remarkable with respect to history of sexual victimisation. The overwhelming majority of the female offenders (78%) had experienced sexual victimisation, compared to only 34 per cent of their male counterparts. Furthermore, relative to the males, the females in the sample were generally victimised beginning at an earlier age, had been targeted by more than one abuser, experienced abuse by both a male and female perpetrator, and were subjected to use of force or aggression during the sexual assault(s). It was noted that the families of the juveniles were disruptive and chaotic, suggesting increased potential for attachment difficulties and a detrimental impact on the development of a sense of self.

In terms of the offence behaviours, both the female and male perpetrators tended to engage in multiple acts of sexually abusive behaviours against multiple victims, primarily younger children of the opposite gender. The female offenders appeared more likely to victimise both genders, although a substantial proportion of the male offenders assaulted victims of both genders as well. For the most part, the victims of both offender groups were relatives or acquaintances. Perhaps not surprisingly, and consistent with previous research, a greater proportion of the female offenders victimised children in the context of babysitting activities. Lastly, although to a lesser extent than the male offenders, many of the female offenders reported having used force during the commission of at least one of their offences.

While recognising that adolescent females who commit sexual offences are a heterogeneous group, Mathews *et al.* (1997) identified three preliminary typologies based on the observed developmental factors, psychological characteristics and offence patterns. The smallest subtype of female offenders tended to have little evidence of prior maltreatment, family dysfunction or psychopathology. The offence behaviours appeared to be very limited and motivated more by experimentation or curiosity. The remaining offenders evidenced more deliberate and repetitive patterns of offending. Girls in the second group appeared to be triggered more by their own early histories of sexual victimisation, with subsequent perpetrating behaviours developing shortly thereafter and paralleling their own victimisation experiences. They tended to evidence mild to moderate levels of family dysfunction and psychopathology. The final proposed typology exhibited more pronounced psychological and family disturbance. More chronic maltreatment and severe sexual victimisation was apparent, with development of disordered arousal in some cases. Given the differences in the typologies, Mathews *et al.* (1997) emphasised the importance of tailoring treatment interventions accordingly.

## System responses

In addition to the previously noted barriers to identifying, reporting and addressing female sexual perpetration, some of the systemic responses to "traditional" adolescent females in the juvenile justice system are worthy of review. It is commonly accepted that for females in particular, adolescence is a period of increased psychological risk (see Brown and Gilligan, 1992; Chesney-Lind, 1995; Chesney-Lind and Shelden, 1998). Behavioural health concerns of juvenile females traditionally centre around the internalisation of societal pressures, environmental concerns, and emotional turmoil manifested through esteem difficulties, body-image concerns, eating disorders, self-mutilation, depression, anxiety and somatic complaints. As these issues are less outwardly aggressive, adolescent females have been commonly perceived as less dangerous than their male counterparts; hence, little emphasis has been placed on disorders of conduct and crimes against persons committed by these females (Chesney-Lind and Shelden, 1998; Office of Juvenile Justice and Delinquency Prevention (OJJDP), 1998). Therefore, it should come as no surprise that adolescent females tend to be largely over-represented in private psychiatric facilities rather than in the juvenile courts and justice agencies (Chesney-Lind, 1995; Poe-Yamagata and Butts, 1996; Weiss *et al.*, 1996). Conversely, policies, court processing, programming efforts and allocation of resources have largely been directed toward managing male offenders in the juvenile justice system.

Although the increase in arrests of adolescent female offenders has led to the accompanying recognition of the need for gender-sensitive responses, inequitable handling of female offenders continues to be the rule rather than the exception in juvenile courts across the nation (Maniglia, 1996; Poe-Yamagata and Butts, 1996). More specifically, it remains less common for delinquency petitions to be filed when a female is the involved party; cases involving females are less likely to be formally processed and adjudicated than cases involving males. From a dispositional perspective, relative to juvenile males, delinquency cases involving juvenile females have been found to be associated with less severe outcomes, in that females are more likely to receive probation, less likely to be placed in short- or long-term custody (either detention or long-term residential programmes) and less likely to be transferred to adult courts for prosecution (Poe-Yamagata and Butts, 1996). However, female offenders have historically been disproportionately detained and sanctioned for status offences and probation violations such as runaway behaviours.

The disparate responses to runaway behaviours warrant particular attention. Given the recognised association between sexual maltreatment, family dysfunction and the delinquent behaviours of adolescent females, running away could represent the need to escape from dangerous and unhealthy circumstances. Sexually abused girls who run away are also at increased risk of further victimisation and drug use, and may steal or engage in prostitution in order to survive on the streets (Chesney-Lind, 1995; 2001). For adolescent females, the ongoing response has been to label runaway behaviours as either trivial or purely delinquent, failing to consider the presence of maltreatment in the environment. Hence, paternalistic systemic responses may inadvertently serve to silence, punish or ignore the needs of these girls. In many instances, these girls are returned to abusive situations, ultimately increasing the likelihood that they may act out in other ways in response to this helpless and hopeless situation (Chesney-Lind, 1995; 2001). With the suggested link between sexual victimisation and sexual perpetration among adolescent females, this begs the question as to the relationship between systemic responses and the exacerbation of existing risk factors which may predispose females to engage in sexually offending behaviours.

The considerable programmatic neglect of females in the juvenile justice system continues to be a significant concern. Whether preventative, community-based or residential, juvenile justice agencies and treatment facilities struggle with the effective and appropriate management of the increasing population of juvenile female offenders (Maniglia, 1996; OJJDP, 1998). Common challenges include the development of comprehensive needs assessments which identify gaps in provision of services for female offenders, the development and implementation of gender-specific services, competition for scarce resources, and a limited understanding of "what works" for female offenders (Maniglia, 1996; Poe-Yamagata and Butts, 1996; Weiss *et al.*, 1996).

A parallel and perhaps more pronounced trend exists in terms of the lack of appropriate systemic responses to juvenile female sexual offending, with little attention to adjudication, specialised programming, and resources for these females. Unfortunately, girls may be inappropriately placed in, and mistakenly believed to be effectively served by, programmes that were designed for adolescent male sexual offenders. However, to design and implement effective and responsive programming for female offenders, the various risk and protective factors associated with *female* offending must be taken into account. The unique needs of girls must be incorporated at all levels, from policy-making and legal decision-making to programme design and service delivery (Chesney-Lind, 1995; 2001; Poe-Yamagata and Butts, 1996; Weiss *et al.*, 1996).

## Gender-specific programming

It is typically the case that the most effective interventions and practices follow from an understanding of the aetiological influences of disorders and subsequent evaluations of treatment efficacy. Much like attempts to understand the development of female delinquency, competing aetiological theories exist with respect to understanding the development of sexually offending behaviours. For both, most contemporary theories suggest a complex and multifaceted interaction of physical and physiological, psychological, social and environmental influences. Hence, the interventions must address these areas, based on a clear understanding of female development, risk and resiliency factors, unique treatment needs, and "what works" with female offenders (Chesney-Lind and Shelden, 1998; Maniglia, 1996; 1998; OJJDP, 1998; Weiss *et al.*, 1996).

It is generally accepted that focusing *exclusively* on the sexual behaviours of adolescent sexual offenders is inadequate and that more holistic, individualised and needs-based programming is essential (see Righthand and Welch, 2001 for a review). Common elements of treatment programmes for juvenile females and others who sexually perpetrate include an emphasis on accountability and responsibility-taking; challenging cognitions which tend to minimise, justify, rationalise or externalise their behaviours; victim impact and empathy enhancement; esteem enhancement; healthy sexual development; social competency; reduction of deviant arousal when warranted; relapse prevention principles; and specialised conditions of supervision (Becker, 1998; Mathews *et al.*, 1997; NAPN, 1993). Other components that may perfunctorily be seen as unique for the young female offender include dispelling misperceptions about sexual offending behaviours, and addressing sexual stereotypes, sexism, and gender roles. Perhaps more important is the need to thoughtfully incorporate the interventions and approaches deemed necessary for effective gender-specific programming for adolescent females in general.

To be effective, gender-specific programming must include a solid foundation at the outset. Staff must be well trained, competent and caring. Ongoing programme evaluative processes must be in place. Structured goals and expectations must be present, and there should exist common theoretical frameworks from which to operate (Maniglia, 1996; OJJDP, 1998). From a female sexual offender management perspective, the foundation should include a multisystemic approach, taking into account the various individual, family, peer, school and community influences (Borduin *et al.*, 1990; Henggeler *et al.*, 1998). The intensive multisystemic interventions should focus on change in the natural environment and utilise the strengths of the youth, family, peers, school and community to foster behavioural improvements.

In addition, recognising the importance of process variables, frameworks that are invitational and utilise therapeutic engagement rather than highly confrontational and shame-inducing approaches (Bumby *et al.*, 1999; Jenkins, 1998; Mathews *et al.*, 1997) may have particular utility with the adolescent female sexual offender population. These approaches allow young offenders to identify their own motivations for change, recognise their own capacity for relating to others, and focus on establishing their own goals and motivations for their achievement (Jenkins, 1998). Treatment occurs in a collaborative, respectful and dignified context, rather than in a punitive and controlling manner. Such a process emphasises the concept of choice, highlights the ability to change behaviours, offers hope, and facilitates self-efficacy (Bumby *et al.*, 1999; Jenkins, 1998).

The overall emphasis on needs-based, individualised and respectful approaches leads to another tenet for effective programming for juvenile female offenders: that programmes reflect the unique needs and differences of young women (Chesney-Lind, 1995; 2001; Maniglia, 1996; 1998; Weiss *et al.*, 1996). Clearly, it is critical that the interventions appropriately reflect adolescent development, but more importantly for this population, adolescent *female* development. Researchers have identified developmental pathways specific to adolescent females, with an increased understanding of risk factors which may impact their healthy development (e.g. Brown and Gilligan, 1992; Chesney-Lind and Sheldon, 1998; Taylor *et al.*, 1995). For example, markedly different from the developmental experiences of adolescent males, young women receive negative societal and cultural messages about their bodies, minds and overall worth, ultimately leading to considerable alterations in self-image and behaviour (Brown and Gilligan, 1992; Taylor *et al.*, 1995). These investigators note that during this "transformation", adolescent females become increasingly confused and disconnected, more withdrawn, less willing and able to assert themselves, and increasingly feel that they are no longer heard by others, all of which contributes to the loss of a sense of self. Hence, treatment must build on the inherent but often unrecognised strengths, skills and creativity to rebuild, and to develop their voices and abilities to assert themselves, while challenging these long-standing influences and barriers (Brown and Gilligan, 1992; Chesney-Lind, 2001; Taylor *et al.*, 1995).

Additional risk factors that tend to be particularly salient for female offenders and must therefore be addressed include the following: academic failure, unmet health and behavioural health needs, pregnancy, family dysfunction and fragmentation, societal influences such as sexism and racism, body image concerns, eating disorders, substance abuse, and exposure to domestic violence within the home and in their own relationships (Chesney-Lind, 1995; 2001; OJJDP, 1998; Weiss *et al.*, 1996). Moreover, as identified in the research, sexual victimisation may play a key aetiological role not only in juvenile delinquency, but also in the development of sexual offending behaviours (Hunter and Figueredo, 2000). Therefore, for these females, interventions should help them to develop an understanding of their own victimisation and to address feelings that may have contributed to later engaging in destructive behaviours (OJJDP, 1998; Weiss *et al.*, 1996). There should be a focus on empowering themselves, recognising that they can choose to not participate in abusive relationships in the future. In addition, these young women need to be afforded opportunities to understand and explore issues of mistrust, while learning to develop and maintain healthy, appropriate boundaries in relationships (OJJDP, 1998). When dealing with personal victimisation, the increased awareness of the impact can also create effective opportunities to engage in perspective-taking exercises and address issues of empathy for the victims of their own offences.

Beyond addressing the risk factors for juvenile female offenders, protective or resiliency factors must also be considered and incorporated (Brown and Gilligan, 1992; Taylor *et al.*, 1995; OJJDP, 1998). A focus on gender identity development and individualism is critical; confidence, assertiveness and a strong sense of self can facilitate healthy relationships with effective boundaries in relationships (Brown and Gilligan, 1992; Chesney-Lind and Shelden, 1998; Maniglia, 1996; 1998). Another key to resiliency is the identification and utilisation of positive female role models and mentors. In homes, schools, neighbourhoods and communities, a young female's relationship with a trusted, caring and supportive adult woman can serve as an influential protective factor by establishing high expectations, providing guidance and modelling skills that can assist in the transition from adolescence to womanhood (Chesney-Lind, 1998; OJJDP, 1998; Taylor *et al.*, 1998; Weiss *et al.*, 1996). Finally, effectively meeting the following needs may increase the likelihood of healthy development among young females: the need for belongingness, physical safety and physical development, and safety to explore sexuality at her own pace for healthy sexual development (Chesney-Lind, 1998; OJJDP, 1998; Weiss *et al.*, 1996).

## Conclusion

Juvenile females who commit sexual offences have been historically under-represented from a policy, programming and research perspective. In part, this has been a reflection of the more global tendency to neglect females within the criminal and juvenile justice systems. However, with increasing numbers of young females coming to the attention of authorities for delinquent and sexually offending behaviours, an increased focus on the gender-specific needs of this population has evolved, and initial progress toward the closing of the gender gap is beginning to emerge. There is much work to be done. The recognition of gender differences among those who commit sexual and other offences should neither be used to imply that females are different from the "norm", nor to exacerbate or support the prevailing inequities in terms of access to resources and services. Assessment tools, workbooks, programmes and other resources must become more sensitive to gender and cultural differences. Increased attention in the empirical arena to gender differences between and similarities among adolescent offenders is needed. Essential outcomes research must be conducted, to identify interventions that are most likely to reduce future victimisation. Lastly, the importance of a victim-centred approach to sexual offender management must be reiterated, with community safety, victim safety and prevention of additional victims remaining paramount (Centre for Sex Offender Management, 2000; D'Amora and Burns-Smith, 1999). The policies and practices designed to address sexually offending behaviours, whether for adults or juveniles, males or females, must never ignore, overlook or override this overarching philosophy and goal, which is the very reason that sexual offender management practices are in place.

## References

Allen, C. M. (1991). Women as perpetrators of child sexual abuse: Recognition barriers. In A. L. Horton, B. L. Johnson, L. M. Roundy and D. Williams (eds), *The Incest Perpetrator: Family Member No One Wants to Treat*. Newbury Park, CA: Sage, pp. 108–125.

Becker, J. V. (1998). What we know about the characteristics and treatment of adolescents who have committed sexual offences. *Child Maltreatment, 3*, 317–329.

Borduin, C. M., Henggeler, S. W., Blaske, D. M., and Stein, R. J. (1990). Multisystemic treatment of adolescent sexual offenders. *International Journal of Offender Therapy and Comparative Criminology, 34*, 105–113.

Brown, L. M., and Gilligan, C. (1992). *Meeting at the Crossroads: Women's Psychology and Girls' Development*. Cambridge, MA: Harvard University Press.

Bumby, K. M., and Bumby, N. H. (1993). *Adolescent Females who Sexually Perpetrate: Preliminary Findings*. Presented at the 12th Annual Research and Treatment Conference of the Association for the Treatment of Sexual Abusers, Boston, MA.

Bumby, K. M. and Bumby, N. H. (1997). Adolescent female sexual offenders. In B. K. Schwartz and H. R. Cellini (eds), *The Sex Offender: New Insights, Treatment*

*Innovations, and Legal Developments*. Kingston, NJ: Civic Research Institute, pp. 10.1–10.16.

Bumby, K. M., Marshall, W. L., and Langton, C. M. (1999). A theoretical formulation of the influences of shame and guilt on sexual offending. In B. Schwartz (ed.), *The Sex Offender: Theoretical Advances, Special Populations, and Legal Developments*. Kingston, NJ: Civic Research Institute.

Centre for Sex Offender Management (2000). *Engaging Victim Advocates and Other Victim Services Providers in the Community Management of Sexual Offenders*. Silver Spring, MD: Author

Chesney-Lind, M. (1995). Girls, delinquency, and juvenile justice: Toward a feminist theory of young women's crime. In B. R. Price and N. Sokoloff (eds), *The Criminal Justice System and Women*. New York: McGraw-Hill, pp. 71–88.

Chesney-Lind, M. (2001). What about the girls? Delinquency programming as if gender mattered. *Corrections Today, 63(1)*, 38–45.

Chesney-Lind, M., and Shelden, R. G. (1998). *Girls, Delinquency, and Juvenile Justice*. Thousand Oaks, CA: Sage.

D'Amora, D., and Burns-Smith, G. (1999). Partnering in response to sexual violence: How offender treatment and victim advocacy can work together in response to sexual violence. *Sexual Abuse: A Journal of Research and Treatment, 11*, 295–306.

Elliott, M. (1993) *Female Sexual Abuse of Children*. New York: Guilford.

FBI (2001). *Crime in the United States, 2000: Uniform Crime Reports*. Washington, DC: Federal Bureau of Investigation.

Fehrenbach, P. A., and Monastersky, C. (1988). Characteristics of female adolescent sexual offenders. *American Journal of Orthopsychiatry, 58*, 148–151.

Henggeler, S. W., Schoenwald, S. K., Borduin, C. M., Rowland, M. D., and Cunningham, P. E. (1998). *Multisystemic Treatment of Antisocial Behavior in Children and Adolescents*. New York: Guilford.

Hunter, J. A., and Figueredo, A. J. (2000). The influence of personality and history of sexual victimization in the prediction of juvenile perpetrated child molestation. *Behaviour Modification, 24*, 241–263.

Hunter, J. A., Lexier, L. J., Goodwin, D. W., Browne, P. A., and Dennis, C. (1993). Psychosexual, attitudinal, and developmental characteristics of juvenile female sexual perpetrators in a residential treatment setting. *Journal of Child and Family Studies, 2*, 317–326.

Jenkins, A. (1998). Invitations to responsibility: Engaging adolescents and young men who have sexually abused. In W. L. Marshall, Y. M. Fernandez, S. M. Hudson and T. Ward (eds), *Sourcebook of Treatment Programs for Sexual Offenders*. New York: Plenum.

Jennings, K. Y. (1994). Female child molesters: A review of the literature. In M. Elliott (ed.), *Female Sexual Abuse of Children*. New York: Guilford, pp. 219–234.

Maniglia, R. (1996). New directions for young women in the juvenile justice system. *Journal of Emotional and Behavioural Problems, 5*, 96–101.

Maniglia, R. (1998). *Juvenile Female Offenders: A Status of the States Report*. Washington, DC: US Department of Justice, Office of Juvenile Justice and Delinquency Prevention.

Margolin, L. (1991). Child sexual abuse by nonrelated caregivers. *Child Abuse and Neglect, 15*, 213–221.

Mathews, R., Hunter, J. A., and Vuz, J. (1997). Juvenile female sexual offenders:

Clinical characteristics and treatment issues. *Sexual Abuse: A Journal of Research and Treatment, 9*, 187–199.

National Adolescent Perpetrator Network (NAPN) (1993). Revised report from the National Task Force on Juvenile Sexual Offending. *Juvenile and Family Court Journal, 44*, 1–120.

Office of Juvenile Justice and Delinquency Prevention (OJJDP) (1998). *Guiding Principles for Promising Female Programming: An Inventory of Best Practices.* Washington, DC: OJJDP.

Poe-Yamagata, E., and Butts, J. A. (1996). *Female Offenders in the Juvenile Justice System: Statistics Summary*. Washington, DC: US Department of Justice, Office of Juvenile Justice and Delinquency Prevention.

Righthand, S., and Welch, C. (2001). *Juveniles who Have Sexually Offended: A Review of the Professional Literature*. Washington, DC: US Department of Justice, Office of Juvenile Justice and Delinquency Prevention.

Taylor, J. M., Gilligan, C., and Sullivan, A. M. (1995). *Between Voice and Silence: Women and Girls, Race and Relationship*. Cambridge, MA: Harvard University Press.

Weiss, F. L., Nicholson, H. J., and Cretella, M. M. (1996). *Prevention and Parity: Girls in Juvenile Justice*. Washington, DC: US Department of Justice, Office of Juvenile Justice and Delinquency Prevention.

# Part V

# Systemic issues

Chapter 15

# Preparing services and staff to work with young people who sexually abuse

## Context, mandate, pitfalls and frameworks

*Tony Morrison*

The central focus of this book is on how to work effectively with young people who sexually abuse others. This chapter however looks at how services and staff can be set up in a manner that will enable them to deliver an effective service. Its underlying premises are simple. Firstly, changing behaviour occurs in the context of empathic, skilled and carefully planned relationships between workers and clients. Secondly, the capacity of workers to create and sustain effective therapeutic relationships is inextricably bound up with the quality of their organisational environments. Thirdly, the majority of young people who exhibit sexually abusive behaviour have multiple and complex needs, therefore the quality of inter-agency collaboration is crucial to the effectiveness of our interventions (Morrison, 2000). Changing their behaviour will require the skills and services of more than one agency or professional discipline. In other words the preparation of staff cannot be separated from the organisational and inter-agency context in which they work. Just as we cannot consider the behaviour of young people without reference to their ecological context, neither can we prepare staff properly without reference to their ecological context. It is these three premises that underpin the approach to this chapter.

The chapter opens with a consideration of the different international contexts in which readers may be operating, before focusing on the UK as the principal context for the discussion that follows. Recent UK legislative and policy developments affecting the management of young people who sexually abuse are highlighted together with an overview of key organisational and system issues facing the field. The core discussion is based on the presentation of an organisational and inter-agency framework for effective service delivery. Throughout, consideration is given to common pitfalls and problems that can arise. The central message is that there are a number of critical conditions to be met if practitioners are to provide an effective and safe service.

The chapter draws from research literature on programme issues and preparation, as well as from my own experience of consulting to programmes and involvement in strategic development work with senior managers and inter-agency groups in the UK and abroad. I also co-run a therapeutic service for the parents of young people who sexually abuse at G-MAP in Manchester (formerly known as the Greater Manchester Abusers Project), and thus also bring a practitioner's perspective to this chapter. Although this chapter loosely focuses on those above the age of criminal responsibility (10 years in the UK), many of its principles are relevant to those running programmes for younger children or for services for adult offenders. The term young people is adopted to refer to those who have engaged in sexually abusive behaviour regardless of whether they have been convicted. The chapter makes reference to the provision of services rather than to the setting up of a specific team. The reason is that although a dedicated team may well be part of the response, it has to be remembered that an effective response requires all services to be engaged, not just specialist sectors. If the wider professional community is not engaged, specialists will be extremely limited in what they can do.

## Comparative contexts

Readers of this book are likely to be drawn from a variety of contexts and jurisdictions, as far apart as the USA, Canada, New Zealand, Australia, the UK and Ireland as well as other European countries. This will have considerable implications for how the material will need to be translated into the reader's own context. There are considerable differences between these countries across a range of domains.

For instance, criminal justice systems in much of Europe and New Zealand follow a restorative justice approach in contrast to the UK, Ireland, North America and Australia, who follow an adversarial system. Within the different criminal justice systems there are wide variations in the powers and disposals available to the courts; for instance, how far parents may be compelled to engage with services. This reflects wider cultural differences about how the problem of young people who sexually abuse is seen at a political and societal level, which is in turn further influenced by public attitudes towards youth crime more generally.

Higher degrees of societal anxiety about youth crime are likely to be reflected in more punitive and less child-centred responses. For instance, Chaffin and Bonner's (1998) editorial in a journal special edition on juvenile sexual offenders was entitled: " 'Don't shoot, we're your children': Have we gone too far in our response to adolescent sexual abusers and children with sexual behaviour problems?" The editorial went on to warn: "We should be on our guard against the potentially punitive aversive and absolutist tone inherent in some of out treatment beliefs. Punitive approaches must be considered within the context of a current political climate that exaggerates our fear of juvenile crime, and energises corresponding movements to punish children and youth as we would do hardened adults" (p. 314). Programmes must be acutely aware of the wider socio-political context in which they work and cannot assume that professionals are unaffected by these wider forces.

There are also major differences in the degree to which services are provided principally through public and voluntary (not for profit) sectors in contrast to private providers financed by either insurance or personal fee systems. In the United States the private provider sector accounts for well over half of all services. In contrast, in the UK this sector accounts for a much smaller proportion of services. This has significant implications for inter-agency working, how specific programmes locate themselves within the wider context, and who are considered to be their key stakeholders.

The UK has a much stronger tradition than most other countries of centrally prescribed guidance on inter-agency collaboration identified in documents such as *Working Together to Safeguard Children* (Department of Health, 1999) and the *Framework for the Assessment of Children in Need and their Families* (Department of Health, 2000a). At the local authority level the UK has a well established system of Children's Service Planning processes and Area Child Protection Committees (ACPCs). The latter are responsible for the coordination at a strategic level of inter-agency policies, services, training and auditing. This is reflected in formal frameworks at an operational level for multi-disciplinary case planning and review that seek to involve parents and young people as fully as possible. Whatever the merits or otherwise of such formal inter-agency systems, from a service development perspective the degree to which such systems exist and work effectively is crucial. Poorer levels of inter-agency collaboration that are over-dependent on individual rather than agency commitment will radically affect the quality of case planning, and the level of resources available to work with these young people. It will also affect the levels of staff anxiety, safety and isolation.

Space permits only this brief exploration of the many important cultural, legislative and policy differences that exist across the readership of a text like this. The author's experience however lies mainly in his work in the UK, and therefore the chapter will take the UK as its principal context. However, my experience of work in Ireland, Australia and New Zealand has shown how many of the issues we face are common across the barriers of land and sea. It is therefore hoped that readers will both recognise the issues raised in this chapter and translate whatever is relevant into their own context. The discussion starts with a brief overview of the current state of services in the UK.

## The UK context: an overview

In the UK the National Children's Home Report (NCH, 1992) provided the first comprehensive picture of how young abusers were being managed in the UK. It painted a gloomy picture by highlighting: conflicts concerning the definition of juvenile sexual abuse; the absence of a coordinated management structure which resulted in individual agencies intervening without reference to others and decisions being made without the involvement of professionals with expertise in sexual abuse issues; an absence of policy; uncertainty about the legitimacy of the work; clashes of philosophy especially between juvenile justice and child protection approaches; inadequate data about the nature, scope and effects of the problem; an absence of internal and inter-agency policy and practice guidance; a lack of clarity about assessment and intervention models; an absence of services for young abusers; placement problems and risks arising from victims and abusers being placed in the same accommodation; inadequate supervision and training; and alienation for frontline workers trying to tackle the problem.

The report suggested that within the management of agencies concerned with the well-being of children, the legal profession and society in general, ignorance, denial, fear, minimisation and collusion were evident in relation to the problem of young people who sexually abuse others. It recommended the need for a comprehensive national strategy. The NCH report was followed by a Department of Health *Strategic Statement* (1992) which stated that young people who engage in sexually abusive behaviour are in need of services because evidence suggests that appropriate and early intervention will bring their difficulties under control. The Department's strategic objectives, which were to be implemented at a local level via ACPCs, were listed as: formulating a coherent policy for the management and treatment of young abusers; building a better understanding of young abusers; viewing sexual abuse as a problem requiring assessment and treatment both for the abuser and for the victim; the promotion of a multi-disciplinary approach to the problem; encouraging the establishment of local and national resources (in recognition of the high demands of the work); and educating the public and professionals about the problem.

## *How far have we come?*

So the stage was set. The problems had been identified by the NCH report, located in the child protection system and a framework for a national policy had been set by the Department of Health's statement. Now nearly a decade later the questions are: How far have we come? and What is the current context into which new services enter?

These questions were in part graphically answered in a recent workshop for practitioners in the UK. Participants from a range of agencies were asked to depict their experience of working with young people who sexually abuse, by making a physical model using a range of craft materials. One model showed a small play-person as the worker walking on a high wire, between two parapets, balanced only by a wide pole. Behind her, waiting to take their turn to attempt this high wire act were several more workers. Prowling around on the ground was a grizzly bear. Indeed, several of the presentations used monsters or crocodiles to depict a sense of danger and threat. In contrast workers were represented by small, isolated figures, in one case, simply by a small piece of play dough. Another group introduced their presentation by throwing a "hot potato" around. The images left a powerful impression. Although the reality may be more differentiated, with some workers operating in more supportive and better organised environments, for a significant proportion these pictures represent an accurate portrayal of their experiences of isolation, anxiety, fear, disempowerment and de-skilling. Few if any of the models included a supportive manager or supervisor.

Nevertheless, there has been progress since 1992. There is undoubtedly a much greater level of professional awareness of the problem, supported by a number of British studies showing that young people and children are responsible for about a third of all child sexual assaults (Horne *et al.*, 1991; Kelly *et al.*, 1991). The facts that the report *Working Together* (Department of Health, 1999) includes guidance on the management of these young people, and that the new Youth Justice Board has funded a number of local projects to develop inter-agency policies and services, are significant. There have also been a number of inter-agency initiatives involving both statutory and voluntary agencies to fund local specialist services. The literature in this field is expanding as the present book testifies, and the UK's first major textbook in this area was published in 1999 (Erooga and Masson, 1999). The National Association for the Treatment of Abusers (NOTA) has also raised the profile of this work through conferences and training events and co-funded a major research project looking to assess current professional attitudes and beliefs about work with these young people (Hackett *et al.*, 2002). Nonetheless these are anecdotal observations as there is no national database or set of national objectives or standards by which it is possible to monitor the real state of affairs. There have, however, been a number of reports on policy, professional attitudes and services which provide a more fine-grained account of how things currently stand.

### *Policy development*

Masson (1996) indicates that some progress has been made in terms of policy development. In her interim report Masson (September, 1995) reported that of 106 ACPCs surveyed, 17 per cent had drawn up inter-agency procedures and a further 43 per cent had working parties examining the issue. Different models were identified designed to integrate child protection and youth justice approaches. Indeed there have been some very good examples of local policy development such as the AIM project (Print *et al.*, 2001). This has created an inter-agency framework for referral, assessment and case planning across ten local authorities, the police and the voluntary sector in Greater Manchester, a population of 4 million people. However, overall it is salutary to note the contrast with policies in respect of adult sexual offenders. A survey of UK Probation Services in 1995 revealed that 98 per cent had strategies for the management of adult sexual offenders. One explanation for this difference lies in the fact that the Probation Service is clearly the lead agency with regard to the management of adult sexual offenders. The question of who the lead agencies are in relation to the management of juvenile sexual abusers remains a key unanswered question. A particular issue is the coordination of child protection and youth justice responses following the new requirements for faster processing of youth crime under the Crime and Disorder Act (1999). There is currently wide variation in the degree to which local police forces are prepared to seek multi-disciplinary input to the assessment of these young people prior to deciding whether to warn, reprimand or prosecute.

These issues of inter-agency coordination were identified in a recent thematic inspection of the Probation Service's work with dangerous offenders. One of its principal findings was the absence of any national strategic framework for the management of these young people (Her Majesty's Inspector of Probation, 1998). Local policy development is being pursued in the absence of any overarching national objectives, which accounts for the fact that so many of the issues identified in the 1992 NCH report remain unresolved. The establishment of a National Youth Justice Board established in 1997, which has responsibility for national standards, a programme of inspections, approving local youth justice team plans, training and disseminating good practice, will hopefully provide a forum in which a national strategy for young people convicted of sexual offences can be built. The Board have already begun to develop papers on effective practice in this area. Nonetheless this leaves unanswered the question of how a strategy for the vast majority of these young people who do not enter the criminal justice system will be forged. The recent creation of an inter-departmental working group on these young people involving both criminal justice and child protection agencies will need to ensure that any strategy targets not just the minority of young people who are convicted, but also the much larger proportion who never enter the criminal justice arena.

### *Philosophy of intervention*

Despite the Government's statement that the management of these young people should be coordinated between child protection and youth justice systems, there remain tensions between and within professional groups as to how this problem should be defined, and over philosophies of intervention. Although there has been a growing recognition that some form of intervention is required, significant debates exist over questions surrounding: whether the young person is seen as victim or perpetrator; the degree to which young abusers should be either placed on child protection registers or subject to public protection registration laws; the degree to which models that have been developed with adult sexual offenders are relevant to juveniles; the degree to which juvenile abusers can be held responsible for their own behaviour; the degree to which the young person or child understands his/her sexuality; the likelihood he/she will grow out of, or into, the abusive behaviour; the need to treat or to punish; and the need for court ordered intervention (Sanders and Ladwa-Thomas, 1997).

However, there is emerging evidence from a current large scale study using a Delphi exercise that practitioner approaches are moving away from "adult-based" intervention models to a more holistic approach in the case of adolescents who sexually abuse (Hackett *et al.*, 2002). For instance, it was found that 97 per cent of respondents agreed with the statement that "children who display sexually harmful behaviour are first and foremost children and should not be regarded as mini sexual offenders" and that "we cannot assume that research models and methods designed for adults can be applied to adolescents". Nonetheless, despite the high degree of consensus on this overall principle, the survey revealed huge variance in treatment approaches.

Much of the difficulty around these debates stems from the paucity of research in this field. As Chaffin and Bonner (1998) observe, reflecting on fifteen years of work with young sexual offenders in the USA, "Not one of the basic critical questions have been answered more than tentatively if at all. There are still no true experimental studies comparing outcomes of treated versus untreated adolescents, and no prospective data on either risk factors or the natural course of the behaviour; there are only the beginnings of empirical typologies and no actuarial risk assessment" (p. 314). It is hardly surprising, therefore, that new services might be faced with major debates about philosophy of intervention, effective risk assessment, choice of treatment and expected outcomes, given the lack of an empirical base for this work, and the fact that the development of adolescent work has largely followed the development of adult sexual offender work.

### *Service provision and delivery*

Probably the easiest thing to say is that we do not know what the current level of provision is, in part because we have no real idea what the level of need is. Anecdotally the picture suggests that services remain extremely patchy, with a predominant focus on working with the young person, and far less emphasis on working with his family. There appear to be massive gaps in the geographical spread of services so that professionals often have to seek treatment and residential provision from services that are at great distances from the young person's home environment. The current research project identified above (Hackett *et al.*, 2002) will helpfully fill some of these gaps in the service mapping work that will be included.

The increase in multi-agency partnership projects since 1992 involving both voluntary and independent sectors has been encouraging. However, Monke and New's (1995) study of eleven treatment centres identified a range of issues in relation to service delivery, including: financial insecurity; difficulty in recruiting experienced staff; uncertainty about service aims; uncertainty concerning which client groups' services ought to be targeted; uncertainty about likely levels of service demand and take-up; a lack of consistent assessment as to suitability of referrals; tensions between how the Social Services department paying for the service and the specialist service see the needs of the case; a pressure to focus on assessment rather than longer-term work; a reluctance by the commissioning authority to include provision for work with other family members; and how to fit existing services to victims alongside new services to young abusers.

In summary the picture since 1992 has been a mixed one in a field still finding its feet. There has undoubtedly been a significant growth in professional awareness and commitment, at an individual level, to address the needs of this population. It also appears that there is a significant shift towards the philosophy of intervention that is more holistic and which incorporates attention not only to risk but also to the needs of these young people. There has been a large increase in the training available, and a gradual increase in the literature. In many parts of the country this has been supported to different degrees by local policy development and inter-agency funding. However, too much remains dependent on short-term funding, and local and individual initiative, leaving too many workers uncertain, isolated and unsupported. This then is the context for which staff and services need to be prepared. For some readers the context will be more benign and robust, while for others an insecure context will be all too recognisable. It is imperative that any preparation starts from how things are, not how one might like them to be. The discussion that follows takes this summary as its starting-point.

## Building effective services

The introduction identified the need to pay as much attention to the inter- and intra-organisational contexts as to the preparation of individual staff. All three levels are important and interrelated. However, before looking at how to address these issues in the field of young people who sexually abuse, it is useful to keep in mind what is known more generally about the requirements for effective teams. Drawing from research across a range of sectors, Larson and Lafasto (1989), Poulton and West (1993), and Woodcock (1988) identify the following factors as important indicators of effective teamwork: having specific agreed and measurable goals; participation, and communication; regular review and feedback; support for innovation; balanced skill mix; balanced roles within the team; competency in team members; high standards; support/openness/trust and ability to confront obstacles; principled leadership including vision, supervision and the management of external boundaries; team-based appraisal; sound inter-team relationships; team development; and positive links with the external world.

Poulton and West (1993), in a wide ranging study of primary health care teams, emphasise the critical need for clear and specific goals. However, these can be particularly difficult to pin down in work with young people, where there are often complex needs, and competing priorities for intervention between funding authorities and service providers. Taking this list as a broad guide, the remainder of the chapter is structured around a service development framework (see Figure 15.1) which explores the organisational and inter-agency building blocks that need to be addressed in developing services for young people who engage in sexually abusive behaviour. Each of the building blocks is important, and readers are invited to consider which are in place and which are missing in their own working context. It may be useful to undertake such an exercise jointly with other professionals or agencies with whom you are involved.

## 1 *Defining and mapping needs*

Defining what is meant by adolescent sexually abusive behaviour is perhaps one of the most important but difficult tasks facing professionals trying to

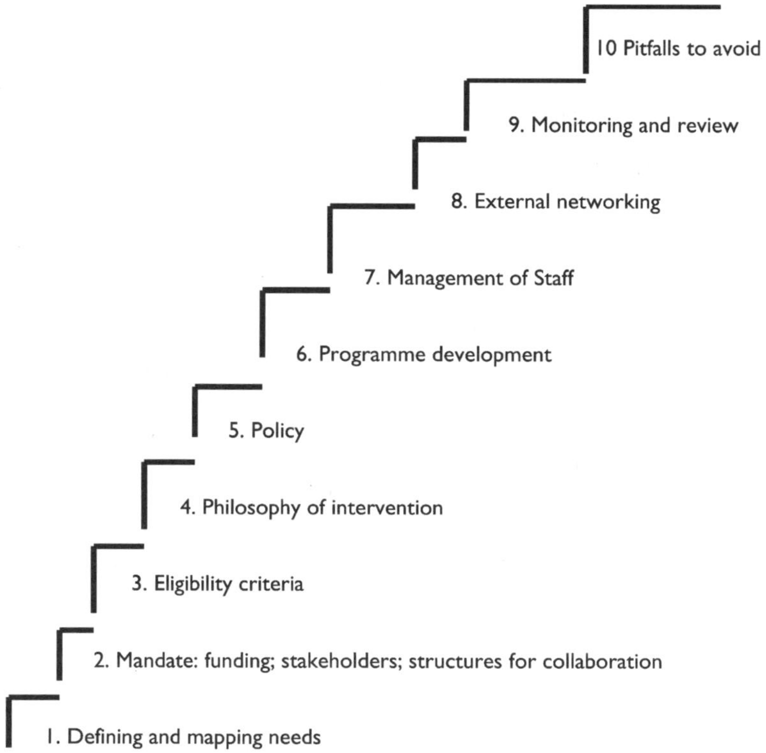


*Figure 15.1* Organisational and inter-agency building blocks for effective services.

deal with this problem. Disagreements over definitions undermine referral, assessment and treatment processes. The capacity of agencies to work together depends upon shared language to describe what professionals are seeing. Thus what to one professional may be explorative behaviour may to another be abusive. Ryan and Lane's (1991) original definition, which has been used by many programmes, states that a juvenile sexual offender is a minor who commits any sexual act with a person of any age against the will of the person victimised; without their consent; and in a way that is aggressive, exploitative or threatening. However, more recently attention has been given to a group who fall somewhere between age appropriate sexual behaviour and clearly abusive behaviours. This group engage in inappropriate but *mutual* sexual behaviour in which it is much more difficult, and possibly not useful, to seek to make clear distinctions between victim and abuser. Nonetheless there is a real need to engage with these situations as there are many risks if the behaviour continues.

A lack of common definition also makes it extremely difficult to map the extent of need in terms of identifying the number of young people in an area requiring services. Without any mapping of need, estimating demand levels and funding requirements may amount to little more than guesswork. It may be unrealistic in the early days of setting up a new service to expect that definitions can be specified too tightly. But there is a need to ensure that key agencies and managers who are involved in funding, running or working alongside treatment services: (a) Have a basic appreciation of research about the nature, scope and significance of the problem of young people who sexually abuse. (b) Recognise the need to develop multi-disciplinary operational definitions of the behaviours that should trigger agreed responses. (c) Identify, even if crudely at first, the size of the problem in their locality by pooling information between social services, police and health. The process of sharing information in mapping need is itself a very positive inter-agency exercise which starts to build shared understanding and commitment around the problem. However, it is essential that crime reports are not used as the principal guide, as the vast majority of these assaults are not reported to the police and even fewer are subject to criminal justice disposals. Schools have not been mentioned in the above list, because for practical reasons gathering information from them is a massive task. However, schools are often informally aware of a much wider pool of cases which they are managing internally. Thus the education sector represents a large source of unmapped need.

## 2 Mandate

### 2.1 Ownership

The work on mapping need leads naturally into establishing the mandate for the provision of services. Essentially establishing the mandate is about ensuring shared ownership of both the problem and the responses to it. This is therefore about more than securing funding, necessary though that is. Mandate flows from managers at a senior level when they: understand the nature and significance of this problem; identify their agency's role and responsibilities towards the problem; get the issue onto their agency's strategic planning agenda; locate it within inter-agency children's planning structures; identify needs, priorities and resources for services to these young people; offer agency leadership and time towards establishing and maintaining a service. In many areas the local ACPC has been a driving force behind the development of services, and increasingly shared forums with local youth offending services are developing. The greater the number of local authorities and other agencies involved, the more complex becomes securing a mandate. Too large a constituency may result in the mandate being reduced to the lowest common denominator: much rhetoric but little real commitment. There is thus a need to identify early on who the key agency stakeholders might be, and how wide a group to involve in the set-up phase.

### 2.2 *Funding*

In terms of funding, many programmes have been established on a three-year initial basis with priming money from the voluntary sector or from central government sources. However, in a climate of increasing demands to meet targets in other sectors, such as child protection and children in care, converting the initial funding into mainstream funding at the end of three years is not always easy. By the end of three years many programmes have only just begun to deliver their service, due to the amount of time it takes to build the infrastructure for an effective service. Even established programmes are vulnerable to spending cuts if their target population does not fit within agencies' priorities, which are increasingly to target the most vulnerable or high-risk groups.

Research (Prentky *et al.*, 2000) suggests that average recidivism runs at between 2 and 14 per cent for those young people who do not commit serious sexual assaults or who do not have a history of associated behavioural problems (conduct disorder, impulsivity, delinquency). Therefore it is very important that service proposals are very clear as to whom the service is targeted (see service eligibility criteria below). The message here is that three-year funding plans are barely enough to get a service up and running, or to act as a small-scale pilot project. To make a significant and measurable impact, funding needs to be for a minimum of five years. It may be that such funding is more likely to be available for the more complex multi-problem young people who pose the highest risks.

### 2.3 *Coordinating structures*

It is essential to sustain initial levels of inter-agency support for the service by establishing at both strategic and operational levels inter-agency structures to ensure continuing ownership, support, resources and a forum for problem-resolution. This may be through a management committee or by creating a reporting relationship to an existing inter-agency forum such as Area Child Protection Committees in the UK, where there has been a recent recommendation that youth offending services should be represented as a matter of course (Department of Health, 2002). These structures will enable the profile and work of the service to be kept alive in the minds of senior managers who have many competing priorities.

## 3 *Service eligibility criteria*

A key issue for services and funding bodies is to identify their target group. Which sort of needs or levels of risk are to be addressed? Accurate assessment is the foundation of an effective service model – research by McKeown (2000) identified the characteristics of the client to be the single most significant influence on the effectiveness of therapeutic interventions, accounting for approximately 40 per cent of the variance in outcome. In contrast, therapeutic method was identified as having only 15 per cent influence on outcome. The more complex and enduring the clients' problems, the worse the prognosis.

There is thus a fundamental difference between services aimed at young people from relatively untroubled family backgrounds, with a stable educational placement who have committed a single non-contact assault, compared with a young man who has committed a similar assault but where there are also long-standing behavioural and emotional difficulties, and where the youngster has experienced several episodes of care placement. The services required to address complex, life-course persistent problem behaviours are entirely different to those for stage-specific/adolescent-limited behaviours. Although for the lower-risk group a brief crisis support and psycho-educational intervention may suffice (Ryan, 1999), for the more complex group, a coordinated package of services focusing on both offence specific and developmental goals delivered by a range of agencies will be required. Services need to clarify and agree with other stakeholders the population they are seeking to target, based on the mapping of needs mentioned above. Clear eligibility criteria can then be established which help to ensure: that the appropriate cases enter the right part of the system so that the appropriate level and intensity of service is offered; that sufficient funding is secured; that expectations of the service are appropriate; that appropriate referrals are made to the service; that boundaries are maintained to prevent the service from being swamped; that other agencies can be clear about their role, so that specialist services do not become a dumping ground for multi-problem cases simply because one of the presenting problems is sexually abusive behaviour; that appropriate outcome measures can be set and monitored.

A "continuum of service" framework (see Figure 15.2) provides a tiered set of responses, linked to levels of need and risk, in order to respond appropriately. In this approach *Level 1* service provision is concerned with responding to an early presentation of sexually problematic behaviour in the context of concerned parents and a reasonably positive functioning family. Intervention aims to be educational and supportive, with the worker helping the parents process their feelings, and providing them with an information and home-counselling pack which they can work through with the child, focusing on issues of consent, empathy and boundaries. One or two follow-up visits would take place to check progress. *Level 2* service provision concerns referral to a psycho-educational group for parents in cases where the young person has had further sexual behaviour problems and there is a need to bolster the parents' skills and commitment. At *Level 3* service provision involves

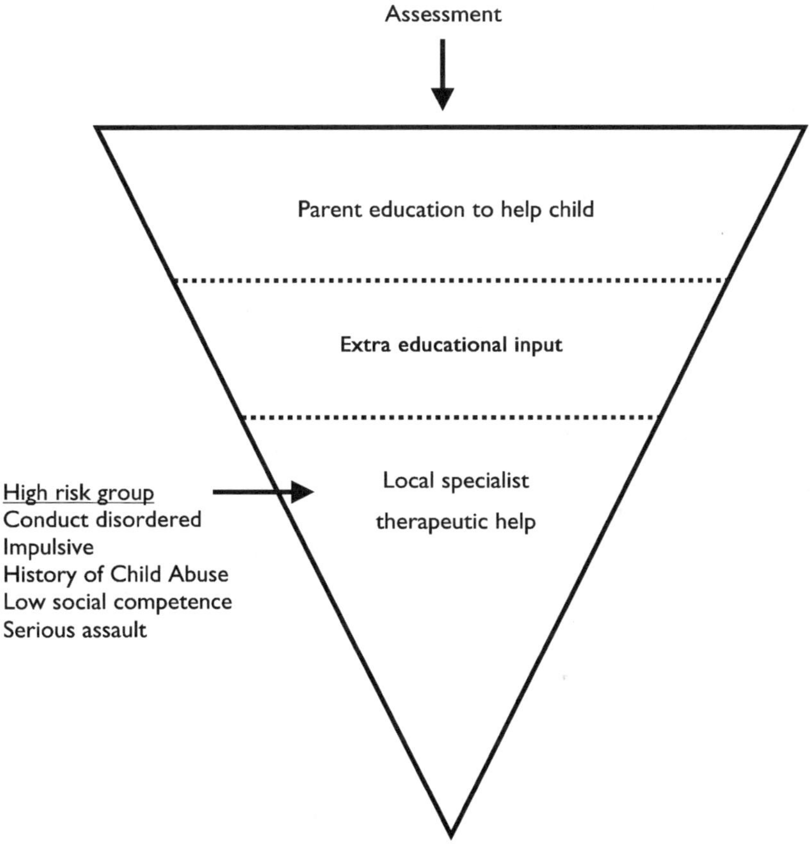


*Figure 15.2* Thresholds for services (based on the ideas of Ryan, 1999).

referral to a community-based treatment programme for the young person and the parents. This service could be run by a mixture of specialist and generalist staff. At *Level 4* service provision would entail referral to a specialist residential/secure programme for a young person identified as belonging to a high risk of re-offending group, who has had multiple problems, engaged in seriously abusive behaviours, and where there is a high public protection concern.

## 4 *Philosophy of intervention*

Although this is still a young field, there has been a rapid expansion of knowledge and understanding in the past decade. Although the drive to work with young offenders came from work with adults, recent research has begun to identify some important distinctions between adults and young people who abuse (Prentky *et al.*, 2000; Ryan, 1999). For instance, the vast majority of adolescent abusers differ from adult offenders in that they do not have deviant urges or fantasies; do not demonstrate specific targeting and selection of victims; have far lower sexual recidivism rates; are much more likely to commit non-sexual offences; are still primarily influenced by their family of origin; and do not have such fixed patterns of thought or behaviour, as they are still in a fluid stage of development. The implications of these findings are that assumptions based on previous models of adult programmes may need significant revision, in favour of a more holistic and developmental approach rather than a forensic and public protection approach. Ryan (1999) summarises this sea change as follows: "Whereas a perspective based on the theory of the criminal personality (Yochelson and Samenow, 1976) views the correction of sexually abusive behaviour as a problem requiring rehabilitation (tearing down and rebuilding) and lifetime management of a propensity for relapse, a developmental perspective hypothesis that the abusive youth may need habilitation (nurturing and growth) to return to a more normative developmental pathway" (p. 427). One immediate implication of this approach is that it is not possible to do effective work with the young person alone, it is essential to work with the parents or carers who create much of the development and affective environment to which Ryan refers.

Programmes need to work out and disseminate clearly their philosophy of intervention, and underpinning values to guide both their own and other staff. Programme philosophy has important practical implications such as: the degree to which parents are included; the extent to which the young person is consulted; and whether developmental considerations are integrated alongside an ethos of accountability for behaviour. An absence of a clear value base will undermine both external credibility and internal consistency. In the worst cases it may result in punitive approaches based on a perception that these young people are first and foremost sexual offenders who simply happen to be adolescents. In contrast, a more preventative ethos will be as concerned to identify assets, capacities, competencies and needs, as well as risks and dangers. It will also have a more systemic and ecological understanding that stresses the role of family and other social systems in changing behaviour, rather than view the issue as an individual pathology that focuses solely on the behaviour of the young person.

## 5 Policy

Many agencies are involved in the identification and management of young people who sexually abuse, all of whom need to work cooperatively if the problem is to be effectively addressed. Simply establishing a specific service will not be enough. Indeed it may result in the other agencies merely dumping cases on the doorstep of the fledgling service. In order to ensure that the service is used appropriately, agencies need to put in place clear multi-disciplinary policies for referral, investigation, assessment, case planning, monitoring and review that specify the ongoing roles and responsibilities of all agencies.

Painful lessons have been learnt from the management of adult sexual offenders that treatment provision is not enough. Effective management must also include monitoring and supervision. There is also a need to ensure, especially with sibling abuse, that the needs and protection of the victim are properly addressed. Without a multi-disciplinary policy framework, service providers can find themselves receiving referrals for treatment where there has been no proper assessment of the child protection or criminal issues involved. To provide treatment in these circumstances may be both dangerous and unethical.

It is especially important that the referral, investigation and early assessment stages are coordinated between criminal justice and child protection responses as they each operate under different legislative, policy and assessment (*Assessment for Children in Need*, Department of Health, 2000a v. ASSETT Home Office, 1999) frameworks with different timescales and requirement in terms of multi-disciplinary consultation. Without some integration of these frameworks at a central government level, it will be left to agencies at a local level to address this. In particular, attention will need to be paid to: ensuring there are common operational definitions of cases to be referred for investigation; clarifying which cases police and social services will investigate, when these will be joint investigations and how each will consult the other throughout the process; establishing an initial assessment framework that addresses both the sexually abusive behaviour and the wider needs of the young person and which includes the parents; identifying who should be involved in doing such assessments; agreeing timescales for the initial assessment that can be accommodated by both child protection and criminal justice agencies. It is highly unlikely that any meaningful initial assessment can be completed within the initial assessment timeframes of either the

Department of Health (7 days) or Home Office (10 days) frameworks. However, local agreements have been forged to extend these timescales, agreeing a multi-disciplinary case planning process for young people who are not subject to child protection conferences. One example is the AIM project in Greater Manchester (Print *et al.*, 2001), which has established assessment frameworks based on the identification not only of risks but also of strengths and needs and agreed an extended period of twenty working days for initial assessment

## 6 Programme development

Once a multi-disciplinary policy framework has been established, and the target population is identified, it is possible to develop services and programmes. In the UK group work, largely based on adult programmes, has until recently been the dominant therapeutic model. This is despite the fact that the vast majority of staff dealing with these young people have no access to group programmes and are working on an individual basis. However, the move to a more holistic approach based on a more developmental understanding will require more attention to individual and family work. Elsewhere in this volume we discuss the importance of and issues surrounding work with parents and other family members. Suffice it to say here that there is a pressing need for funding bodies and providers to recognise that work with parents and key caregivers, regardless of whether the adolescent is living at home, is an essential component of an effective service. Too often it is left as an optional extra when time and money permit.

One final point concerns the importance of writing down programme aims, structures, outcomes, protocols, sessional plans and intervention methods. This is not to make such detail prescriptive but rather to ensure that there is a shared basis of understanding for all workers about how the programme is delivered. Without this, new workers can be left dependent on existing workers to explain these key matters, which can inhibit their integration and induction to the programme, and result in unnecessary mystification and a lack of confidence of new staff. This particularly affects co-workers who may only be co-working on a single case basis.

## 7 Preparation and management of staff

A whole chapter would be required to cover this key area. Therefore, in this section attention is drawn to some critical issues and references to other literature are suggested. Staff are the most precious resource available to the services in which they work. If they are not well managed, their motivation, knowledge, skills and emotional responsiveness will be under-utilised at best and lost at worst. Ensuring that staff can work at their best, requires the establishment of a positive context within which they can perform. Addressing the organisational and inter-agency issues presented here is therefore crucial, alongside the management of individual staff, to which we turn now. Five areas are discussed: recruitment; standards; supervision; training; and staff care.

### 7.1 *Recruitment*

Given how crucial staff are to the delivery and outcomes of any service, good recruitment is essential. It is also one of the hardest elements to get right. In addition to the professional knowledge, skills and experience that are required, attention needs to be paid to the personal capacities and competencies of the individual. This is particularly significant given the emotional demands and potential impact of this work which has been described elsewhere (Morrison, 1997; Ryan and Lane, 1991). In an unpublished doctoral study, Banks (2002) observed workers and young people. The key dynamic was one in which the workers, faced with young people who resisted taking ownership of their abusive sexual behaviour, responded by either engaging in a fight for control during interviews, or adopting a nurturing role to rescue both the worker and the client from this discomfort. In one set of observations Banks found that the workers were talking nearly twice as much as the young people during sessions. Whilst powerful inter-personal processes were clearly in play in the worker's relationship with the young people, there can be no doubt that these are also shaped by the wider context in which the very same "responsibility-avoidance syndrome" is being enacted across government and agencies at national, institutional and inter-agency levels.

Workers must not only have clinical skills, but also organisational, collaborative and self-management skills, and the ability to work constructively within team and multi-disciplinary settings. Goleman (1998) has identified the key role played by emotional intelligence in being effective within the workplace. He describes this under five domains of (a) self-awareness; (b) self-regulation; (c) motivation; (d) empathy; and (e) social skills.

Although not all of these need to be stressed equally, the need to test self-management skills and integrity are essential, and applies every bit as much to managers as to practitioners. Indeed the more powerful the role, the more damaging the absence of these skills becomes. Programmes and teams are far more vulnerable to the corrosive influence of just one member who lacks personal containment or who has no capacity to work with others, than to a colleague who lacks technical knowledge or skills. These issues need to be taken into account in writing job descriptions and person specifications and in designing a selection process that is not oriented simply to the candidate's intellectual or technical prowess but which also explores personal and emotional resilience.

### 7.2 *Standards*

Services need not only multi-disciplinary policies, but also internal policies and standards to ensure role clarity and accountability. Few services will have standards in this new area of work, although some agencies have begun to put these in place. This means a new service is frequently faced with managing new staff who may well be drawn from a range of disciplines, some of whom are working on a seconded basis, without any of the usual performance management structures. This can create anxiety and uncertainty, and needs to be addressed early on. It is particularly important to establish the lines of accountability for seconded staff who may be reporting to two management systems.

It is also useful to bear in mind that the general principles and standards of good practice can be readily translated into this field – for example, evidence-based practice, thorough assessment, clear recording, good planning and review, user-involvement, and a multi-disciplinary approach. Although there may be some specific standards that need to be considered, for instance standards regarding behavioural interventions addressing deviant sexual fantasy, existing child protection or residential child care guidelines are applicable. Written programme protocols, as discussed above, are extremely important in establishing clear standards and expectations.

### 7.3 *Supervision*

It is hard to overestimate the need for good supervision. Every UK child abuse inquiry has stressed the significance of supervision when managing high risk cases, and it is highlighted in *Working Together* (Department of Health, 1999) as being necessary for all disciplines involved in child protection work. Supervision is the helping professional's most essential relationship (Morrison, 1993). The recent Chief Social Services Inspectors Eighth Annual Report (Department of Health, 2000b) stressed the key role played by those who directly manage practice: "What makes a significant difference to the performance of an organisation is the quality and competence of frontline managers. Frontline managers are the keystones of the organisation. They manage the primary tasks and activities of the organisation, they have a key role in determining whether standards of practice are maintained, in supporting staff engaged in complex, personally demanding practice, and ensuring that staff are continually developed in knowledge-based practice" (p. 6).

It is vital to remember that supervision is part of the intervention in the lives of our clients. Furthermore it is not simply having supervision that is important, having *good* supervision is the key to good practice. Poor or negative experience of supervision can be destructive of both workers and their practice, especially if this occurs in the context of work which generates a high degree of anxiety. Good supervision involves some key elements without which the outcomes for both workers and clients are unlikely to be improved. These key elements of supervision are: (a) eliciting accurately the worker's observations and information about the client; (b) processing the worker's emotional responses to and engagement with the client; (c) enabling the worker to use their own and others' evidence and information to analyse the situation with reference to research, theory and agency roles and expectations; and (d) helping the worker to consider the costs and benefits of different options and preparing and supporting the worker in devising and carrying out a plan (Morrison, 2000).

### *7.4 Training*

Many otherwise experienced workers encountering cases of young people who commit sexual assaults suffer an acute loss of confidence and an inability to transfer sometimes considerable professional knowledge and skills to this area. This applies equally to managers as to practitioners, resulting in a knee jerk reaction of seeking immediate and often expensive referral to a specialist, or searching for an external consultant because the work "is so different". Although each may have a role to play, there remains considerable mystique and some unhelpful jargon that further obscures things. In addition there is fear about risk, and anxiety about discussion of sexual matters.

Addressing the areas raised in this chapter will help in reducing these anxieties and providing the infrastructure for practice. The starting-point is a good induction programme for staff. Without this, the transition and joining processes become delayed and staff may quickly lose confidence. Part of the induction process to this work is to enable staff to reflect on the emotional responses and fears they may bring, and to come to terms with the nature of the work itself. The message is one of giving permissions for staff to have difficult and mixed feelings at times, and making this normative. Attention to issues of gender and sexuality is essential, and it can be very helpful to share some of this process in team and supervisory settings.

Early audit of skills, experience and knowledge can then follow, in which it is very important to highlight how skills acquired with other groups of troubled young people and their families are transferable to this work. As Ryan (1999) observes, the more the problem of sexually abusive behaviour in young people is understood developmentally, the greater are the similarities rather than differences across a range of dysfunctions: "Although the manifest behavior problem looks different (e.g.: substance abuse, eating disorders, physical abuse, domestic violence, property destruction and arson, self destructive risk taking), the etiology, dynamics, issues and treatment strategies relevant to abusive behaviors are more similar than specific" (p. 426). Thus, enabling staff to tap into their experience of managing young people with attachment problems, negative coping strategies and poor social skills will constitute a very significant advance in being able to recognise the competencies new staff already possess. After that, identifying some specific training needs can then be undertaken with greater accuracy. A similar process for supervisors is required to help them recognise that what helped staff with child protection or other high risk cases will be exactly what staff in this field require.

### 7.5 *Staff care*

Once the mystique and jargon is peeled away and the similarities with other fields is made manifest, one of the defining differences that remain is that this is a field where staff are asked to address intimate issues about sexual behaviour and identity. For each of us, working in this field will take us on an unavoidable journey that explores the meaning of our own sexuality. For many this may result in personal growth and celebration of the most positive elements of our sexuality, although there may be painful places to visit along the way. But where the journey is avoided, there lies a route not only to personal vulnerability but potentially to a lack of containment, boundaries and mutual trust, which can overwhelm even the strongest of programmes and teams. These observations fit with findings that job satisfaction is lower in professionals where personal or sexual issues intrude into work with clients, or where professionals are preoccupied with work and work related performance to the exclusion of non-work involvements. Therefore, there is a responsibility upon both individuals and agencies to consider the emotional preparation and care of staff. The stronger the organisational framework and professional competence available to the worker, the more possible it will be to negotiate the personal dimensions of this work. For a fuller discussion of these issues and how staff can prepare for this work on a personal level readers are invited to see excellent discussions by Erooga (1994) and Hackett (1999).

However, in terms of stress, we cannot ignore the acutely pressurised context in which we are all working and the effects of this on the emotional capacity and responsiveness of staff. Recent American surveys of child welfare staff (Anderson 2000) found that 62 per cent scored in the high range for both emotional exhaustion and depersonalisation, reflecting a strong trend towards burnout which was appreciably higher than the levels observed among a comparison group surveyed in 1986. The negative implication is clear: staff can carry on performing the task while withdrawing from its emotional demands.

## 8 *External networking*

It will be recalled from the team building framework presented above that the last ingredient cited was positive linkage with the external world. Services that become marginalised or isolated from their external network, within and across agencies, quickly lose credibility. They also lose the capacity to be effective in a field in which multi-disciplinary working is essential. The quality of the individual therapist, however brilliant, is a necessary but never a sufficient condition to be effective with this population.

There is a need therefore for active attention to building networks and having a clear communication strategy at all levels. It is no use having superb communication with senior managers if practitioners and local first line managers do not know who you are, or what you do. The result may be a great service with no referrals. The best multi-disciplinary work occurs when the formal arrangements are built upon strong informal networks. This provides a basis of mutual understanding that will ensure that the service is more likely to be used appropriately, that other agencies play their part, and that the problems and hitches that will inevitably arise can be quickly addressed. Some programmes have found that running regular clinics in different localities where staff can discuss difficult cases can be very useful as well as providing opportunities for non-specialists to co-work. Consultation services are also helpful and allow a wide range of professionals to access the service.

## 9 *Quality assurance and audit*

In recent years there has been an increasing expectation that services will be audited in order to demonstrate outcomes. However, this is far more advanced in work with adult sexual offenders, where there has been Home Office supported research such as that conducted by the Sex-Offender Treatment Evaluation Project (STEP) team. One outcome of this was the development of a number of measures that can be utilised to examine the clinical effectiveness of therapeutic work, in addition to reviewing criminal recidivism. However, in the adolescent field, the picture is much more primitive, with almost no controlled outcome studies and few outcome measures. Although some recidivism studies have been conducted (Sipe *et al.*, 1998) these suffer from a range of methodological problems, and in any event the vast majority of adolescents committing such assaults do not enter the criminal justice system. Moreover, given the complexity and interrelatedness of problems in these young people, auditing effectiveness will require devising measures across a range of social and behavioural functioning. As we become clearer about the distinctions between adults and adolescent offenders, the less it will be safe to rely upon outcome measures that have been traditionally used with adults, such as the reduction in deviant arousal. There will need to be less emphasis on sexual specific areas and more on emotional and behavioural development alongside a reduction in risk. We should not forget too the importance of simply asking young people and their families for feedback on the experience of the services, given that the quality of that relationship is likely to have as much influence on outcomes as the specific methods we use. Thus four levels of audit can be envisioned: (1) Compliance – Did the service deliver against what it promised? (2) User satisfaction – How did young people and their families experience the service? (3) Staff confidence and competence – How equipped do staff feel to deliver the service? (4) Qualitative outcomes – What strengths were enhanced, what risks were reduced, and what needs were met in terms of the overall developmental goals of the young person?

### 10 Pitfalls to avoid

In summarising much of the above there are a number of pitfalls to avoid if services are not to be set up only to fail. Establishing realistic expectations and a viable service mission are crucial to reducing stress and making the job manageable and fulfilling. Here then are ten pitfalls to avoid:

(a) short-term funding;
(b) unclear work and role boundaries;
(c) therapeutic work where child protection and criminal issues have not been addressed.
(d) requests to quantify risk exactly and make impossible predictions;
(e) risk dominated "offence-discrete" approaches which fail to address strengths and needs;
(f) inappropriate use of specialists to carry, rather than share, the anxieties of other agencies, and lack of inter-agency framework for services;
(g) failing to engage parents or caregivers;
(h) over-focus on young people in the criminal justice system, under-focus on other young people "in need";
(i) inappropriate use of models based on work with adult sexual offenders;
(j) lack of attention to unresolved trauma and loss in the young person.

## Conclusions

It was Oscar Wilde who said that a map of the world without Utopia was useless. The intention of this chapter has been to address some of the real world context in which many workers are striving to establish new services and programmes for young people and their families. Although the discussion has been drawn from a UK context, it is hoped that readers from other contexts will be able to translate the core frameworks into their situation. If there is a final message, it is this. As we discover that the sexual offender treatment world is not as narrow as we first thought, that there is a significant cross-over with other types of abusive behaviours, we realise that we have a much wider, richer and deeper pool of knowledge and experience to draw upon. But above all, it will be our persistence and responsiveness that will win the day. As Tonnesmann (1979) reflected at the Fourth Annual Winnicott Conference in London:

> The human encounter in the helping professions is inherently stressful. The stress aroused can be accommodated and used for the good of our clients. But our emotional responsiveness will wither if the human encounter cannot be contained within the institutions in which we work. Defensive manoeuvres will then occur and these will prevent healing . . . by contrast if we can maintain contact with the emotional reality of our clients and ourselves then the human encounter can facilitate not only a therapeutic experience for them, but also an enriching experience for us.

## References

Anderson, D. (2000). Coping strategies and burnout amongst veteran child protection workers. *Child Abuse and Neglect, 24(6)*, 839–848.

Banks, N. (2002). Unconscious Processes in Practitioners who Work Therapeutically with Children and Young People who Sexually Abuse. Unpublished doctoral thesis, University of Sussex.

Chaffin, M., and Bonner, B. (1998). "Don't shoot, we're your children". *Journal of Child Maltreatment*, November, 314–316.

Department of Health (1992). *Strategic Statement on Working with Sex Offenders*. London: HMSO.

Department of Health (1999). *Working Together to Safeguard Children: New Government Proposals for Inter-Agency Collaboration*. London: HMSO.

Department of Health (2000a). *Framework for the Assessment of Children in Need and their Families*. London: HMSO.

Department of Health (2000b). *Modern Social Services: A Commitment to Improve*. 8th Annual Report of Chief Inspector of Social Services. London: HMSO.

Department of Health (2002) *Safeguarding Children: A Joint Chief Inspectors' Report on Arrangements to Safeguard Children*. London: Department of Health.

Erooga, M. (1994). Where the professional meets the personal. In T. Morrison, M. Erooga and R. Beckett (eds), *Sexual Offending against Children*. London: Routledge.

Erooga, M., and Masson, H. (1999). *Children and Young People who Sexually Abuse Others*. London: Routledge.

Goleman, D. (1998). *Working with Emotional Intelligence*. London: Bloomsbury.

Hackett, S. (1999). Empowered practice with young people who sexually abuse. In M. Erooga and H. Masson (eds), *Children and Young People who Sexually Abuse Others*. London: Routledge.

Hackett, S., Masson, H., and Phillips, S. (2002) *Mapping and Exploring Services for Young People who Sexually Abuse*. Funded by NOTA, NSPCC, YJB, in progress.

Her Majesty's Inspector of Probation (1998). *Exercising Constant Vigilance: the Role of the Probation Service in Protecting the Public from Sex Offenders*. Report of a Thematic Inspection. London: Home Office.

Horne, L., Glasgow, D., Cox, A., and Calam, R. (1991). Sexual abuse of children by children. *Journal of Child Law, 3(4)*, 147–151.

Kelly, L., Regan, L., and Burton, S. (1991). *An Exploratory Study of the Prevalence of Sexual Abuse in a Sample of 16–21 year olds*. London: North London Polytechnic Child Sexual Assault Unit.

Larson, C., and Lafasto, F. (1989). *Team Work: What Must Go Right: What Can Go Wrong*. London: Sage.

McKeown, K. (2000). *A Guide to What Works in Family Support Services for Vulnerable Families*. Dublin: Department of Health and Children.

Masson, H. (1996). *Children and Adolescents who Sexually Abuse other Children: An Emerging Problem: Second Interim Report*. UK: University of Huddersfield School of Human and Health Sciences.

Monke, E., and New, M. (1995). *Report of a Study of Sexually Abused Children and Adolescents and of Young Perpetrators of Sexual Abuse who were Treated in Voluntary Agency Community Facilities*. London: HMSO.

Morrison, T. (1993). *Staff Supervision in Social Care*. Brighton: Pavilion.

Morrison, T. (1997). Emotionally competent child protection organisations: Fallacy, fiction or necessity? In J. Bates (ed.), *Protecting Children: Challenges and Change*. Aldershot: Arena.

Morrison, T. (2000). Working together to safeguard children: Challenges and changes for inter-agency co-ordination in child protection. *Journal of Inter-Professional Care, 14(4)*.

Morrison, T. (2001). *Staff Supervision in Social Care: Improving Outcomes for Staff and Users*, 2nd edn. Brighton: Pavilion.

NCH (1992). *Children and Young People who Abuse Other Children and Young People*. London: National Children's Home.

Poulton, B., and West, M. (1993). Effective teamwork in primary health care. *Journal of Advanced Nursing, 18*, 918–923.

Prentky, R., Harris, B., Frizzell, K., and Righthand, S. (2000). An actuarial procedure for assessing risk with juvenile sex offenders. *Sexual Abuse, 12(4)*, 71–89.

Print, B., Morrison, T., and Henniker, J. (2001) An inter-agency assessment framework for young people who sexually abuse: Principles, processes and practicalities. In M. Calder (ed.), *Juveniles and Children who Sexually Abuse: Frameworks for Assessment*, 2nd edn. Lyme Regis: Russell House.

Ryan, G. (1999). Treatment of abusive youth: The evolving consensus. *Journal of Interpersonal Violence, 14 (4)*, 422–436.

Ryan, G., and Lane, S. (1991). *Juvenile Sexual Offending: Causes, Consequences and Corrections*. Lexington, MA: Lexington Books.

Sanders, R., and Ladwa-Thomas, U. (1997). Interagency perspectives on child sexual abuse perpetrated by juveniles. *Child Maltreatment, 2(3)*, 264–271.

Sipe, R., Jansen, E., and Everett, R. (1998). Adolescent sexual offenders grown up: Recidivism in young adulthood. *Criminal Justice and Behaviour, 25(1)*, 109–124.

STRATA (1997). *Policy on Working with Children and Young People who Sexually Abuse Others*. UK: National Children's Home Cymru Wales Office.

Tonnesmann, M. (1979). The human encounter in the helping professions. 4th London Winnicott Conference. In P. Hawkins and R. Shohet (eds), *Supervision in the Helping Professions*. Milton Keynes: Open University Press.

Woodcock, M. (1988). *50 Activities for Team Building*. Aldershot: Gower.

Yochelson, S., and Samenow, S. (1976). *The Criminal Personality*. New York: Aronson.

Chapter 16

# European perspectives on juveniles who sexually abuse

*Ruud Bullens and A. Ph. Van Wijk*

## Introduction

This chapter attempts to provide a European perspective on sexually abusive behaviour perpetrated by juveniles. It has three main sections: a description of the main cultural and contextual differences in European countries with regard to juveniles who sexually abuse; a description of approaches taken by services in various European countries; and a brief review of European research concerning adolescent abusers with particular emphasis given to studies published in languages other than English which consequently do not usually find their way into the mainstream research literature.

## Cultural and contextual differences in European countries

Compared to the decades-old nationwide attention given to juvenile sexual offenders in the USA (Apfelberg *et al.*, 1944; Atcheson and Williams, 1954; Lane and Zamora, 1978; Markey, 1950), it is only in recent years that this topic has received attention in a variety of countries on the European continent. Before addressing the most important cultural and contextual differences within Europe regarding the assessment and treatment of juvenile sexual offenders, we will outline the most important factors that could have hindered the development of this field in comparison to English-speaking countries. In the Netherlands, recognition of juvenile sexual offending has followed from the "discovery" of the phenomenon of sexual abuse in the beginning of the 1980s. The chronological sequence of events related to the recognition of this problem has been that initially attention was concentrated on the victims/survivors of sexual abuse. In the second half of the 1980s there was a recognition of a need for additional focus regarding adult perpetrators of sexual offences. This was followed in the first half of the 1990s by a growing understanding of the needs of non-offending parents and other non-victimised children within a family. It was at this time that the existence of juvenile sexual offenders was also "discovered". Prior to this in the Netherlands sexual abuse by youths was regarded as reflecting a developmentally understandable psychological function for the adolescent during a period of sexual experimentation. This view was altered by research suggesting that many adult sexual offenders have deviant sexual interests in their youth. This raised an awareness of the potential danger to society posed by the juvenile sexual offender.

Without doubt it is interesting from an historical perspective, to trace the slow development of acknowledgement concerning the phenomenon of sexual abuse by juveniles on the European continent. Three factors that have probably played a particularly significant role in delaying awareness are: (1) a lack of a common language on the European continent; (2) socio-cultural differences; and (3) political and historical differences.

### 1 *A lack of a common language*

The availability of a common language is essential for the communication of scientific knowledge. English is the primary language within the USA, thus facilitating general access to scientific findings within the region. This is also true for other English-speaking countries, such as Canada, Australia, New Zealand, South Africa, the Republic of Ireland and the United Kingdom. In these countries an exchange of scientific research findings is easier because they are communicated using a single language. This differs to a large extent on the European continent, where dozens of different languages and dialects stand in the way of a fluid exchange of scientific research findings. In contrast, consider the example of Germany and its neighbours. Germany is bordered by nine different countries with at least nine different languages: the Netherlands (Dutch), Belgium (Dutch/Flemish, French, German), France (French), Switzerland (German, French, Italian), Austria (German), the Chechen Republic (Chechen), the Czech Republic (Czech), Poland (Polish), and Denmark (Danish). This situation of rich linguistic diversity is not conducive to a quick exchange of scientific information in a manner found among the English-speaking countries listed above.

### 2 *Socio-cultural differences*

Undoubtedly the cultural differences among European countries, and the regions within these nations, are great. It seems reasonable to suppose that the cultural heritage of European nations influences the manner in which the phenomenon of sexual abuse is dealt with. For example, Germanic countries tend to be predominantly oriented towards the adoption of psychoanalytical models of psychology. This may in part reflect a recent historical influence promoting a reluctance to adopt a cognitive behavioural model that advocates the changing of "unhealthy" systems of belief. In contrast, after World War II the Netherlands and Scandinavian nations had a significant orientation towards the UK and the USA. Consequently psychological intervention in these countries is more reflective of a cognitive behavioural model of psychology. In the culture of Mediterranean countries such as Italy the family is assigned a particularly important role. This has promoted the adoption of psychological models that emphasise family and systemic factors. These examples illustrate the interaction between different European cultural influences and the adoption of different models of psychology. These different models of psychology promote different ways of understanding and responding to the problem of sexual abuse.

### *3 Political and historical influences*

Not only are the lack of a common language and enormous cultural differences responsible for the delayed development of an adequate approach to juvenile sexual offenders on the European continent, but political and historical differences have also made an important contribution. On the European continent, a great variety of centuries-old traditions, cultures, political systems and perceptions exist concerning many aspects of life, including sexuality and sexual abuse. This greatly complicates the creation of a coordinated vision of a unified assessment and therapeutic approach to juvenile sexual offenders, similar to that which exists in the USA and the United Kingdom.

## Description of approaches to services in various European countries for juveniles who sexually abuse

Given the influences outlined in the previous section that have contributed to a delayed recognition of and response to the problem of juvenile sexual offending, it is not surprising that in many European countries the development of interventions with this population is in its infancy. There are two main types of therapeutic response that have emerged. The first are general individual psychotherapy approaches that are primarily concerned with the development of the young person's well-being. Underlying personality problems are central in these psychoanalytically derived individual treatments whose aim is not so much "control" but "cure". The second type of intervention to emerge in Europe is derived from cognitive behavioural models of intervention which reflect a "no cure but control" paradigm. These approaches to intervention focus on aspects of personality such as self-esteem, locus of control, impulsiveness, assertiveness and social skills, combined with offence related aspects of psychological functioning such as the development of victim empathy, restructuring cognitive distortions, and tackling problems such as experiencing emotional congruence with younger children. There are two aspects of intervention with juvenile sexual offenders that are significantly different from those used with adults. These are the inclusion of information from developmental psychology to inform clinical practice and the recognition that parents play an important role in successful intervention.

In particular, the northern West European countries have followed the USA and the UK in recent years by adopting manualised treatment programmes for juvenile sexual offenders with the aim of ensuring a more structured and transparent approach. "Programme integrity" and "treatment fidelity" have become important concepts. Careful evaluation of treatment programmes based on pre- and post-intervention assessments of young sexual offenders is regarded as one aspect of good practice. As a result of this, we can speak of a more thoughtful approach to the juvenile sexual offender in recent years. Interventions are not simply re-applications of programmes designed for adults. Instead they reflect an understanding of the developmental stage of adolescence. They aim for controlled development informed by educational and occupational needs, the developmental tasks of adolescence, the importance of peer group influence, and the emergence of skills that help a young person avoid the potential negative influence of peer group pressure.

## A brief review of European research concerning adolescent abusers

In this section we will present research on juvenile sexual offenders conducted in the Netherlands, Germany and Sweden. Integrating findings from these studies is difficult because of methodological and other factors. Consequently this review will provide an impression of the current state of non-English-language research from three European countries. This review highlights the early stage of development of research concerning juvenile sexual offenders in these countries and points the direction that future research may take.

### *Dutch research*

There are currently five empirical studies of juvenile sexual offenders available from the Netherlands. The most important results from these studies are discussed below. One of the first people in the Netherlands who brought attention to juvenile sexual offenders was Bruinsma (Bruinsma, 1996). In his psychiatric practice he has studied or treated some three hundred juvenile sexual offenders. From his work a number of basic facts were established, concerning different types of juvenile offenders (Bruinsma, 1996). Fifteen per cent were responsible for hands-off offences; 45 per cent of cases concerned indecent offences with children outside of the family; 15 per cent of the youths had committed incest; and 39 per cent had assaulted or raped a member of their peer group. Almost three-quarters offended alone. The remaining juveniles acted with co-abusers. In two-thirds of the cases, the victims were known by the offender(s). Half of the youths had victimised one person, 15 per cent had two victims, and 35 per cent had more than two. In almost half of the instances the victim was a girl or a woman, in 13 per cent of cases the victim was a boy, and in 9 per cent of cases the victims were boys as well as girls. A psychiatric disorder was present in 30 per cent of cases. About 10 per cent had a personality disorder and about 10 per cent had a severe neurotic disorder. The latter was particularly true of those committing indecency with very young children. Approximately half of the juvenile sexual offenders lived with both natural parents. In 40 per cent of young people there was a query regarding experiences of neglect, in 15 per cent of cases there was suspected physical abuse, and in 14 per cent there was sexual abuse within the family. Thirty-three per cent reported that they had three or more friends, while 22 per cent reported that they had no friends.

Boelrijk (1997) reviewed police records of 182 youths suspected of sexual offences. They found that approximately two-thirds of the suspects were reported to have committed their offence with one or more accomplices. In 75 per cent of cases the offences were reported to be perpetrated on peers. The most extreme cases involved assault and rape. Violation and abuse of small children was less frequently a feature of sexual crimes perpetrated by young people recorded in the police files reviewed. The majority of victims were female (92%). The age range of victims was from three to forty-six years with an average age of fourteen years. In roughly 75 per cent of cases the victim was the same age as the offender. The average age of offenders was fourteen (14.8) years old. In many cases (33%) the offender and the victim came into contact by chance. In one-third of cases the offender had employed some tactics to get access to the victim, such as luring them to a secluded area. In half of the cases the offender knew the victim. Practically none of the alleged offenders used a weapon. However, one-third of the suspects did allegedly use some form of violence. In a small number of cases the alleged offender used alcohol or soft drugs. One-third of the youths had prior non-sexual offences. In contrast, the police records reveal that a small number of youths (4%) had prior sexual offences. Approximately one-quarter of the suspects reoffended after their alleged sexual offence. In most instances their subsequent offence was non-sexual. Half of the alleged offenders lived in two-parent homes and more than half (52%) of the suspects were born in the Netherlands.

Hendriks and Bijleveld (1999) compared solo and group perpetrators of sexual abuse by reviewing 100 psychological assessment files. These files revealed that two-thirds of the juvenile sexual offenders had committed their offences alone. The remainder perpetrated their offences with one or more accomplices. The solo offenders committed rape (55%), sexual assault (35%) and incest (10%). The group offenders committed rape (88%) and sexual assault (12%). The average age of all offenders was fifteen years. The solo offenders were about eight months older than the group offenders. Three-quarters of the solo offenders were recidivists compared to one-quarter of the group offenders. More than half of the recidivists who offended alone perpetrated their offences against different victims. It appeared that the solo offenders were more neurotic and impulsive than the group offenders. In addition they scored more highly on a measure of the need for excitement and scored lower on a measure of sociability. Solo offenders were more often reported to have been the past victim of a sexual offence. Group offenders were reported to have fewer deviant personality traits. Approximately half of the juvenile sexual offenders in Hendriks and Bijleveld's study came from intact families. About 60 per cent were of Dutch ethnicity, 14 per cent Antillian, 6 per cent Surinam, 4 per cent Moroccan and 6 per cent were mixed. Those who offended in a group were predominantly of a Dutch background. About one-quarter of the sample in this study were attending special education. Half were in, or had completed vocational school. Ten per cent had dropped out of further education and the remainder (15%) were in high school or in university preparation.

Van Wijk (1999) reviewed twenty-seven files concerning juvenile sexual offenders randomly chosen from psychological and justice records. The results indicated that there were two groups of juvenile sexual offenders who differed in a number of ways. The two groups were (a) rapists and assaulters of peers or adult women and (b) those who abuse young children. The "rapists and assaulters" offended alone or in groups. Their average age at the time of their offence was fifteen years. They tended to victimise girls of the same age or women who were older. They displayed almost no planning and tended to abuse others opportunistically. Their psychological profile suggested impulsivity combined with an external locus of control. This group committed a variety of sexual and non-sexual offences (including theft and violent assault). In some instances they used alcohol or drugs prior to offending. In contrast, Van Wijk found that those who abused children were solo offenders who tended to be somewhat younger than the rapist group. Their offences were more likely to be characterised by prior planning and manipulation of victims. The victims were both male and female. They tended to minimise the severity of their offending behaviour and displayed deviant sexual fantasies. None of the offenders against children used alcohol or drugs prior to their abusive behaviour.

Van Wijk and Ferwerda (2000) developed a profile of sexual offenders based on a review of 980 police records covering a ten-year period. Thirty-five per cent of these records concerned young people who had perpetrated a sexual crime before their eighteenth birthday. With few exceptions, the offenders were male. They were found guilty of the following types of offences: violation of virtue (6%); rape (36%); assault (41%) and miscellaneous sexual crimes such as lewdness with minors (17%). For almost half of the youths (45%) this was their first offence. The review of police records made clear that juveniles committing sexual offences (n = 338) were also frequently guilty of other non-sexual crimes. On average there were nine crimes per offender, including theft without violence (52%), and public order disturbances and vandalism (11%). The average age that they committed their first offence was fourteen (14.8) years, while the average age of their first registered sexual offence was slightly older (15.4 years). This implies that many juvenile sexual offenders who come to the attention of the police may first commit a non-sexual crime.

### German research

German researchers have also accepted that sexual abuse by juveniles is not just a "puberty phenomenon" or a normal phase in the process of becoming an adult. Data from the Police Criminal Statistics Bureau (Polizeilichen Kriminalstatistik) indicates that juveniles aged between fourteen and twenty years are over-represented in the category "sexual offences" (equivalent to 100 juvenile sexual offenders per 100,000 14–20-year-olds in the general population). This acceptance is further reflected in a thorough article based mostly on English language literature that outlines the necessity for more scientific and therapeutic attention to be given to juveniles who sexually offend (Deegener, 1999).

Hummel (1999) studied the degree to which juvenile sexual offenders differ from each other regarding alcohol abuse in the family. The study compared thirty-eight juveniles who had sexually abused a peer or an adult woman, with thirty-six juveniles that abused young children, and thirty-three juveniles who had committed violent offences. Hummel found that alcohol abuse was most common among fathers of young people who engaged in violent offences and least common among the fathers of those who sexually assaulted peer females and adult women. The level of alcohol use by the juveniles fourteen years of age or older during their offending behaviour was the same for those who sexually offended against peers and adult women as that observed among those who committed violent offences. Alcohol use was rarely a feature of the behaviour of those who sexually offended against young children. The study also suggested the following relationships. Parental alcohol abuse was associated with alcohol abuse by young people who sexually assault peers and adults. Parental alcohol abuse was associated with being expelled from school among those who sexually assault young children. Parental alcohol abuse was associated with alcohol use during offending behaviour among those who were responsible for violent crimes.

In a recent empirical study, Hummel *et al.* (2000) examined the similarities and differences between adolescent sexual offenders against children, with (n = 16) and without (n = 20) a history of sexual abuse themselves. The most important conclusion of this study is that experiences of parental loss or absence were clearly associated with past experiences of sexual abuse. The authors propose that experiencing parental loss, and its related problems, is associated with other problems the abused juvenile sexual offender has, such as inadequate social contact with peers and a lack of assertiveness.

### *Swedish research*

A recent study of juvenile sexual offenders in Sweden was conducted by Långström (1999). He reviewed the records of fifty-six juvenile sexual offenders between the ages of fifteen and twenty years who attended for forensic psychiatric assessment. There were two female offenders in the group. Two-thirds of the total sample of juvenile sexual offenders were of Swedish origin. Family difficulties (such as alcohol or drug use, psychiatric disorder in a family member, and neglect) were apparent in one-third of families. One-third of the young people were diagnosed with neurological or neuropsychiatric disorders. Hyperactivity or attention problems at school characterised two-thirds of the sample. This study highlighted significant language problems among juveniles who sexually offend, with almost half of the sample presenting with speech, reading and writing difficulties. One-third of the youths reported that they had never had a girlfriend or boyfriend, and nine had been members of a criminal group. Almost 50 per cent showed signs of Conduct Disorder before fifteen years of age and nine had a high score (>26) on the revised psychopathy checklist. Ten youths were diagnosed with substance abuse difficulties. More that two-thirds of the sample used force or violence during the sexual offence and the majority (79%) of Långström's subjects penetrated their victims (genitally, orally or anally). Sixteen of the youths were under the influence of alcohol or drugs at the time of their offence. Approximately half of the young people in the study had a prior conviction, usually for a non-sexual offence.

Rates of sexual and general recidivism of 20 and 65 per cent respectively were reported by Långström. Factors predictive of general recidivism were previous criminality, early onset Conduct Disorder, psychopathy, and the use of death threats and weapons during the index sexual crime. Factors correlated with sexual recidivism were sexual deviance (early onset of sexually abusive behaviour, male victims, and more than one victim) and a lack of social skills. Långström reported that the chance of being found to be legally insane during the forensic assessments was, in comparison with juvenile non-sexual offenders and adult sexual offenders, three times higher for juveniles.

## Conclusion

In conclusion it is clear that there have been many factors that have hindered the development of a unified and consistent understanding of the problem of sexual offending by young people across different countries in continental Europe. However, it appears that some countries have begun to recognise this problem and take steps to establish empirical research and suitable therapeutic intervention. These are clearly steps in the right direction, and may yield novel research findings in the future that contribute to the development of more effective intervention programmes.

## References

Andolfi, M. (1982). *La forteresse familiale* [The Family Fortress]. Paris: Dunod.

Apfelberg, B., Sugar, C., and Pfeffer, A. Z. (1944). A psychiatric study of 250 sex offenders. *American Journal of Psychiatry, 100*, 762–770.

Atcheson, J. D., and Williams, D. C. (1954). A study of juvenile sex offenders. *American Journal of Psychiatry, 111*, 366.

Boelrijk, M. (1997). *Minderjarige Zedendelinquenten en Het Strafrecht: De Strafrechtelijke Aanpak van Minderjarige Plegers van Seksuele Delicten* [Minor sex offenders and the penal system: The punitive approach to minors committing sexual offences]. Amsterdam: VU Uitgeverij.

Bruinsma, F. (1996). *De Jeugdige Zedendelinquent* [The juvenile sex offender]. Utrecht: SWP.

Cirillo, S., and Di Blasio, P. (1989). *La famiglia maltrattante* [The bullying family]. Milan: Raffaello Cortina.

Deegener, G. (1999). Sexuell aggressive Kinder und Jugendliche: Häufigkeiten und Ursachen, Diagnostik und Therapie [Sexually aggressive children and youths: Incidence and causes, assessment and therapy]. In S. Höfling, D. Drewes and I. Epple-Waigel (eds), *Auftrag Pravention: Offensive gegen sexuellen Kindesmißbrauch*. Munich: Hans Seidel Stiftung, 352–382.

Hendriks, J., and Bijleveld, C. (1999). Jeugdige zedendelinquenten: Verschillen tussen groeps- en alleenplegers [Youth sexual offenders: Differences between group and solo offenders]. *Delikt en Delinkwent, 29*, 722–736.

Hummel, P. (1999). Familiärer Alkoholmißbrauch im Kontext von Sexual- und Körperverletzungsdelikten durch männliche jugendliche und heranwachsende [Family alcohol abuse in the context of sexual and assault offences by male juveniles and adolescents]. *Praxis der Kinderpsychologie und Kinderpsychiatrie, 48*, 734–750.

Hummel, P., Thömke, V., Oldenbürger, H. A., and Specht, F. (2000). Male adolescent sex offenders against children: Similarities and differences between those offenders with and those without a history of sexual abuse. *Journal of Adolescence, 23*, 305–317.

Lane, S., and Zamora, P. (1978). *Syllabus Materials from Inservice Training on Adolescent Sex Offenders*. Denver, CO: Closed Adolescent Treatment Center, Division of Youth Services.

Långström, N. (1999). *Young Sex Offenders: Individual Characteristics, Agency Reactions and Criminal Recidivism*. Stockholm: Karolinska Institutet, Department of Public Health, Division of Psychosocial Factors and Health, and NEUROTEC, Division of Forensic Psychiatry.

Markey, O. B. (1950). A study of aggressive sex misbehaviour in adolescents brought to juvenile court. *American Journal of Orthopsychiatry, 20*, 731.

Selvini Palazolli, M., Cirillo, S., Selvini, M., and Sorrentino, A. M. (1988). *Giochi Psicotici Nella Famiglia* [Psychotic games in the family]. Milan: Raffaello Cortina.

Wijk, A. Ph. van (1999). *Een Verkennend Onderzoek naar Jeugdige Zedendelinquenten* [An exploratory study of juvenile sex offenders]. Arhem/VU, Amsterdam: Advies- en Onderzoeksgroep Beke.

Wijk, A. Ph. van, and Ferwerda, H. B. (2000). Criminaliteitsprofielen van Zedendelinquenten: Een Analyse van Politiegegevens [Criminal profiles of sex offenders: An analysis of police files]. *Maandblad Geestelijke volksgezondheid, 12*.
Wijk, A. Ph. van, Beckett, R., Bullens, R., and Doreleijers, Th. A. H. (in preparation). *Towards a Preliminary Typology of Juvenile Sex Offenders in the Netherlands*.

Chapter 17

# Ethical and methodological issues in evaluation research with juvenile sexual abusers

*Calvin M. Langton and Howard E. Barbaree*

## Introduction

Children and adolescents who engage in sexually abusive behaviour represent a significant problem in modern western society (Barbaree, Marshall and Hudson, 1993; Ryan and Lane, 1997). Official US data for the year 2000 indicate that 16 per cent of arrests for forcible rape and 19 per cent of arrests for sexual offences (excluding forcible rape) were arrests of juveniles (US Department of Justice, 2002). Data for the years 1991 to 1996 reveal that 23 per cent of sexual offenders against children were themselves under eighteen years of age, with juveniles representing 40 per cent of those offending against victims aged under six and 39 per cent of those offending against victims aged six to eleven (Snyder, 2000). Prevalence rates are similarly disconcerting, with estimates ranging from 1.5 to 16 sexual assaults per 1,000 male juveniles (Ageton, 1983; James and Neil, 1996). Sexually abusive behaviour begins at an early age in these individuals and progresses from less to more serious acts. Burton (2000) found that 45 per cent of his sample of adolescent sexual offenders reported sexual offending before the age of twelve, with progression from less intrusive to penetrative acts. Eighty-seven per cent of juveniles convicted of a contact sexual offence admit to prior non-contact sexual offences (Wieckowski *et al.*, 1998). Importantly, juvenile sexual crimes set the stage for adult sexual crimes, since many adult sexual offenders engaged in sexually abusive behaviour as children or adolescents (Abel *et al.*, 1985; Knight and Prentky, 1993), and many report the onset of paraphilias by the age of eighteen (Abel *et al.*, 1993).

Statistics such as these have provided impetus for the development of preventative interventions and the provision of specialised treatment for adolescent sexual abusers (see Burton and Smith-Darden, 2001, for North American survey data on treatment programmes and models available for adolescent sexual abusers). However, it is disappointing to note that the development of treatment services for young sexual abusers has not been accompanied by an increase in evaluation studies. The lack of evaluation research is disconcerting, not only because of the obvious need for interventions to be informed by empirical research, but also because formal programme evaluations and service accountability should be considered essential components of treatment programmes (National Task Force on Juvenile Sexual Offending, 1993; Swenson *et al.*, 1998).

High quality evaluation research can tell us much about the efficacy of interventions. Such research contributes in important ways to the quality of clinical programmes. It informs the wider audience of clinicians, contributes to scientific knowledge and provides direction as to "best" clinical practices. When clinical programmes are developed and supervised by professionals who are knowledgeable in the relevant evaluation literature, the programme is more likely to conform to standards of practice that are supported by the empirical literature. High quality evaluation research leads to high quality clinical programmes that in turn lead to more desirable outcomes for clients, their families and the community. Peer review can increase the quality of evaluation research, by placing heavy demands on researchers for methodological rigour. Peer review ensures that only the best research gets funded and published.

While this process increases the quality of the research being published, it can have the unfortunate and potentially harmful effect of discouraging data collection of any kind. Often professionals in applied settings shy away from research because they feel they cannot meet the rigorous standards of methodology. However, much evaluation research is conducted in circumstances where exacting standards of methodological rigour cannot be met. A hypothetical example will assist in making this important point. A small agency that has implemented a local treatment programme for juvenile sexual offenders has established a protocol to evaluate the programme's effectiveness. Offenders who participate in the programme are monitored after they leave the programme. Recidivism and other forms of re-offending behaviour are recorded for each participant during a five-year follow-up period. In the mind of the agency's director, this evaluation is necessary to support future requests for financial and other institutional or government support. Her agency is required to seek regular accreditation and she has organised this evaluation project to support her claims that the clinical programme is of a high quality. In this protocol, she has decided to focus on re-offending behaviour because she expects that the first question in the minds of funding bodies and accreditation teams will be whether or not the programme "works" in preventing future sexual abuse.

According to her critics, the evaluation study is methodologically weak and should not have been undertaken. The critics say that the absence of an appropriate comparison (untreated) group makes such a follow-up study worthless as an evaluation of the effectiveness of their treatment. Other critics point out that the numbers of subjects in the ultimate sample will be so small that any future statistical analyses will be compromised. Still others point out that the recidivism rate expected in a short five-year follow-up period is so small that comparisons of these numbers to any benchmark would be essentially meaningless.

Despite these criticisms, the agency continues with the evaluation protocol. While the agency director expects that the results of the evaluation will not be published in a peer-reviewed scientific journal, she feels strongly that the evaluation has an important role to play in the development of her agency and that it will benefit and contribute to the ultimate quality of the programme. Indeed, since establishing the protocol and beginning the data collection, she has noticed that the programme staff have changed in their approach to their work. They think more systematically and strategically about their clinical practice. They focus more on treatments designed to reduce recidivism and failure on release. Programme exercises that had been popular in the past but were not viewed as having an impact on recidivism were being used less frequently. In the words of the programme director, her treatment team was more focused on "results". Further, in regular meetings with referring agencies, her treatment team discussed the outcome data with more and more confidence. While they were unable to attest to the efficacy of the treatment programme in a scientific sense, they were able to communicate the recidivism rate amongst their clientele. The referring agency staff were impressed that the treatment team knew who had re-offended and in what circumstances. Finally, this programme evaluation was credited for securing funding that might otherwise have been lost. In reviewing the recidivism rates as presented in the application for continued funding, the reviewers for the funding agency expressed surprise at how low the rate was. The recidivism rate seemed lower than their general expectations would have predicted.

Often, research projects that begin with compromises to methodological rigour can evolve into research that eventually achieves an acceptable level of methodological rigour. The scientific literature is enriched by the existence of data sets that did not originally meet the standards of scientific rigour. For example, in meta-analyses, such data sets are often sought and combined, leading to important analyses of large sample sizes.

The present chapter will argue that clinical programmes for the juvenile sexual offender should conduct programme evaluations and local research projects to the extent that they can, collecting important data and testing critical hypotheses, even when such research does not and will not meet the standards for peer review publication or grant support. In these circumstances, methodological rigour is achieved to the extent that it is possible, practical and cost-efficient. Everyone accepts that these local research projects may not lead to publication in the peer reviewed literature and cannot lead to the strength of inferences and widespread acceptance that is afforded peer reviewed research. It is important to note here that careful data collection, even within the context of research with methodological weaknesses, is better than no data collection at all.

In this chapter we will consider the literature on young people who sexually offend, focusing specifically on treatment evaluation, with a view to advancing awareness of a number of ethical and methodological issues inherent in the research process. As such, our discussion is intended to apply to both male and female young offenders (although it is worth noting that the research on females who exhibit sexually inappropriate or assaultive behaviour is very limited). Throughout this chapter we will use the terms "young sexual abuser" as well as "child", "adolescent" (developmental constructs), and "juvenile" (a legal term), interchangeably (Barbaree, Hudson and Seto, 1993). This is not to encourage a lax approach to sample description, theoretical specificity or data analysis, but only because it allows us to maintain the emphasis on common methodological and ethical issues in the field. It is also worth noting that while we share with others a concern about the potentially adverse effects of labelling young people who engaged in sexually abusive behaviour as adolescent/juvenile sexual abusers or offenders (Becker, 1998), for the purposes of discussing the literature pertinent to our aims, these are useful and descriptive terms. We will use the terms "intervention", "treatment" and "supervision" to refer to the provision of any programme that represents an independent variable introduced to change sexually abusive behaviour. "Sexually abusive behaviour" as defined by the National Task Force on Juvenile Sexual Offending (1993) refers to "any sexual behavior which occurs 1) without consent; 2) without equality; or 3) as a result of coercion" (p. 11). In the absence of greater specificity in the literature, references to sexually abusive behaviour and sexual offending reflect our use of these terms as general descriptors.

The chapter is divided into two broad sections. In the first section we provide a selected overview of the ethical issues common to research with children and adolescents generally. In the second section we consider a number of methodological issues that have implications for evaluation research with young sexual abusers. By drawing attention to these issues, our intention is to indicate design considerations and foci that researchers can incorporate in their ongoing efforts to advance knowledge in this field.

## Ethical issues

The importance of attending to ethical issues in work with young sexual abusers is becoming increasingly recognised (Becker, 1998; Hunter and Lexier, 1998). Ethical concerns arise in child and adolescent mental health in a number of domains, including clinical practice (O'Rourke *et al.*, 1992), research (Munir and Earls, 1992), and education and training (Sondheimer and Martucci, 1992). Leschied and Wormith (1997) make the important distinction between unethical behaviour and an ethical dilemma. They state, "unethical behavior occurs when one contravenes a principle of practice that has been established by the discipline, an acknowledged specialist body, or the college or registration body of the profession in a specific jurisdiction . . .

[while] ethical dilemmas occur when principles are in conflict and there is no absolute agreement about their resolution" (p. 247). This chapter focuses on ethical dilemmas rather than unethical behaviour. In children's mental health, ethical dilemmas are often complicated, involving the interests and values of societal institutions (e.g. the schools, the police, correctional facilities) and the interests and influence of the child's parents in addition to the interests and perspective of the child. These ethical dilemmas therefore often involve conflicting interests and contrasting interpretations (Sondheimer and Martucci, 1992). This is complicated further in forensic contexts when the professional is confronted with the presence of a supervising authority (e.g. probation, the courts) and the issue of identifying the true client becomes prominent (Leschied and Wormith, 1997).

There are two approaches to ethical dilemmas that will get the practising professional and researcher into difficulty. First, they may try to establish a fixed set of inflexible rules to apply in each and every situation that arises. Fassler (1992) recommends that the practice of ethics remain fluid and evolve with changes in science (the relativist approach), rather than becoming fixed (the absolutist approach) and possibly inapplicable to emerging concerns. The ethical issues that arise come in countless forms and they occur in innumerable different contexts. Finding a set of fixed rules to apply that are effective with each problem in all contexts is simply too much to ask.

Second, when faced with an ethical dilemma, they may try to resolve the issue alone, without advice or input from peers. Professionals should be aware of the influence of their own training, experiences and assumptions on their approach to ethical issues. For example, their training and experience will have emphasised either the principle of rehabilitation in a mental health background, or deterrence in a criminal justice background, and these influences would be expected to quite substantially affect one's perspective (Mulvey and Phelps, 1988). It is almost impossible for any professional to see all aspects or perspectives on an issue. Professionals should utilise the rich source of support and guidance that is available from colleagues in clinical, academic and legal spheres in regard to ethical questions; institutional review boards representing perhaps the most formalised of these available to researchers. Documentation of such consultation is also advisable in order to make explicit the rationale for decisions, especially in the absence of clear direction in professional standards. Finally, there are a number of resources available to the practising professional confronted with these dilemmas, including published guidelines and codes of practice (e.g. American Psychological Association, 1992; Association for the Treatment of Sexual Abusers, 2001; Committee on Ethical Guidelines for Forensic Psychologists, 1991; National Task Force on Juvenile Sexual offending, 1993). Two important sources of ethical dilemmas in conducting research with juvenile sexual offenders have to do with the issues of (1) informed consent, and (2) privacy and confidentiality.

### *Informed consent*

Perhaps the most central ethical issue in research with human subjects concerns the potential subject's informed consent. In research with juvenile sexual offenders, obtaining informed consent from potential research participants presents researchers with particular and important ethical dilemmas. Consider the degree to which consent to participate is truly voluntary and fully informed with correctional clients. There are certainly grounds for questioning whether or not these requirements can be met with juvenile sexual offenders (Hunter and Lexier, 1998; Leschied and Wormith, 1997). Many young sexual abusers will have been mandated to participate in treatment, which, while likely a necessary measure (National Task Force on Juvenile Sexual Offending, 1993; Sheerin, 1998), presents clinicians with a number of ethical dilemmas (Leschied and Wormith, 1997). In research with this population, consent should not be presumed to be voluntary simply because involvement in the research is presented as a choice. In contexts such as mental health and correctional settings, where this treatment and research is often carried out, children and adolescents very likely experience considerable duress, and may feel compelled to consent to research participation due to the ongoing requirement to participate in treatment. Other factors that could contribute to a sense of coercion include the inherent imbalance between the children and staff as well as the children's understandable concern with anticipated costs or benefits resulting from a decision to participate or not (Mulvey and Phelps, 1988). Furthermore, despite the need for full disclosure of the potential risks and benefits of involvement, the ability of the researchers to anticipate these elements may be restricted (especially when they pertain to outcomes outside their control, such as probation and parole), which renders the degree to which the consent is informed rather limited. At a minimum for treatment evaluation research, it would be necessary to discuss the nature of the treatment and the research, the duration, intensity and likely implications of both, as well as the expected outcomes of participation in both (Leschied and Wormith, 1997). It should be emphasised to the youth also that refusal to participate in the research will have no impact on their involvement in treatment, and, of course, it should not.

DeKraai and Sales (1991) set out a number of guidelines that are relevant to the issues of consent and confidentiality with children and adolescents. They suggest that the clinician or researcher first determine whether the child is legally competent to consent. For example, certain children are considered to be emancipated minors under applicable laws. Additionally there may be relevant law that allows a youth of a particular age to consent to treatment or research. Importantly, the child must be able to comprehend the nature and impact of the procedures, and give consent voluntarily based on this understanding (for discussion of minors' capacity to consent generally see Grisso *et al.*, 1987). In cases where the child does not have the legal authority to consent, their assent to participation should be obtained, along with the informed consent of the parents or guardians. In research that has potential therapeutic benefits for the child or adolescent, this should suffice. In research that is not expected to have such a benefit, especially when risks associated with participation are not negligible, the individual's developmental capacity to understand the procedure, associated risks, and the broader benefits of the research should be considered. In such cases, the child or adolescent should be afforded the right to refuse to participate regardless of parental consent (Weinstock, 1999). Furthermore, the importance of the "process" of obtaining consent (e.g. using clear, simple, age-appropriate language, providing sufficient time for discussion and deliberation) should be recognised (National Task Force on Juvenile Sexual Offending, 1993).

Notable among the assessment and treatment tools used routinely by some clinicians and researchers in clinical research with juvenile sexual offenders is the plethysmograph, and arousal conditioning. When conducting research with this population using these intrusive methods, the researcher needs to pay special and detailed attention to the issues of informed consent. For a discussion of similar ethical concerns arising in clinical practice (i.e. assessment and treatment procedures) the reader is directed to Hunter and Lexier (1998).

### *Privacy and confidentiality*

The second central issue that raises ethical dilemmas has to do with the research subject's right to privacy and confidentiality. These rights of research subjects are often pitted against the requirement in criminal justice and forensic mental health settings to communicate important information that relates to potential threats to public safety.

In clinical contexts, consent from both children and their parents should be obtained before confidential information is released. When the parents wish to access information about their child's assessment or treatment, DeKraai and Sales (1991) recommend that the mental health professional first determine if the child can legally consent to the disclosure. If so, access should be denied without the consent, unless the professional believes that the child would benefit from such parental notification. In this case, professionals would be advised to refer to the applicable laws in their jurisdiction. However, if the child cannot legally consent, the professional should determine whether disclosure of the information is in the best interests of the child and whether disclosure would harm the professional relationship. In correctional contexts and with the additional complications of third party involvement, this process becomes more complicated. Becker and Abel (1985) suggest that having the parents and the child sign consent forms prior to assessment and treatment might preclude ethical difficulties in this regard arising later. In the context of research, the intended goals of a project and the methodology to be used should provide the conscientious researcher with an indication of whether or not information may be disclosed in the course of data collection that would invoke ethical dilemmas regarding confidentiality and consent.

There is a need to balance the competing privacy interests of the individual and safety interests of society when considering the limits to confidentiality and reporting with forensic populations (Mulvey and Phelps, 1988). With regard to child abuse, mandatory reporting on the part of the clinician is required across many jurisdictions and is considered crucial for treatment (National Task Force on Juvenile Sexual Offending, 1993). As such, obtaining informed consent to proceed with an assessment or treatment will necessarily involve disclosure of this limit to confidentiality (Committee on Ethical Guidelines for Forensic Psychologists, 1991; Leschied and Wormith, 1997; Rosner, 1999). However, this creates an ethical dilemma with implications for pre-adjudication evaluations, ongoing assessments, the therapist–client relationship, and expectations characteristic of treatments for juvenile sexual offenders such as complete disclosure (Hunter and Lexier, 1998; Thompson-Cooper *et al.*, 1993; see also consensus and dissenting opinions of the National Task Force on Juvenile Sexual Offending, 1993). Becker and Abel (1985) adopt a pragmatic approach in suggesting that clients be cautioned not to disclose specific details of unreported illegal acts, such as identifying information for victims, which would require reporting. This position is likely more straightforward if the clinician or researcher holds a certificate of confidentiality that precludes them from being compelled to testify. However, it does little to allay ethical concerns about the existence of an unidentified victim for whom no assistance can be made available.

From this, an important question then arises concerning whether or not researchers could be held to the same reporting duty imposed on clinicians. Following the well-known Tarasoff case, with regard to anticipated harm to others, mental health professionals have a duty to take whatever action is reasonably necessary to protect potential victims from their patients' violent acts. Appelbaum and Rosenbaum (1989) consider whether a similar duty could be imposed on the researcher and examine the basis on which such a duty might be imposed. Researchers resemble clinicians in regard to special knowledge of interpersonal violence. It might be argued that both the clinician and researcher have an ability to predict violence, and this may become more relevant as advances are made in risk assessment and recidivism prediction (Hanson, 1998). In these circumstances, the imposition on researchers of a duty to protect potential victims may be deemed appropriate. On the other side of this question, however, Appelbaum and Rosenbaum clearly emphasise the importance of protecting the validity of research data through participant confidentiality in all but the most circumscribed of circumstances.

Sieber and Stanley (1988) draw attention to two additional areas in research where ethical dilemmas arise: (a) the formulation of theories and research questions, and (b) the interpretation and application of research findings. As an example of the ethical implications of theory and research focus, consider the long-held beliefs that the sexually abusive acts of minors were merely exploratory or experimental and that few sexual offences of serious consequence were committed by this group (see Finkelhor, 1979, for further discussion). In the absence of more carefully constructed theoretical explanations, the sexually assaultive behaviour of adolescents and prepubescent children was treated as an unimportant area of investigation. This allowed the problem to remain neglected until relatively recently, and serves to remind us that theories have implications for what we choose to research and what we do in clinical practice.

Relating to ethical concerns in the interpretation and application of research findings, we point to the growing body of legislation concerning civil commitment and community notification practices for young sexual abusers (Becker, 1998; Chaffin and Bonner, 1998). These developments have been implemented in the United States, in part because of the alarming figures on incidence and prevalence of sexually abusive behaviour by young offenders. However, the empirical literature affords a poor foundation from which to make the assumptions inherent in these social policies and their judicial applications. There is a notable lack of empirically validated risk assessment tools for child or adolescent sexual abusers, only preliminary conceptions of how to render the heterogeneity characteristic of this population meaningful, and a general paucity of methodologically sound treatment evaluation studies in the literature (Becker, 1998). It is only with further progress in these areas of research that we might be able to reliably identify those for whom interventions can be expected to reduce the risk of re-offence as well as to identify those for whom strategies such as civil commitment and community notification may be warranted. Even assuming that a state of predictive accuracy can be achieved, the effects of these social policies and their efficacy as management strategies will, themselves, need to be investigated. Indeed, their application should be founded on empirical data rather than on misconceptions about their value as panaceas (Berliner, 1996). As Sieber and Stanley (1988) observe, "sensitive research topics are more likely to have applications in the 'real' world that society will enthusiastically embrace, irrespective of the validity of the application. Hence, caution is needed" (p. 53).

## Methodological issues

When local agencies establish programmes of treatment for sexual offenders, the ultimate evaluation question has to do with whether or not the programme has the beneficial effect of reducing recidivism. This is an extremely difficult question to answer, and fully understanding the difficulties requires specialised knowledge of statistics, experimental design and research methodology. Even considering and understanding these complexities, there is little consensus amongst the experts in the field concerning the ultimate answer to the question as to whether or not sexual offender treatment "works" in reducing recidivism (Hanson *et al.*, 2002). Despite the controversy, most authorities agree that there is sufficient promising evidence supporting the effectiveness of treatment to justify the establishment and running of treatment programmes.

The present chapter is intended to provide enough knowledge to local sexual offender treatment programmes to allow them to establish an effective programme evaluation that will stand up to scrutiny and provide useful guidance on the improvement of treatment. At the same time, it is hoped that the present chapter will provide an appreciation of the methodological complexities that impair our ability to evaluate the effects of treatment on recidivism. In the remaining sections of the chapter, we will concentrate on three important methodological issues: (1) the requirements of adequate experimental design, including whether or not there is a need for random assignment of subjects to treatment groups; (2) the problems caused by treatment dropouts; and (3) the difficulties of using recidivism as the outcome measure. We conclude with an overview of the best available evidence directly addressing the efficacy of sexual offender treatment. For discussion of additional methodological issues in evaluation research, the reader is directed to Brown and Kolko (1998); Henggeler *et al.* (1994); and Kazdin (1991).

## Research design

Research designs are adequate when they ensure internal validity (Cook and Campbell, 1979). Internal validity allows the researcher to ascribe causal effects of an observed reduction in recidivism (the dependent variable) to treatment (the independent variable). In the typical research design, a group of offenders who have been treated are compared in their rates of recidivism with a group who have not received treatment. Threats to internal validity are referred to as confounding or extraneous variables. Any differences between the groups apart from the treatment intervention that might explain the differences in outcome are confounding variables. Hanson and Nicholaichuk (2000) describe an excellent example of a potentially confounding variable. These authors pointed to a subtle methodological bias in an outcome study reported by Nicholaichuk *et al.* (2000) that may have inflated a reported treatment effect. The untreated group was released earlier than the treatment group, and records of the non-recidivists were more likely to go missing from the untreated group than from the treatment group.

There are many other potential threats to internal validity. For example, the process by which subjects are selected and included in the various groups can ensure or threaten internal validity, and any systematic difference between groups being compared except for the treatment variable threatens internal validity. The groups may be different prior to treatment in levels of risk for sexual recidivism. Attrition of subjects during or after treatment or after release from custody (i.e. participants who die or are removed or drop out from a study prior to completion) can affect outcomes and threaten internal validity. More about this particular confounding variable will be presented below. Confounding variables may show up after treatment and release from custody. For example, policing or supervision policies may differ between groups since the treated offenders might be considered to be lower risk. Besides confounding, uncontrolled variables represent a problem for researchers because they add to the within-group variability and so reduce the sensitivity of the statistical test designed to detect real effects between groups (leading to a Type II error).

There are a number of ways in which researchers can control for extraneous variables and ensure group equivalence. From a purely research design and statistical perspective, the preferred method of control is randomisation. A description of randomisation can be found in all introductory texts on research design, and is accomplished through any procedure of assignment of subjects to groups that ensures randomness (toss of a coin; selecting from a hat). Systematic biases due to confounding variables are thereby controlled by distributing the influence of confounding variables equally between the two groups. While randomisation ensures equivalent expected population values, it does not necessarily ensure equivalent obtained sample values (Cook and Campbell, 1979). In other words, randomisation does not always preclude the occurrence of extraneous differences between groups, as when the higher risk subjects were, by chance, assigned to one of the experimental groups in the well-known Sex Offender Treatment and Evaluation Project (SOTEP, Marques, 1999). Nevertheless, compared with all other methods of subject assignment, causal inferences are least undermined when random assignment of participants to conditions is employed. Randomisation is the conceptual basis of statistical hypothesis-testing procedures, permitting the researcher to make statistical statements about the role of chance factors versus the effects of treatment. The randomised controlled trial is the preferred method for establishing the efficacy of any psychological or medical treatment (McConaghy, 1999; Shadish and Ragsdale, 1996).

Becker and Abel (1985) note that especially when young sexual abusers are mandated to receive treatment, there is an ethical obligation to ensure that they receive the most efficacious treatment available. In order to demonstrate the efficacy of treatment for the juvenile sexual offender, it would be expected that research designs would have used random assignment to conditions as the optimal strategy to control potential confounding factors (Boruch *et al.*, 2000; Henggeler *et al.*, 1994). Despite this, random assignment has rarely been employed in treatment evaluation studies with sexual offenders. In the most recent review of the sexual offender treatment outcome literature, Hanson *et al.* (2002) report that only three of forty-three treatment outcome studies employed randomisation as a control procedure, and only one of these involved juvenile offenders.

It has been argued that the use of randomised controlled trials in the evaluation of treatment for sexual offenders is unethical (Marshall *et al.*, 1991; Marshall and Pithers, 1994). To be specific, it is not the randomisation procedure that is considered to be unethical. A randomised controlled trial requires the systematic and long-term withholding of treatment from sexual offenders. Certainly, given the potential for serious harm to others posed by sexual offenders, one could argue for a professional obligation to intervene in all cases where possible, especially where the offender is seeking treatment. Whereas in the clinical aspects of treatment research, the protection of the safety of the public and potential victims is paramount, in the traditional ethics review of treatment research, the protection of participants' rights has been seen to be paramount. However, here it is argued that the rights of the potential victim should be protected by the deliberations of institutional Review Ethics Boards (REBs). In the context of treatment evaluation research with sexual offenders, the persons who suffer the risks of withholding treatment (potential victims) would not have the opportunity to give informed consent to the research procedure. Therefore, most REBs would have difficulty giving approval to a proposal involving the withholding of treatment for sexual offenders who were seeking treatment. In addition, there are legal liability issues. Assigning offenders who seek treatment to a no-treatment control group and later enforcing the no-treatment condition is a serious and understandable liability risk for government ministries that fund such treatment, or agencies or institutional corporate interests that provide treatment services. Victims and families of victims (and perhaps the offender as well) could bring legal action seeking financial damages against agencies or institutions that were responsible for withholding treatment from a sexual offender who was seeking treatment and later re-offends.

Besides the ethical and legal concerns, there are practical issues involved in withholding treatment. It is difficult, if not impossible, to ensure that no-treatment subjects do not get treatment at some time during the follow-up period. This is especially true when you consider the length of the follow-up period, which is generally deemed to require more than five years to provide an adequate baseline of recidivism. Of course, the longer the follow-up, the greater the chance that the untreated subject in the study will seek and receive some kind of treatment.

While these ethical, legal and practical concerns would preclude the use of no-treatment conditions, random assignment to alternative treatment conditions would seem reasonable. For example, when a novel treatment that can be supported on theoretical or empirical grounds is compared with some currently accepted treatment or intervention, random assignment to these conditions would not be ethically improper, especially where there is no withholding of later services to which the comparison group subjects would otherwise be entitled. In these designs, it is the relative impact of the experimental intervention compared with what otherwise would have been the treatment or management of the sample that should be assessed (Metcalf and Thornton, 1992). The comparison of two or more treatment models is sometimes referred to as a dismantling design (in which components of a treatment are varied across conditions to identify the active elements), and these represent viable research designs in which random assignment would be ethically justified. However, it is unlikely that recidivism studies would provide the statistical power or sensitivity to detect differences between different treatments in dismantling designs (Barbaree, 1997). Perhaps this has led to Miner (1997) noting, "there is no strong support, either within this field or in the general population for conducting such [random assignment] experiments" (p. 102).

As the field has evolved, there has been a greater recognition of the role of research designs that permit a reasonable degree of causal inference but that do not require the withholding of treatment from offenders. Hanson *et al.* (2002) make a distinction among three kinds of research designs: (a) designs in which pre-existing group differences would not be expected (randomised controlled designs); (b) designs in which prior equivalence of groups was not assured, but where there were no obvious reasons to expect group differences; and (c) designs in which prior group differences would be expected. Hanson *et al.* (2002) refer to designs in (b) above as incidental assignment designs in which group assignment has been predetermined through some kind of administrative convenience, but where there has been no systematic bias in group assignments. In contrast, the designs in (c) above would include designs in which the comparison group is made up of persons who refused the treatment offered or who dropped out of the treatment. For the purposes of the following discussion, we will refer to designs described in (a) above as *experimental designs*, in (b) above as *quasi-experimental designs*, and in (c) above as *convenience designs*.

In evaluation studies, using quasi-experimental designs, the researcher has the further option of choosing amongst the available subjects in order to match participants on important variables (for example, actuarial risk to re-offend, victim gender, victim age) or those variables that are expected to have a relationship with the outcomes of interest on theoretical or empirical grounds. Indeed, matching groups on selected variables is a strategy often employed when randomisation is either not possible (cf. Worling and Curwen, 2000) or the integrity of the randomisation assignment has been compromised, as often occurs in applied contexts (Dunford, 1990).

In summary and to conclude with respect to research design, *Convenience designs* common in the literature do not provide convincing evidence of treatment efficacy. *Experimental designs* are extremely difficult to implement and some acceptable alternative design(s) must be sought. *Quasi-experimental designs* which control for potentially confounding variables may offer an acceptable alternative. *Quasi-experimental designs* may be the design of choice and these should control for a number of potentially confounding variables, including treatment readiness and motivation.

It is worth noting that withholding treatment from the comparison group is not always inappropriate from an ethical perspective. In the much heralded and well-respected longitudinal SOTEP outcome study, Marques *et al.* (1994) used a randomised controlled trial. The treatment programme being evaluated was a state-of-the-art cognitive-behavioural therapy programme with an emphasis on the principles of relapse prevention. The programme was well funded, with strong support from the Californian government. It involved detailed assessment and evaluation components. Treated subjects moved from a correctional setting to a secure mental health facility to receive the programme of treatment over a period of approximately two years. Untreated volunteers and non-volunteers stayed in their correctional settings. Treatment did not affect release dates. The rationale for its ethical acceptability was the fact that treatment was not generally available to any of the approximately 6,000 sexual offenders incarcerated in the state. Therefore, randomly assigning a few hundred volunteers to treatment or no-treatment conditions would not involve withholding of treatment in the usual meaning of these terms, since without the treatment programme being evaluated, none of the offenders would receive institutional treatment.

### Loss of subjects

The SOTEP outcome research carried by Marques and her colleagues (Marques, 1999; Marques *et al.*, 1994) illustrates the problem that subject drop-out poses for programme evaluation. Marques *et al.* (1994) presented recidivism rates (%) for a number of groups in their sample for a mean follow-up period of thirty-four months. The groups included: sexual offenders who volunteered but were randomly assigned to the no-treatment condition; sexual offenders who volunteered and were randomly assigned to treatment but who dropped out before completing a year in the programme; and sexual offenders who volunteered and were randomly assigned to treatment, and who completed one year or more of the programme. Initial inspection of the recidivism rates in the first three rows presented in Table 17.1 suggests that treatment had a positive effect on sexual recidivism.

The rate of recidivism for the treated group was the lowest of the groups shown. Because the time for which each group was at risk after release differed, Marques *et al.* (1994) employed survival analysis to statistically compare the groups (survival analysis takes into account the varying times at risk between groups and the decline in sample size as the follow-up period increases, see Wright, 2000). The authors found that while the difference in failure rates between the treated and untreated groups approached significance,

*Table 17.1* Reoffence rates for matched groups in the SOTEP

| | *n* | *Recidivism (%)*[a] |
|---|---|---|
| *Volunteer control (untreated)* | 97 | 13.4 |
| *Ex-treatment (drop-outs)* | 8 | 37.5 |
| *Treatment* | 98 | 8.2 |
| *Treatment (including drop-outs)*[b] | 106 | 10.3 |

Source: The data in rows 1 to 3 are from Marques *et al.*, 1994, p. 46. Copyright 1994 by the American Association for Correctional Psychology. Adapted with permission.

Notes

[a] Recidivism represents the percentage of sexual recidivists in each group at a mean follow-up time of 34.2 months.

[b] All sexual offenders who volunteered and were randomly assigned to treatment, and began the programme (treatment plus ex-treatment groups).

the failure rate for the drop-outs was significantly higher (i.e. they reoffended at the fastest rate).

In support of removing the drop-outs from the treated group, it could be argued that the inclusion of data for drop-outs would obscure detection of an actual treatment effect because these individuals would not have participated in sufficient treatment to reasonably test hypotheses. Worth noting here is the lack of empirical data to assist us in determining what "sufficient treatment" might be (although preliminary work is under way with adult sexual offenders, see Gordon and Packard, 1999).

Unfortunately, removing drop-outs in this way undermines the internal validity of the research design. Keppel (1991) has stated that "Most experiments begin with the expectation that the various treatment and control conditions will have equal *n*s. This is so each condition contributes equally to the outcome of the data analysis. . . . Often, . . . the data reflect a loss of subjects. There are two kinds of loss of subjects, including (1) inadvertent, accidental loss, and (2) loss due to the effects of the independent variable. . . . In each situation, we have to determine whether the reason for the loss of subjects is in any way associated with the experimental treatments . . . if the loss of subjects is related to the phenomenon under study, randomness is destroyed and a systematic bias may be added to the differences among the means, which cannot be disentangled from the influence of the treatment effects" (pp. 280–282). The problem of drop-outs from experimental groups has been studied in its own right (Baekeland and Lundwall, 1975).

It is clear to all who have had experience with the treatment of the sexual offender that dropping out of treatment is rarely inadvertent or accidental. The demands of treatment have specific effects on particular participants that lead to their withdrawal from treatment. Barbaree and Seto (1998) report a number of variables that were associated with dropping out of sexual offender treatment. For example, (1) younger offenders, (2) offenders who had no previous experience in treatment, and (3) offenders who expressed more negative attitudes toward treatment were more likely to drop out of treatment. It is not unreasonable to draw a connection between the personal characteristics that lead to dropping out of treatment and those that place an offender at higher risk for reoffence, and research supports this (Browne *et al.*, 1998). Therefore, it is likely that treatment as a demand on participants has the effect of removing individuals from the treatment group who are at higher risk to recidivate. Of course, since no treatment demands are placed on individuals in matched comparison groups, the individuals with characteristics associated with "dropping out" of treatment remain in the comparison group and likely increase the rate of recidivism for the group. Removal of the drop-outs from the treatment group, combined with the retention of individuals sharing the same characteristics in the comparison group, would lead to group differences that might result in an inflated treatment effect. This is a clear confound that threatens the internal validity of the evaluation design.

From a statistical point of view, drop-outs should be retained, as assigned, in the treatment group and analyses first reported using this grouping. Returning to Table 17.1 and the SOTEP data, the recidivism rate for the treated group, including the drop-outs originally assigned to it, is shown in the fourth row. As can be seen, the apparent difference between percentage of recidivists in this group and the untreated group is attenuated. Indeed, Marques *et al.* (1994) reported that the survival analysis comparing these two groups revealed no significant difference in failure rates at the end of the first follow-up period.

In evaluation research, following presentation of results for groups as assigned, secondary analyses can be carried out to determine whether there were systematic differences between drop-outs and completers, from which hypotheses for further investigation can be generated (Day and Marques, 1998; Marques, 1999). Indeed, to better understand treatment failure it is necessary to study those individuals who refuse, are removed, or drop out of treatment, as well as those that reoffend following completion of treatment so that we can identify associated factors, and revise interventions in order to address these factors (Hunter and Figueredo, 1999; Proulx *et al.*, 1999).

### Recidivism as an outcome measure

Recidivism studies are not sensitive to the effects of treatment. This lack of sensitivity is due to the low power of the statistical tests, which is in turn due to the low base rates of recidivism. Barbaree (1997) examined the sensitivity of recidivism studies to treatment effects and reported that the power of the statistical tests depends on $n$ (the total sample size), the size of the treatment effects, and the base rate of reoffence. At low base rates, the power of the statistical tests is low. In actuality, the base rates for known sexual reoffences are low. For example, Hanson and Bussière's (1998) meta-analysis of recidivism studies has reported an overall reoffence rate of 13 per cent. Additionally, the reality is that, for sexual offender treatment, treatment effects are probably less than 50 per cent (the percentage reduction in recidivism due to treatment). Hanson *et al.* (2002) suggest a 40 per cent reduction in recidivism due to treatment. For programme evaluations to show a significant effect of treatment, the requirements for $n$ are high. Given a base rate of .30, a (conservatively estimated) treatment effect of 30 per cent, and a required power of .80, in order to detect a significant treatment effect ($p < .05$), the local programme would require an $n$ of 1,000. Unfortunately, in sexual offender treatment evaluation research, especially at the local treatment programme level, the $n$ (combined treated and untreated sample) is generally small.

Therefore, studies of treatment efficacy require very large samples such as can be obtained using multi-site designs or meta-analysis (Durlak, 1995). Randomised cross-site studies have their own problems, including concerns with site-specific variability, which can decrease statistical power (Metcalf and Thornton, 1992). As Hanson (1997) notes, meta-analytic procedures are practical approaches that can be adopted to increase sample size.

The evaluation of sexual offender treatment is a recent scientific activity. In 1989 Furby *et al.* reviewed forty-two published studies of sexual offender recidivism. Of six studies that compared treated with untreated offenders, four showed lower rates among the untreated offenders. These reviewers noted many confounds and methodological difficulties among these studies, and suggested that even tentative conclusions about treatment efficacy for sexual offenders would be inadvisable. Following this review, considerable discussion in the literature ensued (see Day and Marques, 1998; Hanson, 1997; Marshall *et al.*, 1991; Marshall and Pithers, 1994; McConaghy, 1998; 1999; Quinsey *et al.*, 1993).

More recently, three comprehensive reviews using quantitative techniques have been published. First, Hall (1995) conducted a meta-analysis of twelve studies of treatment with sexual offenders (combined $n = 1,313$). A small but robust effect size was found for treatment versus comparison conditions. Cognitive-behavioural and hormonal treatments were reported to be significantly more effective than behavioural treatments. However, Rice and Harris (1997) re-examined the results of the Hall meta-analysis and argued against Hall's conclusions. In seven of the twelve studies, the research designs involved *convenience designs* in which all or most of the control group were men who had refused or dropped out of treatment. The other five studies employed *experimental designs* with random assignment, or *quasi-experimental designs.* Rice and Harris (1997) report that for the studies using convenience designs, mean effect size (Cohen's $d$) = 0.49 ($p < .05$), but for the studies using experimental or quasi-experimental designs, mean effect size (Cohen's $d$) = –0.01 (*ns*). Rice and Harris argued, cogently, that when potential confounding variables were adequately controlled for, such as in the experimental and quasi-experimental designs, no treatment effect was evident. These authors concluded that treatment efficacy for the sexual offender had not been demonstrated in the Hall meta-analysis.

Second, Gallagher *et al.* (1999) conducted a meta-analysis of twenty-five studies in the treatment outcome literature. These authors concluded that there was a significant treatment effect for cognitive-behavioural treatments, but unlike Hall (1995), they found no treatment effects for medical/hormonal treatments. As Hanson *et al.* (2002) observe, although Gallagher *et al.* made some effort to restrict their analysis to well controlled studies, they nevertheless included a number of studies (6 out of 25) in which a pro-treatment bias could be expected (comparison groups made up of drop-outs and refusers). These inclusions serve to weaken the conclusions that can be drawn.

Finally, in 1997, in an attempt to resolve this controversy, a small group of members of the Association for the Treatment of Sexual Abusers launched the Collaborative Outcome Data Project. The project team included some of the most well respected authorities in the area, from both sides of the debate. Hanson *et al.* (2002) reported the first set of conclusions as a result of a meta-analysis of forty-three studies of sexual offender recidivism (combined $n$ = 9,454). In addressing the criticism levelled by Rice and Harris (1997) against the earlier Hall (1995) meta-analysis, Hanson *et al.* coded treatment studies as to the adequacy of their research designs to control for potentially confounding variables as described above. Combining experimental with quasi-experimental designs, Hanson *et al.* found a significant treatment effect. Amongst current psychological treatments (those programmes initiated after 1980 or those initiated before 1980 but still in operation) the authors report a significant effect in reducing rates of both sexual and general recidivism by approximately 40 per cent. Current treatments were described as cognitive-behavioural therapies (or systemic therapy with juveniles), most often with an emphasis on relapse prevention. Older forms of treatment (prior to 1980) were found to have little effect. Importantly, the treatment effect remained significant when considering only studies in which drop-outs were explicitly included with the treatment group. On the face of it, this study encourages the conclusion that sexual offender treatment can be effective in reducing recidivism amongst sexual offenders.

## Summary and conclusions

The present chapter has recommended that treatment providers conduct programme evaluation research in order to ensure programme quality. In addition to the value of such work at the local level, small-scale evaluation studies can contribute to the wider knowledge base through inclusion in meta-analytic research. In planning and conducting programme evaluations, local programme staff require an understanding of some basic but important principles guiding the evaluation research. The present chapter focused on ethical and methodological issues. It was recommended that local programme staff adopt a flexible, evolving approach to the resolution of ethical dilemmas that will arise from time to time in the conduct of evaluation research, and that programme staff consult widely when seeking resolutions to such dilemmas. Programme staff were encouraged to seek and obtain informed consent from participants and their parents or guardians for their involvement in research and for any transmission of information. The present chapter also recommended that local programme staff refrain from attempts to conduct randomised controlled trials that involve a no-treatment condition, since the systematic withholding of treatment from offenders who seek treatment invites severe criticism on ethical grounds and potential civil liability. Quasi-experimental designs can be used in which the comparison group is made up of individuals who sought treatment but did not receive treatment due to some incidental factor or administrative convenience. Convenience designs in which the comparison group is composed of individuals who have dropped out of treatment or refused treatment should be avoided due to lack of internal validity. The most recent meta-analysis of the sexual offender treatment outcome literature has indicated that, based on the combination of experimental and quasi-experimental designs, treatment leads to a reduction of sexual recidivism of approximately 40 per cent. Such findings provide justification for the continuing treatment of sexual offenders in institutional and community settings, and the establishment of new programmes in response to offender needs.

## References

Abel, G. G., Mittelman, M. S., and Becker, J. V. (1985). Sex offenders: Results of assessment and recommendations for treatment. In M. H. Ben-Aron, S. J. Hucker and C. D. Webster (eds), *Clinical Criminology: The Assessment of Criminal Behavior*. Toronto: M and M Graphics, pp. 207–220.

Abel, G. G., Osborn, C. A., and Twigg, D. A. (1993). Sexual assault through the life span: Adult offenders with juvenile histories. In H. E. Barbaree, W. L. Marshall and S. M. Hudson (eds), *The Juvenile Sex Offender*. New York: Guilford Press, pp. 25–63.

Ageton, S. (1983). *Sexual Assault among Adolescents*. Lexington, MA: Lexington Books.

American Psychological Association (1992). Ethical principles of psychologists and code of conduct. *American Psychologist, 47*, 1597–1611.

Appelbaum, P. S., and Rosenbaum, A. (1989). Tarasoff and the researcher: Does the duty to protect apply in the research setting? *American Psychologist, 44*, 885–894.

Association for the Treatment of Sexual Abusers (2001). *Association for the Treatment of Sexual Abusers Professional Code of Ethics*. Beaverton, OR: Author.

Baekeland, F., and Lundwall, L. (1975). Dropping out of treatment: A critical review. *Psychological Bulletin, 82*, 738–783.

Barbaree, H. E. (1997). Evaluating treatment efficacy with sexual offenders: The insensitivity of recidivism studies to treatment effects. *Sexual Abuse: A Journal of Research and Treatment, 9*, 111–128.

Barbaree, H. E., Hudson, S. M., and Seto, M. C. (1993). Sexual assault in society: The role of the juvenile offender. In H. E. Barbaree, W. L. Marshall and S. M. Hudson (eds), *The Juvenile Sex Offender*. New York: Guilford Press, pp. 1–24.

Barbaree, H. E., Marshall, W. L., and Hudson, S. M. (eds) (1993). *The Juvenile Sex Offender*. New York: Guilford Press.

Barbaree, H. E., and Seto, M. C. (1998). *The Ongoing Follow-Up of Sex Offenders Treated at the Warkworth Sexual Behavior Clinic*. Research Report prepared for the Correctional Service of Canada.

Becker, J. V. (1998). What we know about the characteristics and treatment of adolescents who have committed sexual offenses. *Child Maltreatment, 3*, 317–329.

Becker, J. V., and Abel, G. G. (1985). Methodological and ethical issues in evaluating and treating adolescent sexual offenders. In E. M. Otey and G. D. Ryan (eds), *Adolescent Sex Offenders: Issues in Research and Treatment*. Rockville, MD: National Institute of Mental Health, pp. 109–129.

Berliner, L. (1996). Community notification: Neither a panacea nor a calamity. *Sexual Abuse: A Journal of Research and Treatment, 8*, 101–104.

Boruch, R., Snyder, B., and DeMoya, D. (2000). The importance of randomized field trials. *Crime and Delinquency, 46*, 156–180.

Brown, E. J., and Kolko, D. J. (1998). Treatment efficacy and program evaluation with juvenile sexual abusers: A critique with directions for service delivery and research. *Child Maltreatment, 3*, 362–373.

Browne, K. D., Foreman, L., and Middleton, D. (1998). Predicting treatment drop-out in sex offenders. *Child Abuse Review, 7*, 402–419.

Burton, D. L. (2000). Were adolescent sexual offenders children with sexual behavior problems? *Sexual Abuse: A Journal of Research and Treatment, 12*, 37–48.

Burton, D. L., and Smith-Darden, J. (2001). *North American Survey of Sexual Abuser Treatment and Models Summary Data*. Brandon, VT: Safer Society Press.

Chaffin, M. C., and Bonner, B. (1998). "Don't shoot, we're your children": Have we gone too far in our response to adolescent sexual abusers and children with sexual behavior problems? *Child Maltreatment, 3*, 314–316.

Committee on Ethical Guidelines for Forensic Psychologists (1991). Specialty guidelines for forensic psychologists. *Law and Human Behavior, 15*, 655–665.

Cook, T. D., and Campbell, D. T. (1979). *Quasi-Experimentation, Design and Analysis for Field Issues*. Boston: Houghton Mifflin.

Day, D. M., and Marques, J. K. (1998). A clarification of SOTEP'S method and preliminary findings: Reply to Nathaniel McConaghy. *Sexual Abuse: A Journal of Research and Treatment, 10*, 162–166.

DeKraai, M. B., and Sales, B. D. (1991). Liability in child therapy and research. *Journal of Consulting and Clinical Psychology, 59*, 853–860.

Dunford, F. W. (1990). Random assignment: Practical considerations from field experiments. *Evaluation and Program Planning, 13*, 125–132.

Durlak, J. A. (1995). Understanding meta-analysis. In L. G. Grimm and P. R. Yarnold (eds), *Reading and Understanding Multivariate Statistics*. Washington, DC: American Psychological Association, pp. 319–352.

Fassler, D. (1992). Ethical issues in child and adolescent psychiatry. *Journal of the American Academy of Child and Adolescent Psychiatry, 31*, 392.

Finkelhor, D. (1979). What's wrong with sex between adults and children? Ethics and the problem of sexual abuse. *American Journal of Orthopsychiatry, 49*, 692–697.

Furby, L., Weinrott, M. R., and Blackshaw, L. (1989). Sex offender recidivism: A review. *Psychological Bulletin, 105*, 3–30.

Gallagher, C. A., Wilson, D. B., Hirschfield, P., Coggeshall, M. B., and MacKenzie, D. L. (1999). A quantitative review of the effects of sex offender treatment on sexual offending. *Corrections Management Quarterly, 3*, 19–29.

Gordon, A., and Packard, R. (1999). *Testing Treatment Assumptions: The Effects of Open Versus Closed-Ended and Shorter Versus Longer Term Treatment*. Paper presented at the 18th annual conference of the Association for the Treatment of Sexual Abusers (ATSA), Buena Vista, Florida.

Grisso, T., Miller, M. O., and Sales, B. (1987). Competency to stand trial in juvenile court. *International Journal of Law and Psychiatry, 10*, 1–20.

Hall, G. C. N. (1995). Sexual offender recidivism revisited: A meta-analysis of recent treatment studies. *Journal of Consulting and Clinical Psychology, 63*, 802–809.

Hanson, R. K. (1997). How to know what works with the sexual offenders. *Sexual Abuse: A Journal of Research and Treatment, 9*, 129–145.

Hanson, R. K. (1998). What do we know about sex offender risk assessment? *Psychology, Public Policy, and Law, 4*, 50–72.

Hanson, R. K., and Bussière, M. T. (1998). Predicting relapse: A meta-analysis of sexual offender recidivism studies. *Journal of Consulting and Clinical Psychology, 66*, 348–362.

Hanson, R. K., and Nicholaichuk, T. (2000). A cautionary note regarding Nicholaichuk *et al.* (2000). *Sexual Abuse: A Journal of Research and Treatment, 12*, 289–293.

Hanson, R. K., Gordon, A., Harris, A. J. R., Marques, J. K., Murphy, W., Quinsey, V. L., and Seto, M. C. (2002). First report of the collaborative outcome data project on the effectiveness of psychological treatment for sex offenders. *Sexual Abuse: A Journal of Research and Treatment, 14*, 169–194.

Henggeler, S. W., Smith, B. H., and Schoenwald, S. K. (1994). Key theoretical and methodological issues in conducting treatment research in the juvenile justice system. *Journal of Clinical Child Psychology, 23*, 143–150.

Hunter, J. A., and Figueredo, A. J. (1999). Factors associated with treatment compliance in a population of juvenile sexual offenders. *Sexual Abuse: A Journal of Research and Treatment, 11*, 49–67.

Hunter, J. A., and Lexier, L. J. (1998). Ethical and legal issues in the assessment and treatment of juvenile sex offenders. *Child Maltreatment, 3*, 339–348.

James, A. C., and Neil, P. (1996). Juvenile sexual offending: One-year period prevalence study within Oxfordshire. *Child Abuse and Neglect, 20*, 477–485.

Kazdin, A. E. (1991). Effectiveness of psychotherapy with children and adolescents. *Journal of Consulting and Clinical Psychology, 59*, 785–798.

Keppel, G. (1991). *Design and Analysis: A Researcher's Handbook*. Englewood Cliffs, NJ: Prentice Hall.

Knight, R. A., and Prentky, R. A. (1993). Exploring characteristics for classifying juvenile sex offenders. In H. E. Barbaree, W. L. Marshall and S. M. Hudson (eds), *The Juvenile Sex Offender*. New York: Guilford Press, pp. 45–83.

Leschied, A. D. W., and Wormith, J. S. (1997). Assessment of young offenders and treatment of correctional clients. In D. R. Evans (ed.), *The Law, Standards of*

*Practice, and Ethics in the Practice of Psychology*. Toronto: Emond Montgomery, pp. 233–258.

McConaghy, N. (1998). Neglect of evidence that relapse prevention is ineffective in treatment of incarcerated sexual offenders. *Sexual Abuse: A Journal of Research and Treatment, 10*, 159–162.

McConaghy, N. (1999). Methodological issues concerning evaluation of treatment for sexual offenders: Randomization, treatment dropouts, untreated controls, and within-treatment studies. *Sexual Abuse: A Journal of Research and Treatment, 11*, 183–193.

Marques, J. K. (1999). How to answer the question "Does sex offender treatment work?" *Journal of Interpersonal Violence, 14*, 437–451.

Marques, J. K., Day, D. M., Nelson, C., and West, M. A. (1994). Effects of cognitive-behavioral treatment on sex offender recidivism: Preliminary results of a longitudinal study. *Criminal Justice and Behavior, 21*, 28–54.

Marshall, W. L., and Pithers, W. D. (1994). A reconsideration of treatment outcome with sex offenders. *Criminal Justice and Behavior, 21*, 10–27.

Marshall, W. L., Jones, R. L., Ward, T., Johnston, P., and Barbaree, H. E. (1991). Treatment outcome with sex offenders. *Clinical Psychology Review, 11*, 465–485.

Metcalf, C. E., and Thornton, C. (1992). Random assignment. *Children and Youth Services Review, 14*, 145–156.

Miner, M. H. (1997). How can we conduct treatment outcome research? *Sexual Abuse: A Journal of Research and Treatment, 9*, 95–110.

Mulvey, E. P., and Phelps, P. (1988). Ethical balances in juvenile justice research and practice. *American Psychologist, 43*, 65–69.

Munir, K., and Earls, F. (1992). Ethical principles governing research in child and adolescent psychiatry. *Journal of the American Academy of Child and Adolescent Psychiatry, 31*, 408–414.

National Task Force on Juvenile Sexual Offending (1993). Revised report. *Juvenile and Family Court Journal, 44*, 1–61.

Nicholaichuk, T., Gordon, A., Gu, D., and Wong, S. (2000). Outcome of an institutional sexual offender treatment program: A comparison between treated and matched untreated offenders. *Sexual Abuse: A Journal of Research and Treatment, 12*, 139–153.

O'Rourke, K., Snider, B. W., Thomas, J. M., and Berland, D. I. (1992). Knowing and practicing ethics. *Journal of the American Academy of Child and Adolescent Psychiatry, 31*, 393–397.

Proulx, J., Ouimet, M., Pellerin, B., Paradis, Y., McKibben, A., and Aubut, J. (1999). Posttreatment recidivism in sexual aggressors: A comparison between dropout and nondropout subjects. In B. K. Schwartz (ed.), *The Sex Offender: Theoretical Advances, Treating Special Populations and Legal Developments*, vol. 3. Kingston, NJ: Civic Research Institute, pp. 15.1–15.13.

Quinsey, V. L., Harris, G. T., Rice, M. E., and Lalumière, M. L. (1993). Assessing treatment efficacy in outcome studies of sex offenders. *Journal of Interpersonal Violence, 8*, 512–523.

Rice, M. E., and Harris, G. T. (1997). The treatment of adult offenders. In D. M. Stoff, J. Breiling and J. D. Maser (eds), *Handbook of Antisocial Behaviour*. New York: John Wiley, pp. 425–435.

Rosner, R. (1999). Forensic psychiatry for adolescent psychiatrists: An introduction.

In A. H. Esman, L. T. Flaherty and H. A. Horowitz (eds), *Adolescent Psychiatry: Developmental and Clinical Studies*, vol. 24. Hillsdale, NJ: Analytic Press, pp. 135–142.

Ryan, G. D., and Lane, S. L. (eds) (1997). *Juvenile Sexual Offending: Causes, Consequences, and Correction*, 2nd edn. San Francisco: Jossey-Bass.

Shadish, W. R., and Ragsdale, K. (1996). Random versus nonrandom assignment in controlled experiments: Do you get the same answer? *Journal of Consulting and Clinical Psychology, 64*, 1290–1305.

Sheerin, D. (1998). Legal options in Ireland for getting adolescent sex offenders into treatment programmes and keeping them there. *Irish Journal of Psychology, 19*, 181–189.

Sieber, J. E., and Stanley, B. (1988). Ethical and professional dimensions of socially sensitive research. *American Psychologist, 43*, 49–55.

Snyder, H. N. (2000). *Sexual Assault of Young Children as Reported to Law Enforcement: Victim, Incident, and Offender Characteristics*. Bureau of Justice Statistics report, NCJ 182990.

Sondheimer, A., and Martucci, L. C. (1992). An approach to teaching ethics in child and adolescent psychiatry. *Journal of the American Academy of Child and Adolescent Psychiatry, 31*, 415–422.

Swenson, C. C., Henggeler, S. W., Schoenwald, S. K., Kaufman, K. L., and Randall, J. (1998). Changing the social ecologies of adolescent sexual offenders: Implications of the success of multisystemic therapy in treating serious antisocial behavior in adolescence. *Child Maltreatment, 3*, 330–338.

Thompson-Cooper, I., Fugere, R., and Cormier, B. M. (1993). The child abuse reporting laws: An ethical dilemma for professionals. *Canadian Journal of Psychiatry, 38*, 557–562.

US Department of Justice (2002). *OJJDP Statistical Briefing Book*. Retrieved 3 August, 2002, from http://ojjdp.ncjrs.org/ojstatbb/html/qa251.html

Weinstock, R. (1999). Competence in adolescents. In A. H. Esman, L. T. Flaherty and H. A. Horowitz (eds), *Adolescent Psychiatry: Developmental and Clinical Studies*, vol. 24. Hillsdale, NJ: Analytic Press, pp. 159–173.

Wieckowski, E., Hartsoe, P., Mayer, A., and Shortz, J. (1998). Deviant sexual behavior in children and young adolescents: Frequency and patterns. *Sexual Abuse: A Journal of Research and Treatment, 10*, 293–303.

Worling, J. R., and Curwen, T. (2000). Adolescent sexual offender recidivism: Success of specialized treatment and implications for risk prediction. *Child Abuse and Neglect, 24*, 965–982.

Wright, R. E. (2000). Survival analysis. In L. G. Grimm and P. R. Yarnold (eds), *Reading and Understanding More Multivariate Statistics*. Washington, DC: American Psychological Association, pp. 363–407.

Chapter 18

# Treatment outcome with juvenile sexual offenders

*William L. Marshall and Yolanda M. Fernandez*

The provision of treatment for juvenile sexual offenders has lagged behind the provision and development of treatment for adult offenders. For many years it was assumed that young people who committed sexual offences were simply experimenting and, left alone, their problematic behaviours would disappear (Maclay, 1960; Roberts *et al.*, 1973). It is now clear that many of these juvenile offences do not reflect simple transitory experimentation but rather are signs of a persistent problem behaviour in need of treatment. Estimates indicate that 20 per cent of rapes and 50 per cent of sexual assaults of children are committed by juveniles (Barbaree and Cortoni, 1993). Furthermore, in some studies 50 per cent of adult offenders say their deviant sexual behaviour began during childhood or adolescence (Abel *et al.*, 1985; Longo and Groth, 1983). Obviously providing treatment for juvenile sexual offenders is both necessary and socially valuable but only if such treatment is effective.

Demonstrating that treatment for sexual offenders is beneficial requires a researcher/clinician to operate a programme long enough to generate a sufficient number of graduates released into the community for sufficient time to conduct a proper evaluation. It also requires that some agency provide the funds to do the study, and very few agencies have believed their responsibilities extend beyond funding treatment if, indeed, they can be persuaded to do even that. The fact that the United States spends over $125 million on studies of depression and yet only $1 million on research of sexual offenders (Goode, 1994) tells us that society is not fully ready to accept the extent of sexual offending and the damage it does to so many innocent people; not just the victims, although for them the damage is extensive, but also the victim's family, the offender's family, and the offender him/herself. Most of the money that is spent on sexual offender research goes to the study of adult offenders.

The increase in treatment programmes for juvenile sexual offenders over thirteen years from twenty programmes in the USA in 1982 (United States National Adolescent Perpetrator Network, 1988) to over six hundred in 1995 (Freeman-Longo *et al.*, 1995), reflects the dedication of many treatment providers given the evident lack of funding. This devotion on behalf of treatment providers is evident in numerous other countries as well and stands as a tribute to these dedicated workers. With this proliferation of programmes there has not, as yet, been a corresponding flood of evaluations of treatment for juvenile sexual offenders. However, there are some studies and there is a more extensive literature on the treatment of adult sexual offenders from which we might infer some relevance for the effectiveness of treatment of juveniles. In any event this is all that is available, so our review will necessarily be limited in scope.

Since there are arguments about what should be addressed in treating juvenile sexual offenders, and particularly whether such treatment should simply be a match for adult offender programmes (Friedrich and Chaffin, 2000), the meaning of the results of our review will necessarily be constrained. The only data available at present involve adult offender programmes and eleven reports (Becker, 1990; Borduin *et al.*, 1990; Brannon and Troyer, 1995; Bremer, 1992; Hagan and Cho, 1996; Kahn and Chambers, 1991; Kahn and Lafond, 1988; Lab *et al.*, 1993; Mazur and Michael, 1992; Smith and Monastersky, 1986; Worling and Curwen, 2000) of evaluations of juvenile offender programmes. Of these eleven evaluations of juvenile programmes eight did not include a comparison with untreated offenders, ten were conducted in the United States (which, as we will see, limits their meaning), and most had a limited follow-up period. The reader should, therefore, interpret the present review with caution. What we will do, since we wish to strongly encourage the development of good evaluations, is first review what we think is essential, and obtainable, in treatment evaluations and then turn to what limited evidence is available.

## Features of treatment evaluation

### *Interpretation of the evidence*

Until quite recently those who read the available literature on the efficacy of treatment with sexual offenders could interpret the evidence as either suggesting beneficial effects (Marshall *et al.*, 1991) or as indicating that treatment had not been shown to be useful (Furby *et al.*, 1989). Some, in fact, claimed the evidence demonstrated that treatment was ineffective and should be abandoned (Quinsey *et al.*, 1996). This latter perspective requires some comment. At the time Quinsey *et al.* made this claim (i.e. that treatment had been shown to be ineffective) there were at least twelve reports evaluating sexual offender treatment with eight showing significantly lower reoffence rates among the treated subjects while four found no differences between treated and untreated offenders; two of these four failures were reports in which Quinsey was a co-author.

The first point to be made about these data is that it is unreasonable to expect all treatment programmes for all sexual offenders to demonstrate effectiveness. For one thing there is a statistical limitation on detecting statistically significant treatment effects imposed by the known low base-rates of reoffending among sexual offenders. When base rates (i.e. the recidivism rates of untreated offenders) are sufficiently low then very large numbers of treated subjects discharged for lengthy periods of time, are required to have the statistical power necessary to be able to demonstrate effectiveness even when treatment is, in fact, effective (Barbaree, 1997). Hanson and Bussière (1998), for example, report that on average only 10–15 per cent of the sexual offenders in the studies they reviewed committed a new crime over the four- to five-year follow-up. This leaves little room for treatment to reduce reoffence rates to a level that is significantly lower than an untreated comparison.

Second, since treatment programmes differ somewhat in content (i.e. in the issues that are targeted in treatment), and the client group who are treated differ across studies, it would be unreasonable to expect all programmes to be equally effective. In the primary study (Rice *et al.*, 1991) upon which Quinsey's conclusions depend, very deviant and dangerous sexual offenders made up the treated and untreated samples. While it would be gratifying to learn that it was possible to effectively treat these very difficult clients, it should not surprise us to find that treatment produced no benefits. In addition, treatment involved electric aversive therapy aimed at reducing deviant sexual arousal (no procedure was used to enhance appropriate arousal) along with some social skill training (received by 40 per cent of the clients) and sex education (again only 40 per cent received this). Quite clearly this was a very limited treatment programme for very difficult clients and it should not surprise anyone that it was ineffective.

Third, even if treatment content (i.e. the target problems addressed) was the same for all programmes, which is far from true, the manner in which treatment is delivered can reasonably be assumed to influence effectiveness. In a recent review of the therapy process literature (Marshall *et al.*, 2003), we found clear and compelling evidence that the therapeutic alliance accounted for a reasonably substantial amount of the variance in behaviour change and treatment outcome across a broad range of disorders. This was equally true for more traditional approaches to treatment and for cognitive behavioural therapy. In addition, Beech and Fordham (1997) demonstrated that the group environment, generated by the therapist's style and the clients' perceptions of that style, significantly influenced the magnitude of treatment-induced changes. Our (Marshall *et al.*, 2001) recent analyses of behavioural and attitudinal changes within sexual offender treatment across several English Prison programmes revealed that various features of the therapists' style enhanced or reduced treatment changes. This was true despite the fact that treatment providers in these programmes all followed a carefully detailed manual and their adherence to this manual was continuously monitored. Thus, differential effectiveness of different treatment programmes for sexual offenders may, in part at least, be due to different therapist characteristics.

To conclude that treatment is ineffective is one thing, but to recommend, as Quinsey *et al.* (1996) did, that treatment for sexual offenders should be abandoned and replaced by extensive (ten years or more) and intensive community supervision, is to go well beyond the data. One or two, or even more, treatment failures cannot justify abandoning our efforts. Cancer researchers have never given up treating these diseases despite years of repeated failures and for that we are grateful now that many cancers may be slowed and others cured. Furthermore, as we have seen, treatment successes outnumbered failures even when Quinsey made his recommendations. Finally, there is no evidence at all that would encourage the belief that supervision (no matter how extensive or intensive) will have an impact on the likelihood of reoffending. Either we are guided by evidence in our pronouncements or not; there is no logic to abandoning one strategy because there is no evidence of its utility and then advocating an alternative for which there is also no evidence. At any rate, as we will see, there is evidence that treatment for sexual offenders is effective.

### *Procedural aspects of treatment evaluation*

The first thing to consider is, what is it we should be using as an index of treatment effectiveness? Since therapists are likely to overestimate their effectiveness, and clients understandably want to report themselves as problem-free, we can dismiss studies relying on these two sources. Some objective index of long-term outcome is required. Official sources of reoffending seem to be best although they are not without their problems. They are, no doubt, underestimates of the true rate of offending, but this may not be sufficient grounds for rejecting them as there is no obvious reason to suppose such underestimates differentially affect treated and untreated samples.

The main limitation on official records concerns how complete they are. For example, in the United States there is not a satisfactory national crime tracking system. Individual offences in any state are unlikely to be entered into the poorly managed US national data system; this means that when a researcher is doing a follow-up study in the USA, he/she can expect to be able to track offences committed in his/her own state but will be unlikely to identify reoffences committed by those clients who left their home state after discharge. Janice Marques' otherwise very sophisticated follow-up study (Marques, 1999), appears to have suffered from this lack of a satisfactory tracking system. For example, only 6 per cent of her non-volunteer, untreated rapists had been identified as recidivists (Marques, personal communication, March 1998). Unless California rapists are an exceptionally non-problematic group, which stretches credibility, these have to be inaccurate data reflecting an underestimate of the untreated base rate. This low base rate makes it impossible to show effects for treatment.

In our view, satisfactory treatment evaluations cannot be done in jurisdictions like the United States where effective national tracking systems are lacking. These problems are not evident in Canada or New Zealand where the national tracking systems are legally mandated and accurately enacted. Thornton (personal communication, June 2000) reports that there are also base-rate problems in the tracking system in England, and this may limit the value of outcome studies there as well. These are unfortunate facts, but we must face things as they are, not as we would wish them to be.

Using recidivism as the index of treatment effects is one reason base rates are low because it simply counts any or all reoffences as one (i.e. recidivism is simply the percentage of clients who reoffend). Harm reduction advocates (Laws, 1996; 1999) would point to the value of other indices of treatment effectiveness such as the number of reoffences, the number of victims, the delay in onset of reoffending, or the viciousness and harm of offences. Let us take as an example a sexual offender who prior to treatment was offending several times each year against numerous victims and had beaten or killed some of his victims. If this offender, subsequent to treatment, committed just one offence of a relatively minor nature over a four-year follow-up period, then surely we should judge him to have been improved by the programme. Unfortunately indices that would track these features are rarely employed in outcome studies. Hopefully increased respect for the harm reduction viewpoint will change this.

Perhaps the primary issue in outcome studies concerns the actual design of the evaluation. The main point here has to do with the need for an untreated comparison group. Quinsey *et al.* (1993) declare that the only basis upon which treatment effectiveness can be inferred involves an outcome study in which volunteers for treatment are randomly assigned to treatment or no treatment. Aside from the limitation that random assignment does not guarantee good matches between groups on important features (e.g. offence histories, degree of risk, etc.), most would agree that this constitutes close to an ideal design. There are, however, very serious limitations to the implementation of this ideal design. We (Marshall, 1993; Marshall *et al.*, 1999; Marshall and Pithers, 1994) have delineated these problems before, so we will only briefly note them here. We will consider a prison-based programme as illustrative of these problems.

It is unlikely that prison authorities (or any other organisation funding treatment for sexual offenders) would countenance deliberately withholding treatment from men who constitute a danger to the public and then release them to see if more reoffend than a treated group. At the very least this has the potential to be a public relations disaster, an experience most organisations go out of their way to avoid. If the administration did, however, approve of such a study, would all the offenders feel free to volunteer? In Canadian penitentiaries well over 50 per cent of incarcerated sexual offenders express a strong desire to enter treatment and may not, on this account, volunteer for a study in which they have a 50–50 chance of not being treated. Second, in the Canadian system if the sexual offenders in such a study were unfortunate enough to be randomly allocated to no treatment, they would not be released as early as would those who received treatment. This would, of course, generate a fatal confound in the design. Finally, ethics committees who approve treatment evaluation studies typically demand that as soon as the study is complete the untreated clients must be given treatment. This demand is attainable in disorders such as anxiety or depression where a relatively brief follow-up period is sufficient to discern treatment effects, but not so with sexual offenders where a minimum of four years is empirically necessary. In the random design (or ideal) study, then, the comparison group would remain untreated for at least four years while at risk. This certainly puts a lot of innocent people at risk to be victimised, such that a likely public outcry might very well terminate the study before the data are in hand.

The best alternative to the random design is to compare the treated group with a group that either did not enter treatment or withdrew at an early stage. This is referred to as the "incidental assignment design" (Hanson, 2000). In these incidental assignment studies the comparison group should be selected from the same setting as the treated group and should be chosen so that they are approximately matched on those features that might be expected to influence the likelihood of future reoffending (e.g. offence history, psychopathy, sexual deviance). However, using the particular form of the incidental design that compares treated subjects with those who withdrew from treatment (i.e. drop-outs), is not the best choice, since there is evidence (Hanson, 2000) that drop-outs have higher recidivism rates than those who refused, or otherwise did not enter, treatment; using drop-outs would, therefore, bias the study in favour of finding a treatment effect.

## Treatment evaluations

### *The ATSA collaborative study*

In 1997 the Association for the Treatment of Sexual Abusers (ATSA), a North American based international organisation of sexual offender treatment providers and researchers, formed a committee to evaluate the effectiveness of treatment (see Hanson, 2000). After some discussions they settled on the following criteria for selecting among available studies to include in a review of effectiveness: studies using random designs, studies using incidental designs, reports of programmes that targeted a range of criminogenic needs (e.g. cognitive distortions, victim empathy, social skills deficits, attitudes tolerant of sexual offending, deviant sexual interest), and reports that based reoffending on data independent of the therapists' and clients' reports. A total of forty-two studies (twenty published and twenty-two unpublished) were reliably identified as meeting the criteria for entry into a meta-analytic study. Unfortunately, twenty of the studies were American and we have already expressed our reservations about these studies. However, it is important to note that their inclusion should prejudice against finding treatment effects since the inability to comprehensively track discharged clients should generate low base rates and thereby limit the power of statistical tests to detect real benefits for treatment. Thus, if the ATSA study demonstrates a treatment effect the inclusion of the American studies would increase our confidence in the finding.

The ATSA study did, indeed, reveal statistically reliable benefits of treatment. Across all studies almost 18 per cent (17.7%) of the comparison subjects sexually reoffended over the follow-up period (Median = 46 months) whereas only 12 per cent (12.3%) of the treated group were recidivists. Similar, but stronger, results were evident for general recidivism (28.7% of treated subjects versus 41.7% of untreated clients). Greater effects were evident for more current treatment programmes, most of which followed a cognitive-behavioural, relapse prevention model. The overall benefits demonstrated by the ATSA study were equally evident for institutionally based programmes and for those run in the community. Most importantly for the present chapter was the observation that the three identified programmes for juvenile offenders were no less effective than those for adults. It is important to note that the adolescent programmes did not, on their own, show a statistically significant effect, which Hanson (2000) attributed to the small sample size (three programmes and 205 subjects), although this should not obscure the fact that at least one of these programmes was clearly effective (see Worling and Curwen report below).

### *Direct appraisals of juvenile treatment*

Since all of the currently available reports of treatment outcome with juvenile sexual offenders have serious problems that limit their value, we will consider only one here in order to demonstrate how a good study can be done and what its effects are.

Worling and Curwen (2000) evaluated the Sexual Abuse: Family Education and Treatment Programme (SAFE-T), which is a Canadian specialised, community-based programme for juveniles who have committed sexual offences. This programme involves both the young offenders and their families in individually tailored treatment that typically runs for twenty-four months. Worling and Curwen identified fifty-eight of these youngsters who had completed twelve or more months of treatment between 1987 and 1995, and a comparison group of ninety untreated juvenile sexual offenders. The untreated offenders were from three groups: those who dropped out before twelve months of treatment ($n$ = 27), those who refused treatment ($n$ = 17), and forty-six who were referred for assessment only. Of these latter forty-six, thirty were receiving treatment elsewhere, so if we add these to the drop-outs, 67 per cent of the so-called untreated subjects had received some form of treatment. This, of course, should reduce the chances of detecting a treatment effect. The follow-up period ranged from two to ten years (Mean = 6.2 years). As their index of recidivism, Worling and Curwen counted charges rather then simply convictions, and they distinguished sexual offences from violent nonsexual offences, and from non-violent nonsexual offences.

All subjects and their families were interviewed and the juveniles completed a comprehensive battery of tests. On the basis of the data from these initial assessments, and an examination of the official records, the three comparison groups were contrasted with the treatment group. No differences were found on demographic factors (age and socio-economic status), offence histories (number of victims, delinquent, and aggressive behaviours), and responses to eight psychological tests. Thus the groups were essentially matched prior to treatment.

The results of the evaluation revealed recidivism rates for the treatment group as follows: 5 per cent committed a further sexual offence, 19 per cent another violent offence, and 21 per cent committed another nonsexual non-violent offence. This produced an overall recidivism rate of 35 per cent. Since the three untreated groups (drop-outs, refusers, and assessment only subjects) did not differ on any recidivism index, their data were combined to reveal the following recidivism data: 18 per cent for sexual offences, 32 per cent for violent offences, 50 per cent for nonsex non-violent offences, and an overall rate of 54 per cent. On each of these different offence categories, and on the overall category, the treated group had statistically significantly lower reoffence rates, thereby demonstrating a strong and positive treatment effect.

Sexual recidivists across all groups were more likely to report past or present sexual fantasies of children, more extensive grooming of their victims, and more intrusive sexual acts with their victims. They were less likely to have nonsexual delinquent behaviours. The nonsexual recidivists were more likely to be psychopathic, and to have a more extensive history of offending and aggressive behaviour, and low self-esteem. Economic disadvantage and a history of childhood sexual victimisation also characterised the nonsexual recidivists.

## Need for more studies

While it is usual to note at the end of almost all reports that further research is needed, in the present case this call should be writ bold. There is a poverty of evaluation studies of treatment with adolescent sexual offenders, and none at all with children under age twelve years, despite the fact that such children pose problems for their own and others' lives (Johnson, 1998). The evaluation by Worling and Curwen (2000) presents a model for how the efficacy of treatment can be examined within the constraints of operating a clinically sound, and socially responsible, treatment programme.

We strongly encourage clinicians who provide treatment for young sexual offenders to attempt an evaluation of their programme and report the results in publications accessible to other clinicians and researchers. Evaluating treatment is not technically daunting, although the process takes a long time and can be fraught with obstacles. Working with sexual offenders is not easy, but it is easy to become discouraged by the failures that necessarily occur. Having completed an evaluation that shows positive effects can serve to remind clinicians of their effectiveness when a failure is brought to their attention. Even with minimally effective treatment, the number of innocent people who are saved from suffering at the hands of sexual offenders is enough to justify continuing the arduous task of providing treatment. Beyond this Marshall (1992) demonstrated that effective treatment also saves thousands, and may even save millions, of dollars (or pounds) that would otherwise be incurred for recidivists in subsequent investigations, prosecutions and incarceration of these reoffenders. In this examination of costs Marshall did not include the untold costs to health services to care for the victims.

We believe, as we have persistently said for years now, that the outcome literature on the treatment of sexual offenders encourages the view that our work can be effective. Effective treatment of these offenders can save considerable human suffering not only in terms of victims but also in terms of the lives of our clients. Sexual offenders are not diabolical people who simply decided one day to harm others. They too are victims of their histories, none of which are histories any reasonable person would have chosen (Starzyk and Marshall, 2003). Helping sexual offenders change their lives not only prevents others from being victims, it gives offenders a chance to be productive and happy prosocial members of society. This surely is a laudable goal.

## References

Abel, G. G., Mittleman, M. S., and Becker, J. V. (1985). Sex offenders: Results of assessment and recommendations for treatment. In M. H. Ben-Aron, S. J. Hucker and C. D. Webster (eds), *Clinical Criminology and the Assessment and Treatment of Criminal Behavior*. Toronto: M&M Graphics, pp. 207–220.

Barbaree, H. E. (1997). Evaluating treatment efficacy with sexual offenders: The insensitivity of recidivism studies to treatment effects. *Sexual Abuse: A Journal of Research and Treatment, 9*, 111–128.

Barbaree, H. E., and Cortoni, F. A. (1993). Treatment of the juvenile sex offender within the criminal justice and mental health systems. In H. E. Barbaree, W. L. Marshall and S. M. Hudson (eds), *The Juvenile Sex Offender*. New York: Guilford Press, pp. 243–263.

Becker, J. V. (1990). Treating adolescent sexual offenders. *Professional Psychology: Research and Practice, 21*, 362–365.

Beech, A., and Fordham, A. S. (1997). Therapeutic climate of sexual offender treatment programs. *Sexual Abuse: A Journal of Research and Treatment, 9*, 219–237.

Borduin, C. M., Henggeler, S. W., Blaske, D. M., and Stein, R. J. (1990). Multisystemic treatment of adolescent sexual offenders. *International Journal of Offender Therapy and Comparative Criminology, 34*, 105–113.

Brannon, J. M., and Troyer, R. (1995). Adolescent sex offenders: Investigating adult commitment-rates four years later. *International Journal of Offender Therapy and Comparative Criminology, 39*, 317–326.

Bremer, J. F. (1992). Serious juvenile sex offenders: Treatment and long-term follow-up. *Psychiatric Annals, 22*, 326–332.

Freeman-Longo, R. E., Bird, S., Stevenson, W. F., and Fiske, J. A. (1995). *1994 Nationwide Survey of Treatment Programs and Models*. Brandon, VT: Safer Society Press.

Friedrich, W. N., and Chaffin, M. (2000). *Developmental-Systemic Perspective on Children with Sexual Behavior Problems*. Paper presented at the 19th Annual Research and Treatment Conference of the Association for the Treatment of Sexual Abusers, San Diego, November.

Furby, L., Weinrott, M. R., and Blackshaw, L. (1989). Sex offender recidivism: A review. *Psychological Bulletin, 105*, 3–30.

Goode, E. (1994). Battling deviant behavior. *US News and World Report*, November, 74–75.

Hagan, M. P., and Cho, M. E. (1996). A comparison of treatment outcomes between adolescent rapists and child sexual offenders. *International Journal of Offender Therapy and Comparative Criminology, 40*, 113–122.

Hanson, R. K. (2000). *The Effectiveness of Treatment for Sexual Offenders: Report of the ATSA Collaborative Data Research Committee*. Paper presented at the 19th Annual Research and Treatment Conference of the Association for the Treatment of Sexual Abusers, San Diego, November.

Hanson, R. K., and Bussière, M. T. (1998). Predicting relapse: A meta-analysis of sexual offender recidivism studies. *Journal of Consulting and Clinical Psychology, 66*, 348–362.

Johnson, T. C. (1998). Children who molest. In W. L. Marshall, Y. M. Fernandez, S. M. Hudson and T. Ward (eds), *Sourcebook of Treatment Programs for Sexual Offenders*. New York: Plenum Press, pp. 337–352.

Kahn, T. J., and Chambers, H. J. (1991). Assessing reoffense risk with juvenile sexual offenders. *Child Welfare, 70*, 333–345.

Kahn, T. J., and Lafond, M. A. (1988). Treatment of the adolescent sexual offender. *Child and Adolescent Social Work, 5*, 135–148.

Lab, S. P., Shields, G., and Schondel, C. (1993). Research note: An evaluation of juvenile sexual offender treatment. *Crime and Delinquency, 39*, 543–553.

Laws, D. R. (1996). Relapse prevention or harm reduction? *Sexual Abuse: A Journal of Research and Treatment, 8*, 243–247.

Laws, D. R. (1999). Harm reduction or harm facilitation? A reply to Maletzky. *Sexual Abuse: A Journal of Research and Treatment, 11*, 233–241.

Longo, R. E., and Groth, A. N. (1983). Juvenile sexual offenses in the histories of adult rapists and child molesters. *International Journal of Offender Therapy and Comparative Criminology, 27*, 150–155.

Maclay, D. T. (1960). Boys who commit sexual misdemeanors. *British Medical Journal, 11*, 186–190.

Marques, J. K. (1999). How to answer the question, "Does sex offender treatment work?" *Journal of Interpersonal Violence, 14*, 437–451.

Marshall, W. L. (1992). The social value of treatment for sexual offenders. *Canadian Journal of Human Sexuality, 1*, 109–114.

Marshall, W. L. (1993). The treatment of sexual offenders: What does the outcome data tell us? A reply to Quinsey et al. *Journal of Interpersonal Violence, 8*, 524–530.

Marshall, W. L., and Pithers, W. D. (1994). A reconsideration of treatment outcome with sex offenders. *Criminal Justice and Behavior, 21*, 10–27.

Marshall, W. L., Jones, R., Ward, T., Johnston, P., and Barbaree, H. E. (1991). Treatment outcome with sexual offenders. *Clinical Psychology Review, 11*, 465–485.

Marshall, W. L., Anderson, D., and Fernandez, Y. M. (1999). *Cognitive Behavioral Treatment of Sexual Offenders*. Chichester: John Wiley.

Marshall, W. L., Serran, G. A., and Mulloy, R. (2001). *The Effect of Therapist Style on Treatment-Induced Changes with Sexual Offenders*. Submitted for publication.

Marshall, W. L., Fernandez, Y. M., Serran, G. A., Mulloy, R., Thornton, D., Mann, R. E., and Anderson, D. (2003). Process variables in the treatment of sexual offenders: A review of the relevant literature. *Aggression and Violent Behaviour, 8*, 205–234.

Mazur, T., and Michael, P. M. (1992). Outpatient treatment for adolescents with sexually inappropriate behaviour: Program description and six-month follow-up. *Journal of Offender Rehabilitation, 18*, 191–203.

Quinsey, V. L., Harris, G. T., Rice, M. E., and Lalumiere, M. L. (1993). Assessing treatment efficacy in outcome studies of sex offenders. *Journal of Interpersonal Violence, 8*, 512–523.

Quinsey, V. L., Khanna, A., and Malcolm, P. B. (1996). *A Retrospective Evaluation of the Regional Treatment Centre Sex Offender Treatment Program*. Paper presented at the World Congress of Psychology, Montreal, August.

Rice, M. E., Quinsey, V. L., and Harris, G. T. (1991). Sexual recidivism among child molesters released from a maximum security psychiatric institution. *Journal of Consulting and Clinical Psychology, 59*, 381–386.

Roberts, R. E., Abrams, L., and Finch, J. R. (1973). Delinquent sexual behavior among adolescents. *Medical Aspects of Human Sexuality, 7*, 162–183.

Smith, W. R., and Monastersky, C. (1986). Assessing juvenile sexual offenders' risk for reoffending. *Criminal Justice and Behaviour, 13*, 115–140.

Starzyk, K. B., and Marshall, W. L. (2003). Childhood Family and Personological Risk Factors for Sexual Offending. *Aggression and Violent Behaviour, 8*, 93–105.

US National Adolescent Perpetrator Network (1988). Preliminary-report from the National Task Force on Juvenile Sexual Offending. *Juvenile and Family Court Journal, 39*, 1–67.

Worling, J., and Curwen, T. (2000). Adolescent sexual offender recidivism: Success of specialized treatment and implications for risk prediction. *Child Abuse and Neglect, 24(7)*, 965–982.

# Index